D1702021

Differential Diagnosis in Conventional Gastrointestinal Radiology

Excerpt from
Differential Diagnosis in Conventional Radiology

Francis A. Burgener, M.D.
Professor of Radiology
University of Rochester
Medical Center
Rochester, USA

Martti Kormano, M.D.
Professor and Chairman
Department of Diagnostic Radiology
University Central Hospital
Turku, Finland

521 Illustrations
 41 Tables

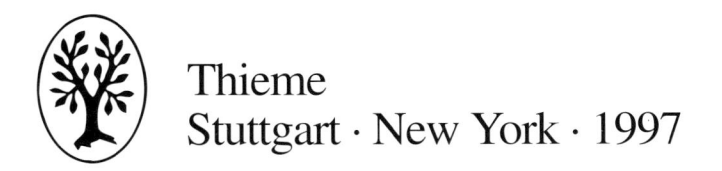

Thieme
Stuttgart · New York · 1997

Francis A. Burgener, M.D.
Professor of Radiology
University of Rochester
Medical Center
Rochester, N. Y. 14642, USA

Martti Kormano, M.D.
Professor and Chairman
Department of Diagnostic Radiology
University Central Hospital
20520 Turku, Finland

Library of Congress Cataloging-in-Publication Data

Burgener, Francis A.:
Differential diagnosis in conventional gastrointestinal radiology : excerpt from Differential diagnosis in conventional radiology / Francis A. Burgener ; Martti Kormano. – Stuttgart ; New York : Thieme, 1997

NE: Kormano, Martti:

Important Note: Medicine is an ever-changing science undergoing continual development. Research and clinical experience are continually expanding our knowledge, in particular our knowledge of proper treatment and drug therapy. Insofar as this book mentions any dosage or application, readers may rest assured that the authors, editors and publishers have made every effort to ensure that such references are in accordance **with the state of knowledge at the time of production of the book.**

Nevertheless this does not involve, imply, or express any guarantee or responsibility on the part of the publishers in respect of any dosage instructions and forms of application stated in the book. **Every user is requested to** examine carefully the manufacturers' leaflets accompanying each drug and to check, if necessary in consultation with a physician or specialist, whether the dosage schedules mentioned therein or the contraindications stated by the manufacturers differ from the statements made in the present book. Such examination is particularly important with drugs that are either rarely used or have been newly released on the market. **Every dosage schedule or every form of application used is entirely at the user's own risk and responsibility.** The authors and publishers request every user to report to the publishers any discrepancies or inaccuracies noticed.

Any reference to or mention of manufacturers or specific brand names should not be interpreted as an endorsement or advertisement for any company or product.

Some of the product names, patents and registered designs referred to in this book are in fact registered trademarks or proprietary names even though specific reference to this fact is not always made in the text. Therefore, the appearance of a name without designation as proprietary is not to be construed as a representation by the publisher that it is in the public domain.

This book, including all parts thereof, is legally protected by copyright. Any use, exploitation or commercialization outside the narrow limits set by copyright legislation, without the publisher's consent, is illegal and liable to prosecution. This applies in particular to photostat reproduction, copying, mimeographing or duplication of any kind, translating, preparation of microfilms, and electronic data processing and storage.

© 1991, 1997 Georg Thieme Verlag, Rüdigerstraße 14, D-70469 Stuttgart, Germany
Thieme Medical Publishers, Inc., 381 Park Avenue South, New York, N.Y. 10016
Typesetting by Druckhaus Götz GmbH, Ludwigsburg
Printed in Germany by Grammlich, Pliezhausen

ISBN 3-13-107621-6 (GTV, Stuttgart)
ISBN 0-86577-676-8 (TMP, New York)   2 3 4 5 6

About This Book

This book presents a section taken from one of *the* standard works on radiographic diagnosis—Burgener and Kormano's *Differential Diagnosis in Conventional Radiology*. It allows doctors involved in the radiographic diagnosis of the gastrointestinal system to access and make use of the vital information they need, in a *targeted* and therefore cost-effective way.

By presenting original illustrations of almost all the conditions mentioned in the book alongside tables showing the most important additional differential diagnostic information, the book points to the correct diagnosis even in difficult situations.

Preface to *Differential Diagnosis in Coventional Radiology,* Second Edition

Conventional radiographs remain the backbone of our specialty despite the advent of new, fascinating imaging techniques such as ultrasonography, computed tomography and, most recently, magnetic resonance imaging. In contrast to many of these newer methods, conventional radiology is practiced not only by radiologists but also by a large number of clinicians and surgeons. With each film, one is confronted with radiologic findings that require interpretation in order to arrive at a general diagnostic impression and a reasonable differential diagnosis. To assist the film reader in attaining this goal our book is based upon radiographic findings, unlike most other textbooks in radiology that are disease-oriented. Since many diseases present radiographically in a variety of manifestations, some overlap in the text is unavoidable. To minimize repetition, the differential diagnosis of a radiographic finding is presented in tabular form whenever feasible. The tables list not only the various diseases that may present radiologically in a specific way, but also describe in a succinct form the characteristically associated radiographic findings and pertinent clinical data. Radiographic illustrations and drawings are included to demonstrate visually the radiographic features under discussion.

This book is meant for physicians with some experience in radiology who wish to strengthen their diagnostic acumen. It is a comprehensive outline of radiographic findings, and we expect it to be particularly useful to radiology residents preparing for their specialist examinations. Any physician involved in interpreting radiologic film images should find this book helpful, in direct proportion to his curiosity.

The positive response to our textbook has prompted us to update the first edition, while keeping to the same basic concept. Conventional radiographic findings are described and their differential diagnostic possibilities analyzed. The lists of diseases presenting with similar radiographic abnormalities are complemented by descriptions of other associated radiographic findings and relevant clinical data characteristics for specific conditions.

It is our hope that the second edition will be as well received by medical students, residents, radiologists and physicians—all of those practicing radiology—as the first one was.

Francis A. Burgener, M.D.
Martti Kormano, M.D.

Contents

Chapter 1
Abnormal Gas Pattern 1

Chapter 2
Abdominal Calcifications 31

Chapter 3
Displacement of Abdominal Organs 55

Chapter 4
Dilatation and Motility Disorders in the
Gastrointestinal Tract 83

Chapter 5
Abnormal Mucosal Pattern in the
Gastrointestinal Tract 105

Chapter 6
Narrowing in the Gastrointestinal Tract 135

Chapter 7
Filling Defects in the Gastrointestinal Tract . . . 161

Chapter 8
Ulcers, Diverticula, and Fistulas in the
Gastrointestinal Tract 195

Chapter 9
Gallbladder and Bile Duct Abnormalities 215

References 228

Index 229

Abbreviations

AP	Anteroposterior
ASD	Atrial septal defect
BCG	Bacille Calmette-Guérin
BIP	Bronchiolitis obliterans and diffuse interstitial pneumonia
BOOP	Bronchiolitis obliterans with organizing pneumonia
CID	Cytomegalic inclusion disease
CPPD	Calcium pyrophosphate dihydrate
CRST	Calcification, Raynaud's phenomenon, sclerodactyly, and telangiectasia
CT	Computed tomography
DD	Differential diagnosis
DIC	Disseminated intravascular coagulation
DIP	Desquamative interstitial pneumonitis
DISH	Diffuse idiopathic skeletal hyperostosis
GIP	Giant-cell interstitial pneumonia
HADD	Hydroxyapatite deposition disease
IV	Intravenous
IVC	Inferior vena cava
IVP	Intravenous pyelogram
MRI	Magnetic resonance imaging
PMF	Progressive massive fibrosis
POEMS	Polyneuropathy, organomegaly, endocrinopathy, skin changes
TAPVR	Total anomalous pulmonary venous return
UIP	"Usual" interstitial pneumonia
UPJ	Ureteropelvic junction
VSD	Ventricular septal defect

Chapter 1 Abnormal Gas Pattern

Abnormalities of the abdominal gas pattern are most commonly associated with an acute abdomen, with the usual question being whether a surgical emergency exists or not. For the proper evaluation of such a case, the following films are required:
1 Supine anteroposterior radiograph of the abdomen that includes the pelvic floor.
2 Upright radiograph of the abdomen after the patient has been in a sitting position for a few minutes. This allows free air to rise to the diaphragm.
3 Lateral radiograph of the abdomen.
4 Posteroanterior and lateral chest radiographs.
5 Lateral decubitus radiographs will replace the upright view (2) if the patient is unable to stand. They are also particularly useful in cases of questionable air–fluid levels of the colon.

An inverted lateral radiograph for the demonstration of rectal gas is used in newborn infants with bowel obstruction.

In the normal adult, varying amounts of gas and stool are seen in the large bowel. An additional air–fluid level is constantly present in the stomach and frequently in the duodenal bulb and/or terminal ileum. The small bowel is essentially gasless. Most of the gas is swallowed, but some is produced by bacteria in the large bowel.

At birth, the abdomen is gasless, but normally air reaches the large bowel by three hours and the whole alimentary tract is usually filled with gas within 6–12 hours. The normal gas pattern of an infant is totally different from the adult: both the small and large bowel contain gas (Fig. **1**). Increased amounts of gas in the bowel are also seen in edentulous patients who must eat by sucking. Impaired intestinal blood supply in elderly patients may be partly responsible for increased gas content of the bowel.

Gas in the bowel, whether normal or abnormal, serves as a natural contrast agent and allows various segments of the bowel to be identified by their wall patterns (Fig. **2**). Small bowel loops wider than 3 cm in diameter are considered distended. Differentiation between widely dilated ileum and colon may be difficult, but the fixed

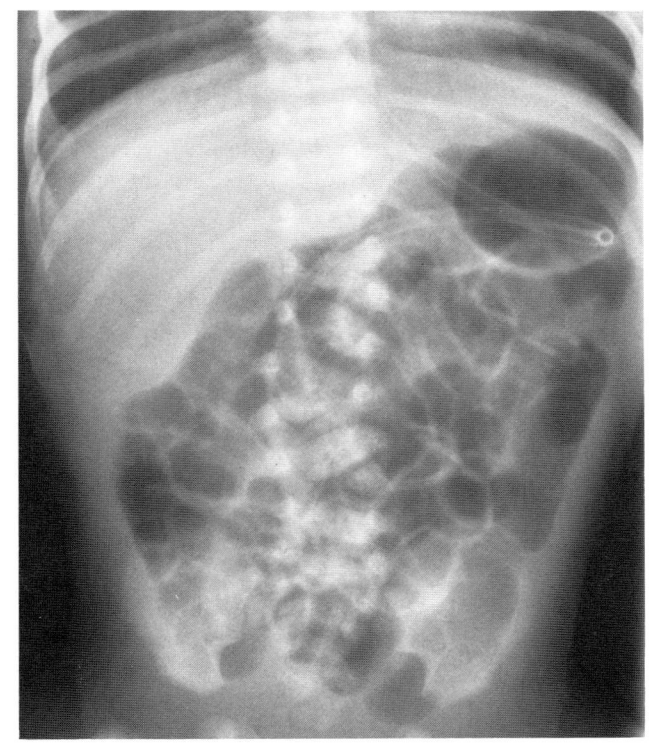

Figure **1** **Normal abdominal gas pattern** of an infant: both small and large bowel contain gas. Small bowel loops have polyhedral pattern.

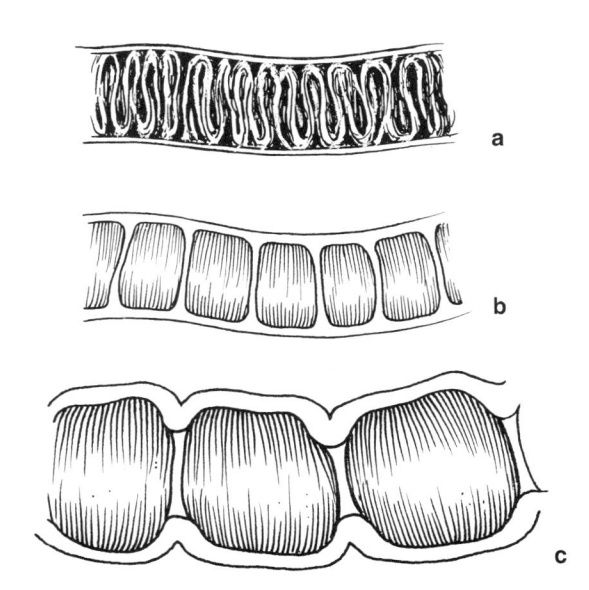

Figure **2** **Wall patterns** of **a** jejunum, **b** ileum, and **c** colon.

lateral position of the ascending and descending colon as well as stool in the colon are helpful. The watch spring appearance of the valvulae conniventes of the small bowel and the interrupted haustral pattern of the large bowel, which are characteristic in adults and older children, are not evident in the neonate. In neonates, the translucent air shadows within the bowel are relatively compressed so that a polyhedral (honeycomb) pattern results, but normally the bowel is not distended and no continuity of bowel loops is discernible.

Gastrointestinal glands produce 4–10 liters of fluid per day. In bowel transport failure the fluid production continues, but absorptive function of the bowel diminishes. Fluid accumulation in the bowel thus indicates an impairment in transport (either obstruction or absence of peristalsis) or mucosal inflammation responsible for the additional fluid. More than two air–fluid levels in the distended small bowel or any in the large bowel are therefore considered abnormal, unless caused by a water enema prior to filming.

Absence of gas in a failure of intestinal transport (e.g., in the presence of increased intestinal fluid) merely means failure to swallow, unless caused by vomiting or nasogastric suction. In the absence of gas the evaluation is difficult. An almost gasless abdomen is frequently seen in *strangulation, acute pancreatitis, mesenteric infarction,* and *esophageal or pyloric obstruction.*

The radiological diagnosis of *mechanical large or small bowel obstruction* is dependent on finding dilatation of the bowel to a point of obstruction beyond which the bowel collapses. All other findings are secondary to this. A mechanical obstruction may be complicated by a *reflex (adynamic) ileus,* which alters the appearance. *Postoperative abdomen* is particularly difficult to interpret, since postoperative mechanical obstruction may be masked by a postoperative adynamic ileus pattern. Since the colon is usually involved in the adynamic ileus, the greater the collapse of the colon and the greater the dilatation of the small bowel, the more likely is the presence of mechanical obstruction.

Dilatation of the small bowel secondary to colonic obstruction depends on the action of the ileocecal valve. If the ileocecal valve is closed both ways or allows reflux from the colon, small bowel dilatation with air–fluid levels occurs.

A loop of bowel paralyzed by adjoining inflammation in the absence of generalized bowel paralysis is called a *sentinel loop.* It may help in localizing abdominal infections.

Tables **1** and **2** present conditions with predominantly small bowel and large bowel dilatation, respectively. Bowel disorders that may be associated with abnormal gas pattern in a newborn are often different from the causes common in adults and older children. Therefore, they are presented separately in Table **3**. Table **4** is a collection of conditions that are most commonly associated with abnormal gas collections outside the bowel.

The presence of gas outside the bowel lumen (in bowel wall, peritoneal cavity, extraperitoneal space, or within the parenchymal organs) is always abnormal, with the rare exception of free intraperitoneal gas in females following vigorous intercourse. Whereas gas in the peritoneal space moves according to body position, intramural or retroperitoneal gas is fixed and often present as small bubbles that do not coalesce. Extraperitoneal gas may be difficult to detect without CT.

A localized air–fluid level outside the bowel lumen is indicative of an *abscess*. In a plain film, the intra-abdominal abscess may be radiologically manifested by demonstrating (1) a soft-tissue mass, (2) a collection or pattern of extraluminal gas, (3) viscus displacement, (4) loss of normally visualized structures, or (5) fixation of a normally mobile organ. Secondary signs include scoliosis, elevation or splinting of a diaphragm, localized or generalized ileus, and pulmonary basilar changes. If a localized gas collection with fluid level is lacking, diagnosis of an abscess on plain films is difficult and usually requires ultrasonography or CT.

The transverse mesocolon (Fig. **3**) constitutes the major barrier dividing the abdominal cavity into supramesocolic and inframesocolic compartments. The obliquely oriented root of the small bowel mesentery further divides the inframesocolic compartment into the smaller right infracolic space and the larger left infracolic space. The latter is open toward the pelvis. Consequently, the intraperitoneal abscess can be classified into supramesocolic (right subphrenic, right subhepatic, left subphrenic, and lesser sac) and inframesocolic (right and left paracolic, right and left infracolic, and pelvic) abscesses (Fig. **3**).

The major fascial marginations of the retroperitoneal space (Fig. **4**) include:

1 The anterior pararenal space, a potential space between the posterior parietal peritoneum to the anterior renal fascia.
2 The perirenal space, which encompasses the kidney and contains the perirenal fat and has no communication across the midline.
3 The posterior pararenal space extends from the posterior renal fascia to the transversalis fascia. This space is potentially in communication bilaterally via the properitoneal fat of the anterior abdominal wall, and is radiologically visualized as the "flank stripe".

Since some compartments of the retroperitoneal space are in communication with each other, and some are not, the distribution of retroperitoneal gas and fluid can be helpful in diagnosing the location of a retroperitoneal process.

Extraperitoneal gas following perforation has a mottled appearance and the gas bubbles do not move according to posture. The extraperitoneal collection of gaseous lucencies is oriented with a general vertical axis, sometimes as linear lucencies, tracking along the fascial planes. In the absence of gas, extraperitoneal abscesses are difficult to diagnose without ultrasound or CT. Radiologically, loss of visualization of the lateral margin of the psoas muscle has been considered a hallmark of extraperitoneal effusions, but 25% of normal individuals show unequal visualization of the psoas borders. The radiographic signs of extraperitoneal abscesses demonstrable on plain radiographs are usually late and

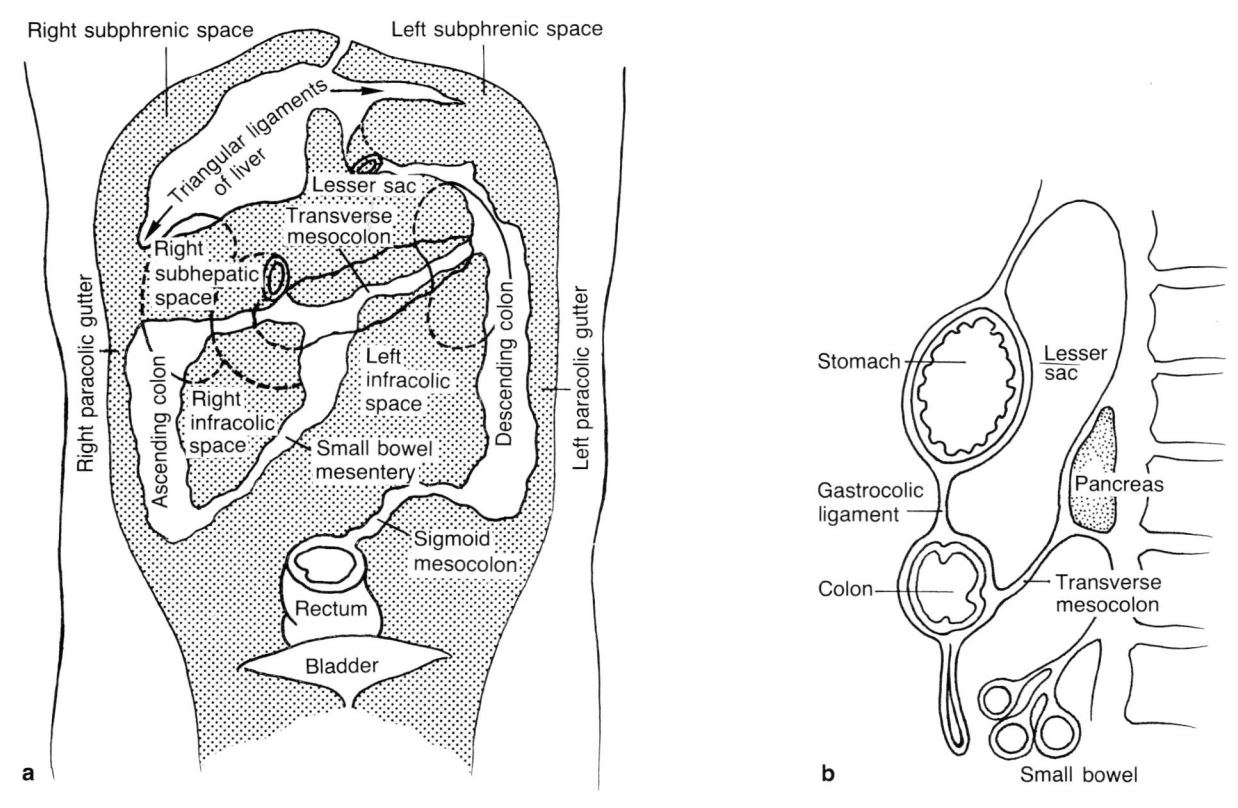

Figure 3 **Compartments of the abdominal cavity** (after Meyers 1988).

unreliable. Whenever possible, the diagnosis should be confirmed using ultrasound, CT or MRI. The anterior pararenal space is the most common site of extraperitoneal infection. Most abscesses arise from primary lesions of the alimentary tract, especially the colon, extraperitoneal appendix, pancreas, and duodenum. They originate from perforating malignancies, inflammatory conditions, penetrating peptic ulcers, and accidental or iatrogenic trauma (including endoscopy).

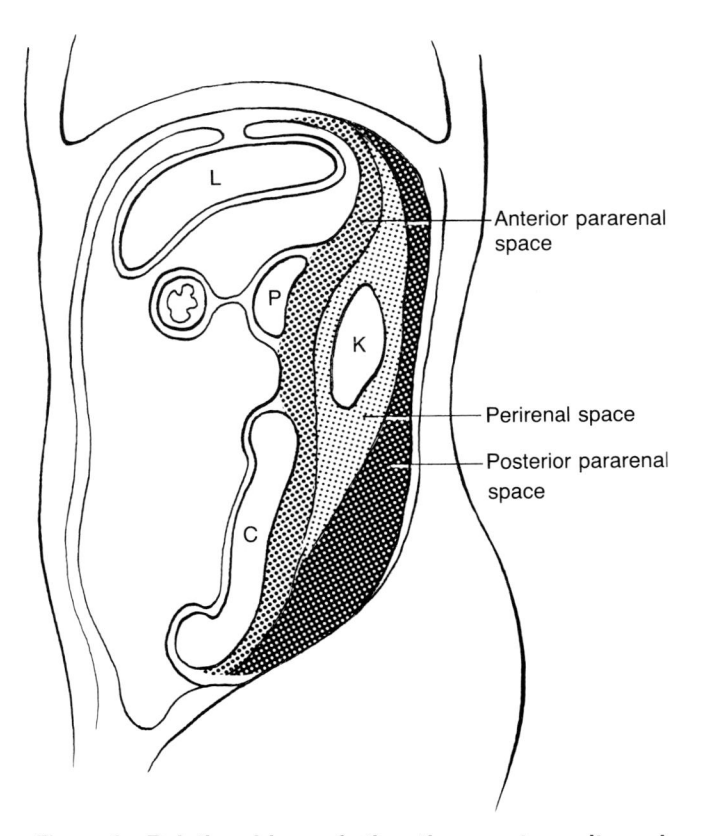

Figure 4 **Relationships of the three retroperitoneal compartments** in the sagittal plane (after Meyers 1988).

Table 1 Predominantly Small-Bowel Distension

Disease	Radiographic Findings	Comments
Meteorism (aerophagia) (Fig. 5)	Gas-filled loops of small and large bowel, without air–fluid levels. Small-bowel loops are angular (not spherical) when seen end on, and take a sinuous course through the abdomen.	Underlying conditions include: Lack of teeth (infants, edentulous patients). Pain: postoperative, fractures, ureteral calculi. Crying. Apprehension. Postoperative.
Mechanical small-bowel obstruction (Fig. 6)	Dilated small-bowel loops containing gas and fluid occupy the mid-abdomen. The proximal loops are high arched and spherical, arranged one above the other. A minimal amount of gas is present in the colon without air–fluid levels. A change of gas pattern occurs in subsequent films. In partial obstruction, significant amounts of gas but no fluid levels may be present distal to the obstruction.	The most common cause is small-bowel *adhesions,* usually postoperative. Other causes: Partial small-bowel obstruction occurs in (ileal) *inflammatory bowel disease* (Crohn's disease) and tumors (*carcinoid,* usually in ileum; *adenocarcinoma,* usually in duodenum or jejunum). If gas in the biliary tract and large amounts of intestinal fluid are present, a *gallstone ileus* should be considered. *Intussusception* of Meckel's diverticulum, tumor with or without an underlying lesion may manifest as nonspecific small-bowel obstruction. For *hernias,* see page 6. Small-bowel distension that may mimic mechanical obstruction may occur in lower lobe pneumonia, pancreatitis, appendicitis, urinary retention, gastroenteritis, hypokalemia, and after saline cathartics.
Carcinoma of the cecum	Signs of total or partial distal small-bowel obstruction as in mechanical small-bowel obstruction.	Carcinoma in the cecum and in the ileocecal valve may cause obliteration, and is an unusual cause of small-bowel distension.
Strangulation (volvulus) of the small bowel (Fig. 7)	Typical roentgenologic appearances include: *Coffee bean sign:* a loop of dilated small bowel containing variable amounts of gas. If filled by fluid only, it appears as a *pseudotumor.* *Fixation of bowel loop:* unchanging position of a gas or fluid-filled loop of bowel in multiple projections. *Absence of valvulae conniventes* in the closed loop due to edema, hemorrhage, or decreased blood supply. *Absence of bowel gas* is often seen even in low small-bowel strangulation.	Secondary to *small-bowel volvulus* about adhesions or *herniation,* which cause impairment of the circulation to the obstructed intestine. Occlusion of the mesenteric artery and vein tends to fill the bowel with fluid. The radiological diagnosis of strangulation is often difficult, since at times very little gas is present in the bowel loops proximal to a strangulating obstruction, resulting in a gasless (or normal-looking) abdomen in the presence of clinical suspicion of bowel obstruction.

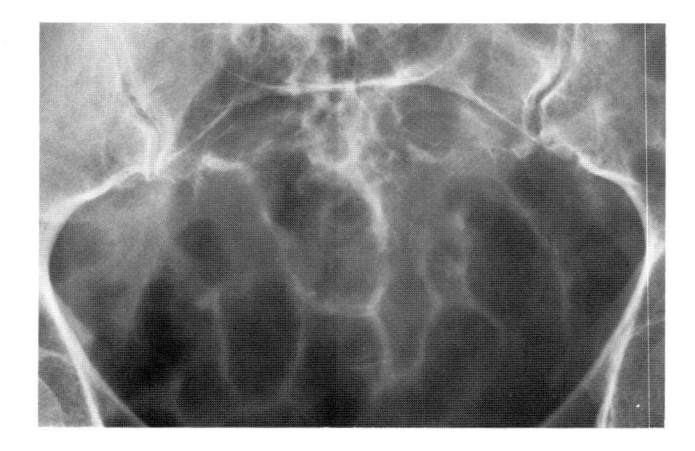

Figure **5** **Meteorism.** Coned-down view of meteoristic small-bowel loops. The loops are angular when seen end on (and without air–fluid levels).

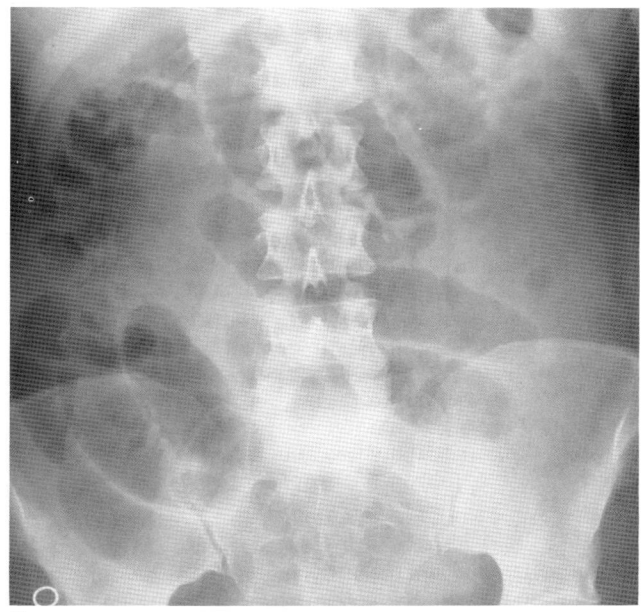

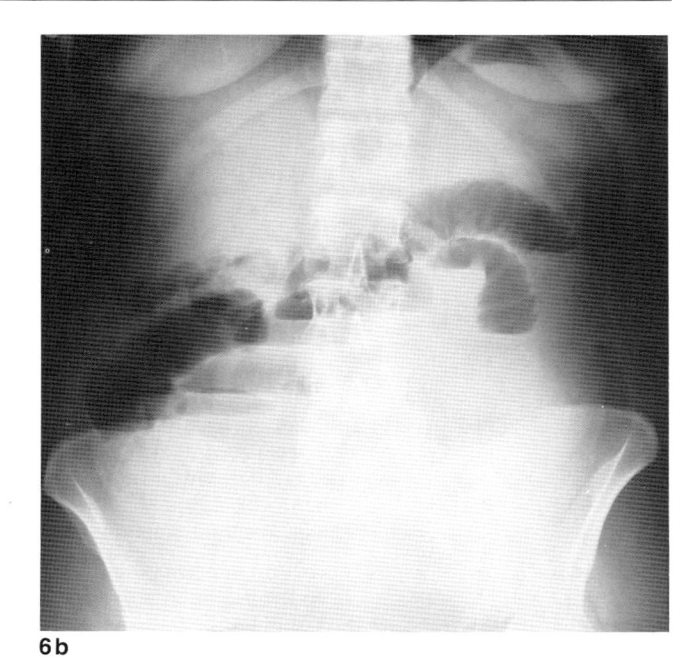

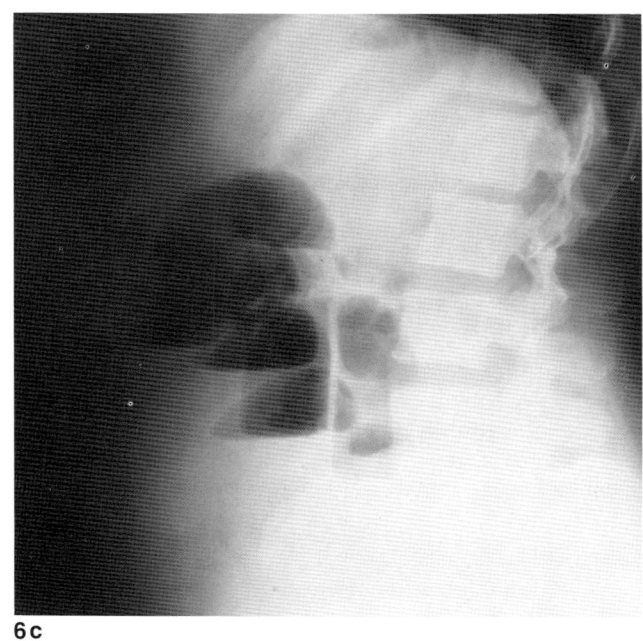

Figure **6a–c Mechanical small-bowel occlusion.** Proximal loops are high-arched, spherical, and distended. Distal small-bowel loops contain a few short air–fluid levels. The colon is essentially gasless. **a** Supine anteroposterior, **b** upright anteroposterior, **c** lateral upright radiograph.

Figure **7a, b Strangulation of the small bowel. a** A strangulated loop of jejunum with thickened folds and dilatation is seen left of the spine. Minimal jejunal dilatation in the left upper abdomen, otherwise the gas content of the abdomen is unremarkable. **b** Strangulation of ileum. A "coffee bean" sign is seen (arrows), otherwise the pattern is normal.

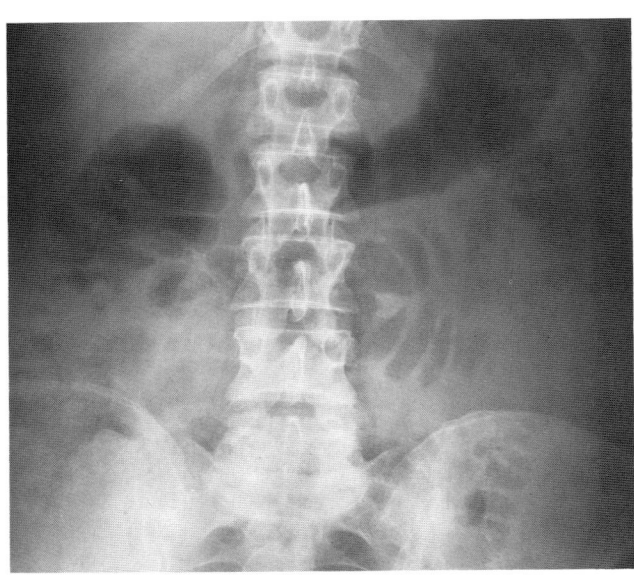

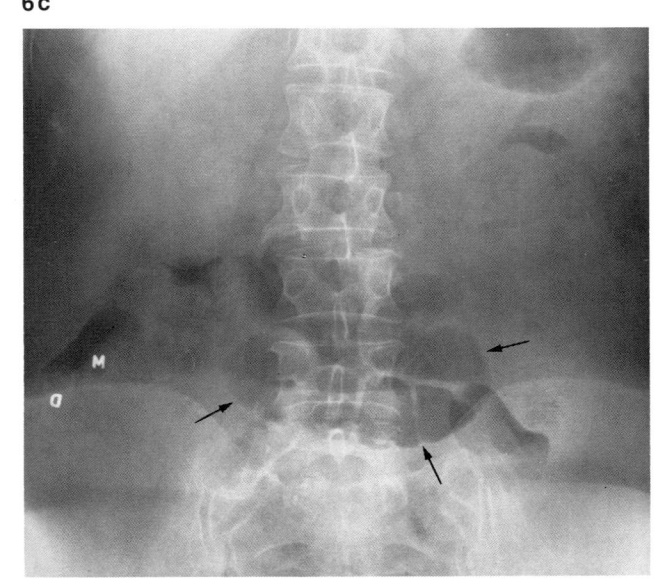

Table 1 (Cont.) Predominantly Small-Bowel Distension

Disease	Radiographic Findings	Comments
Intussusception (Fig. 8)	*Ileocolic:* The normal outline of the proximal colon that contains the intussusceptum is not identified, but a vague right-sided mass may be seen. In the adult the leading tumor of the intussusception is occasionally outlined by colonic gas. The degree of small-bowel distension (and air–fluid levels) depends on the amount of obstruction. A barium enema is diagnostic and often therapeutic in the absence of significant obstruction. *Ileoileal or jejunoileal:* The radiographic appearance is identical to other forms of low small-bowel obstruction (mechanical obstruction).	Most common in white males (3:1) between 6 months and two years. 90% are *ileocolic* or ileoileocolic. The probability of a surgical lesion such as Meckel's diverticulum or polyp producing intussusception rises significantly after 2 years of age, and hydrostatic reduction should not be attempted in these patients. In adults, duodenal or jejunal polypoid tumors (especially leiomyoma, leiomyosarcoma, polyp) lead to the intussusceptum and present as a high mechanical small bowel obstruction. Mechanical small bowel obstruction secondary to intussusception is frequently the presenting problem in *Peutz–Jeghers syndrome*.
Incarcerated hernia (Fig. 9)	Gas-containing small-bowel loops within the hernia. Distended proximal small-bowel with air–fluid levels, e.g., mechanical small bowel obstruction.	Hernias of the groin and anterior abdominal wall are the most common and clinically obvious. Radiologic studies are a primary diagnostic measure in the evaluation of diaphragmatic and internal hernias.
Umbilical hernia (Fig. 9)	Tumor-like density of the hernia and signs of mechanical small-bowel obstruction. Gas-filled loops within the hernial sac indicate the likelihood of incomplete obstruction.	Umbilical hernias are common in middle-aged women and often associated with obesity, history of multiple pregnancies or with cirrhosis and ascites. They are particularly prone to incarceration and strangulation.
Indirect inguinal hernia	Massively distended small-bowel loops converge toward the hernia. The afferent loop of the hernia may be recognized as tapering toward the groin and showing relatively fixed position. A bulging groin mass with a possible gas–fluid level overlies the obturator foramen.	The most common hernia, 50% of all hernias; affects predominantly males. Indirect inguinal hernias are a major cause of small bowel obstruction and strangulation. A gas-filled loop of bowel overlying the obturator foramen and associated bowel distension indicate the presence of *an incarcerated* inguinal hernia. When the obturator foramen on the affected side is occupied by a soft-tissue mass, a *strangulation* must be suspected.
Femoral hernia	Similar to incarcerated or strangulated indirect inguinal hernia.	Femoral hernias occur predominantly (84%) in women. Strangulation occurs ten times as frequently as it does in inguinal hernias. *Richter's hernia* contains only the antimesenteric bowel wall and does not cause radiographic intestinal obstruction.
Internal abdominal hernia	The following patterns may be diagnostic: *Foramen of Winslow hernia* (8%): Mechanical small bowel obstruction in a middle-aged patient. Gas-containing intestinal loops within the lesser sac medial and posterior to the stomach. *Pericecal hernia* (13%): Mechanical small bowel obstruction. A portion of gas-filled ileum may be seen in the right paracolic gutter. *Transmesenteric hernia* (8%): Mechanical small-bowel obstruction with a single distended closed loop in a patient with severe periumbilical pain (similar to small-bowel volvulus).	The majority of internal abdominal hernias are associated with anomalies of rotation and peritoneal attachment. Their incidence is under 1% in autopsies, but most are small and easily reducible. Plain films are taken when they are complicated by small bowel obstruction. In barium studies they may be noted as incidental findings. The most common is *paraduodenal hernia* (53%). It has no characteristic features on plain films. If incarceration of the pericecal hernia is chronic, it may clinically resemble a periappendicular abscess, Crohn's disease, or intestinal obstruction due to adhesions. The transmesenteric hernia is the most common internal hernia in children. The mesenteric defect may be near the ligament of Treitz or near the ileocecal valve. The incidence of strangulation is relatively high and intestinal gangrene is frequent.

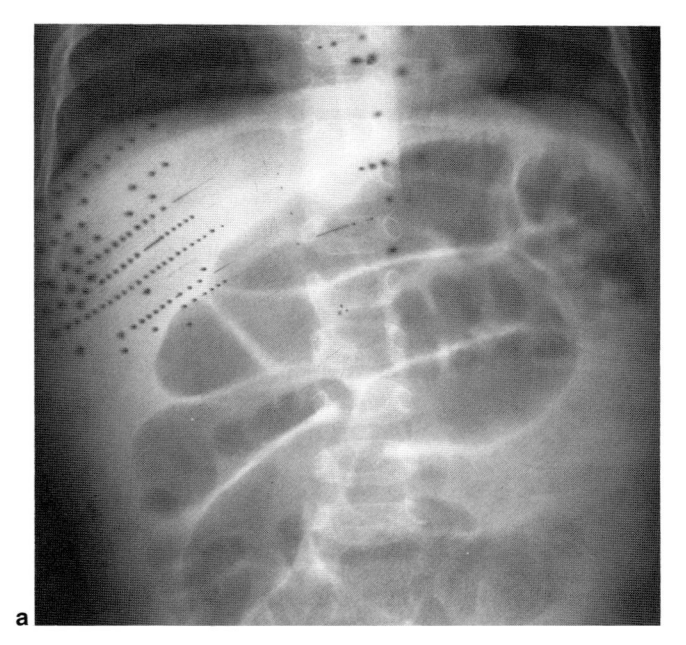

Figure **8a, b Ileocolic intussusception,** age 1. The outline of the proximal colon is not identifiable, the distal colon appears normal. Dilated small bowel loops with air–fluid levels are seen. Valvulae conniventes are not visualized, a common finding in infants and small children.

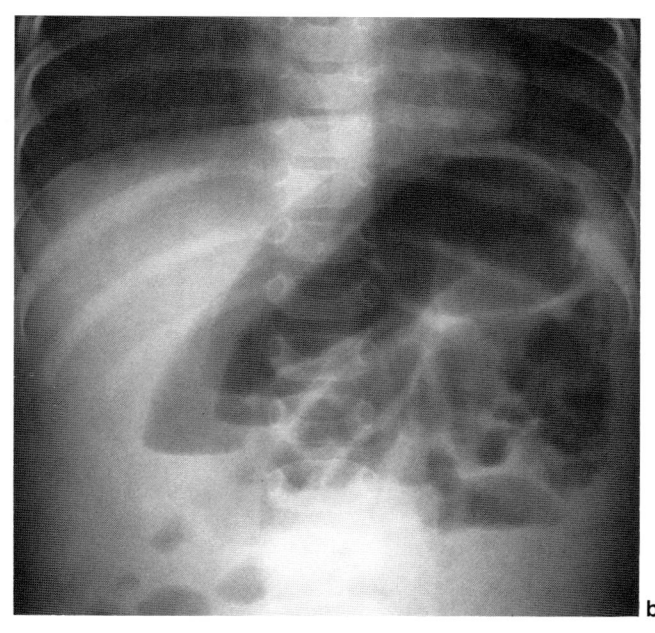

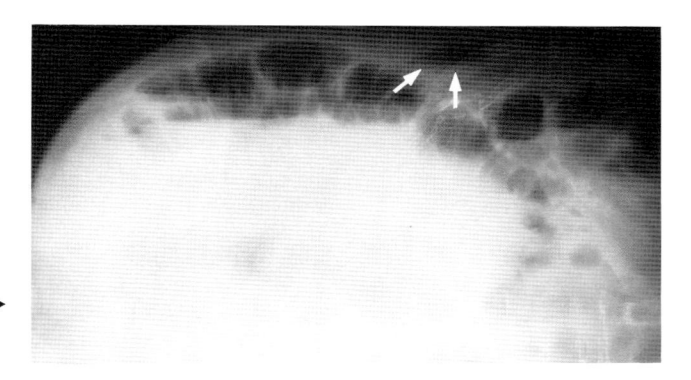

Figure **9 Incarcerated umbilical hernia.** The small bowel ▶ contains multiple air–fluid levels. An air–fluid level is seen in the hernia sac (arrow).

Table 1 (Cont.) Predominantly Small-Bowel Distension

Disease	Radiographic Findings	Comments
Paraesophageal hernia (Fig. 10)	An air–fluid level behind the heart. Symptoms of obstruction without bowel dilatation.	An *obstructed paraesophageal hernia* contains dilated and often twisted stomach whereas *foramen of Bochdaleck* and *foramen of Morgagni hernias* contain large bowel, producing dilatation of the proximal colon if obstructed.
Acquired (traumatic) diaphragmatic hernia (Fig. 11)	A left-sided central or posterior mass above the diaphragm containing stomach and bowel loops or with possible signs of bowel obstruction.	Bochdalek's hernia and acquired diaphragmatic defect appear in the same location. Bochdalek's hernia often contains left kidney and fixed portions of colon, whereas traumatic hernias contain stomach and mobile bowel. 90% of strangulated diaphragmatic hernias are traumatic in origin.
Intestinal pseudo-obstruction (Fig. 12)	Clinical and radiologic evidence of small-bowel obstruction with patent bowel lumen. A barium study is necessary to distinguish this condition from obstruction, unless associated findings of disease are present.	Occurs in generalized diseases with decreased motor function of the bowel, e.g., *pancreatitis, renal failure, lower lobe pneumonia, scleroderma, myxedema, systemic amyloidosis, congestive heart failure, trauma, nontropical sprue* or can be idiopathic.
Postoperative	*Pelvic surgery* that involved manipulation of the small-bowel often causes radiographic changes indistinguishable from mechanical small bowel obstruction between the second and fifth postoperative day. *Gastric surgery* may be complicated by stasis of food and secretions in the afferent loop and present as distension of a jejunal loop. *Ileostomy* dysfunction may present as dilated distal ileum.	*Narcotic analgesia* during the operation commonly causes temporary small-bowel distension. Bowel dilatation may be secondary to *postoperative hypokalemia*.
Localized ileus (sentinel loop) (Fig. 13)	An isolated loop of intestine distended with air due to adjoining inflammation. *Duodenum:* acute pancreatitis, acute cholecystitis, trauma. *Left upper quadrant:* acute pancreatitis *Right lower quadrant:* acute pancreatitis *Terminal ileum:* acute appendicitis *Small bowel around pelvic floor:* acute salpingitis.	Only the most common causes and patterns are mentioned here. Any segment of bowel can be paralyzed due to adjoining inflammation. In pancreatitis, the whole small bowel may be paralyzed. Also the ascending and transverse colon may be dilated in pancreatitis (colon cut-off sign). Cecum is usually involved in appendicitis. Perforation of appendicitis may cause true distal small bowel obstruction or paralytic ileus secondary to peritonitis.

Abnormal Gas Pattern

Figure **10 Incarcerated paraesophageal hernia** containing a twisted stomach (mesenteroaxial volvulus) and an air–fluid level. The gas pattern is otherwise unremarkable. Barium is seen in the distal esophagus.

Figure **11a, b Traumatic left diaphragmatic hernia** with bowel obstruction. The stomach is displaced into the left hemithorax. It is dilated and contains an air–fluid level.

Figure **12 Scleroderma with intestinal pseudo-obstruction.** Multiple dilated loops with air–fluid levels in the small bowel. There is plenty of colonic gas but no air–fluid levels in the colon.

Figure **13 Localized ileus** (sentinel loop) in traumatic perforation of the descending duodenum, a left lateral decubitus projection. The duodenal loop is slightly dilated and edematous. Retroperitoneal gas is present as small air bubbles above the duodenum (arrows).

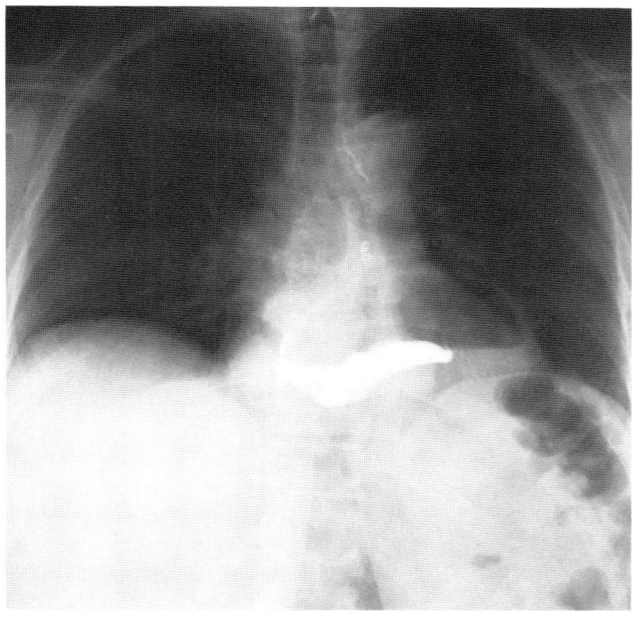

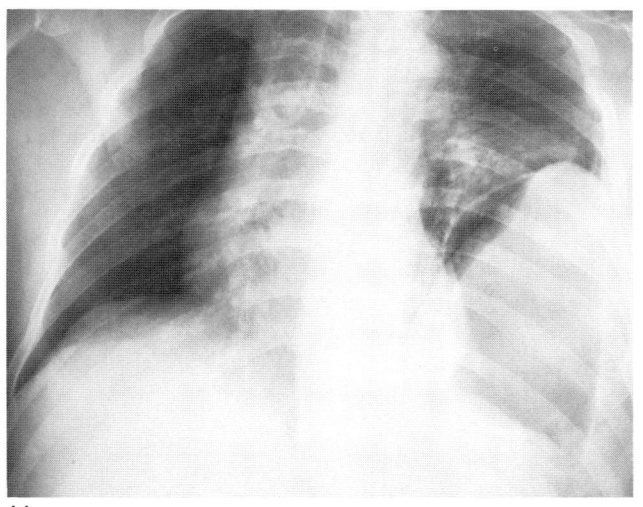

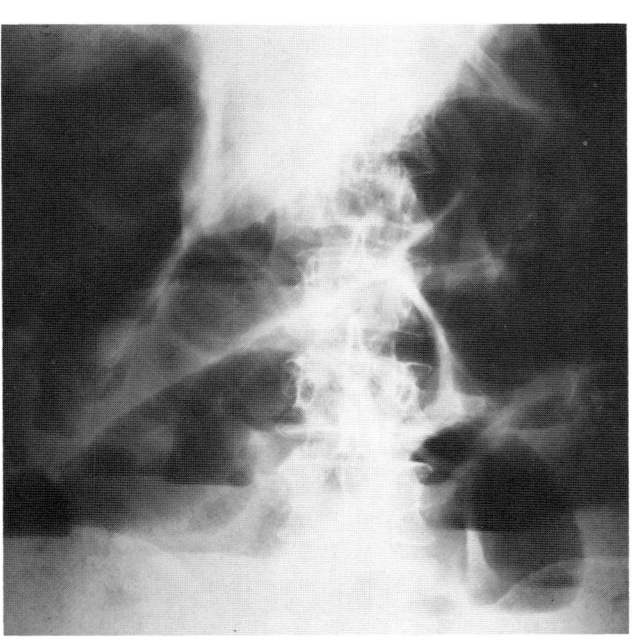

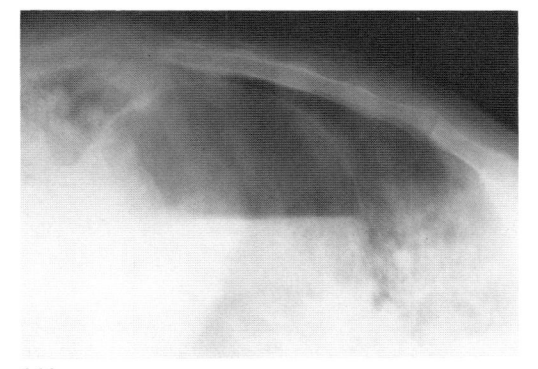

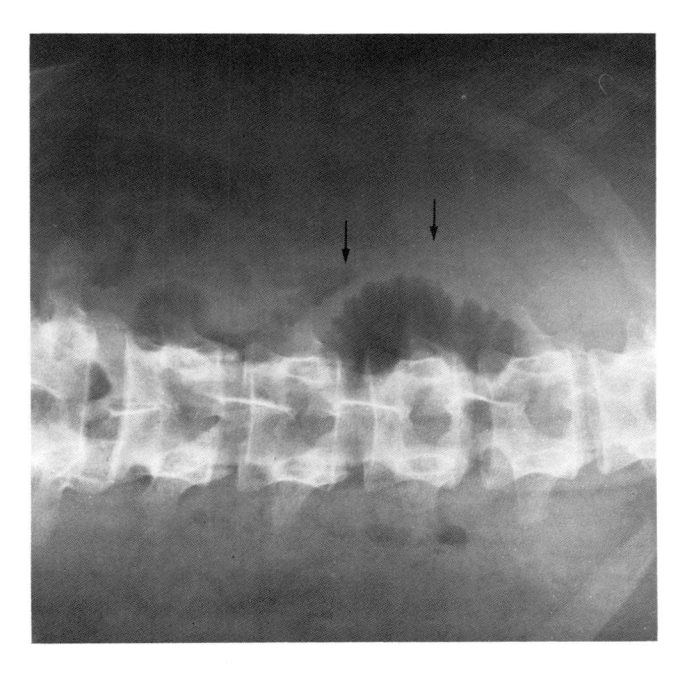

Table 2 Large Bowel Distension

Disease	Radiographic Findings	Comments
Obstructive lesions		
Simple mechanical occlusion of colonic lumen (carcinoma of colon, diverticulitis, stricture due to colitis, radiation or trauma) (Figs. 14–16)	Three radiographic patterns may be present: 1 Closed-loop obstruction with competent ileocecal valve: colon dilated to the level of obstruction, minimal or no dilatation of distal ileal coils. Distended cecum. 2 Closed-loop obstruction with competent ileocecal valve and obstruction pattern in small bowel: colon dilated to the level of obstruction with marked dilatation of cecum and dilatation of loops of small bowel proximal to cecum. 3 Closed-loop obstruction with incompetent ileocecal valve: colon dilated to the level of obstruction, moderately dilated cecum, moderately distended loops of ileum. Fluid levels in colon and small bowel.	The majority of simple colonic occlusions are due to carcinoma. The sigmoid region is the usual site of obstruction in both carcinoma and diverticulitis, which is the second most common cause. Rare causes of simple colonic obstruction include *sarcoma, benign tumor, lymphogranuloma, actinomycosis, dysentery, hematoma, pancreatic pseudocyst, huge urinary bladder.* If obstruction is incomplete, the pattern may be less characteristic on plain films.
Sigmoid volvulus (Fig. 17, p. 11, Fig. 23, p. 16)	Markedly distended sigmoid loop with loss of haustral margins ascending from the pelvis in a vertical or oblique direction, overlapped by the distended proximal colon. Small-bowel distension is not significant in the early phase. Air–fluid levels are present in the ascending and descending colon proximal to the volvulus. Three lines formed by bowel wall converge downward to the point of twisting.	The most common colonic volvulus (over 50%). Twisting of a long and freely movable sigmoid loop, usually in a counterclockwise direction from 180° to 720°. Air in the wall of the bowel is suggestive of gangrene. *Pseudovolvulus* is produced by a dilated redundant ptotic transverse colon in simple obstruction of the sigmoid. It simulates sigmoid volvulus radiographically.

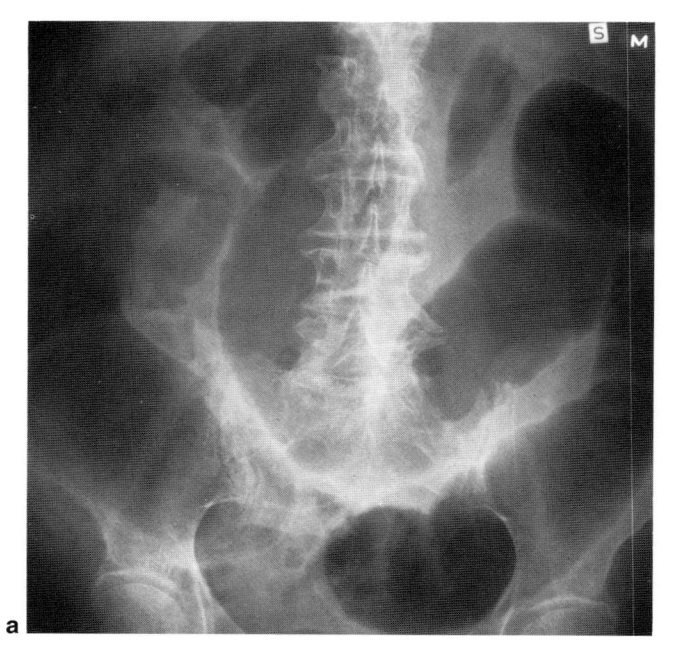

Figure **14a,b** **a** Supine and **b** upright. **Distal colonic occlusion** (carcinoma of the sigmoid colon). Dilatation of colon with air–fluid levels. Minimal dilatation of distal ileum.

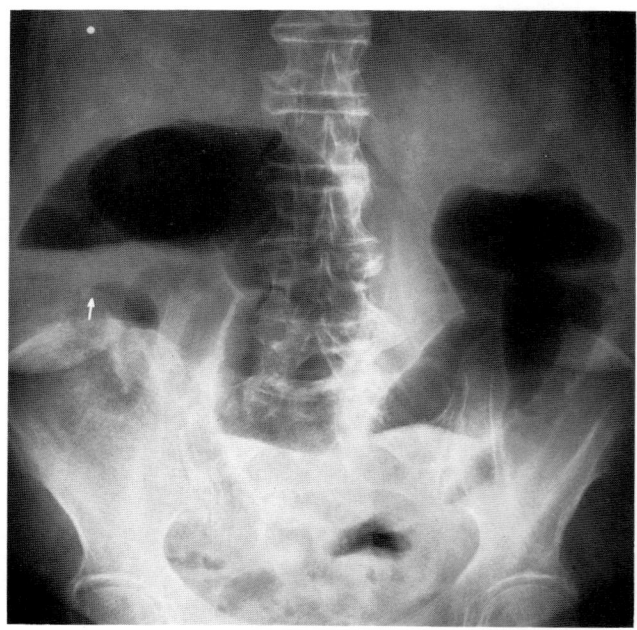

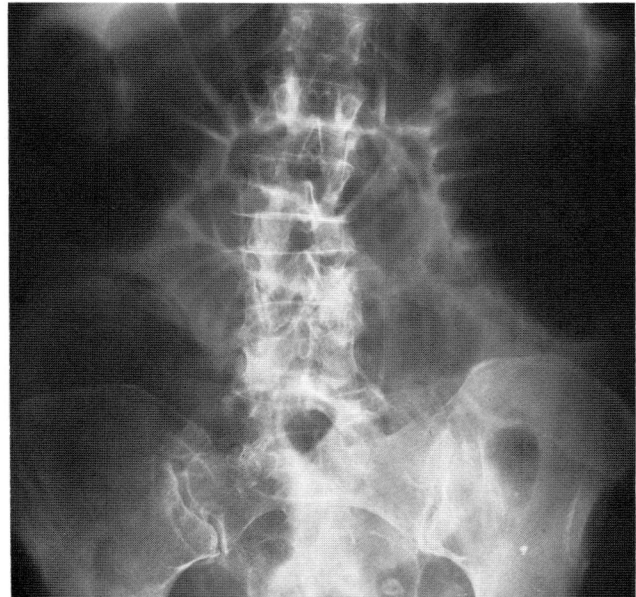

Abnormal Gas Pattern

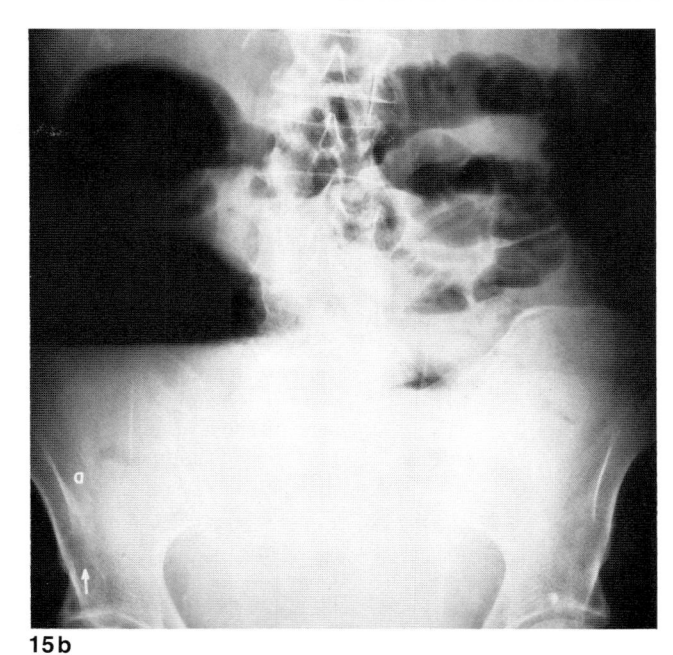

Figure **15a, b a** Supine and (**b**) upright. **Distal colonic occlusion** (carcinoma of the distal descending colon). Dilated colon with air–fluid levels proximal to the obstruction and dilated small bowel loops with air–fluid levels, as well.

Figure **16** Supine. **Carcinoma of the transverse colon** with partial occlusion. The right transverse colon is dilated, the left colon contains only little gas.

Figure **17a, b a** supine and **b** upright. **Sigmoid volvulus.** Massively distended sigmoid loop with air–fluid levels and loss of haustral markings. Little distension of the feces-containing colon proximal to the obstruction. The sigmoid loop creates a "coffee bean" sign.

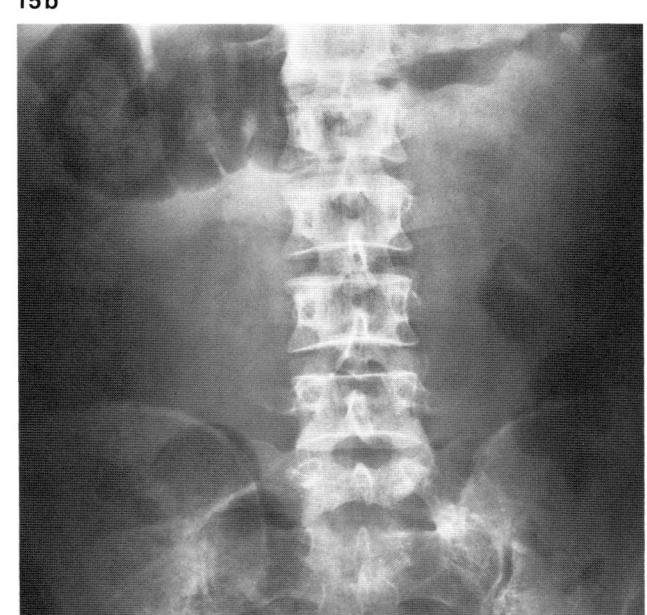

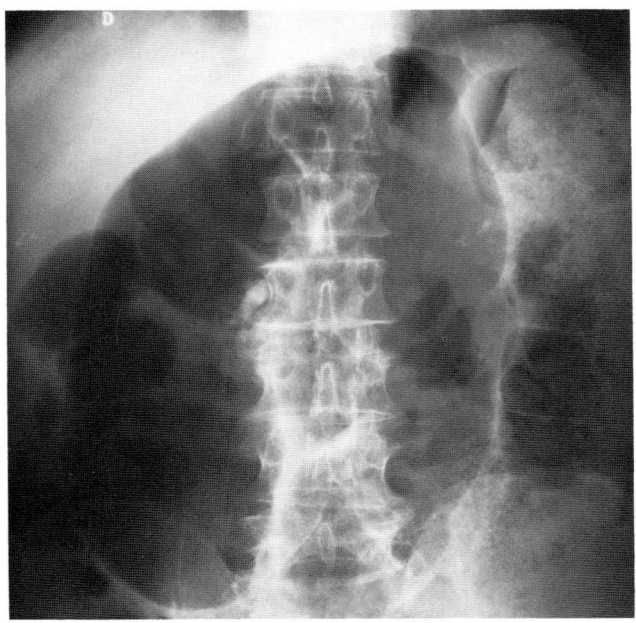

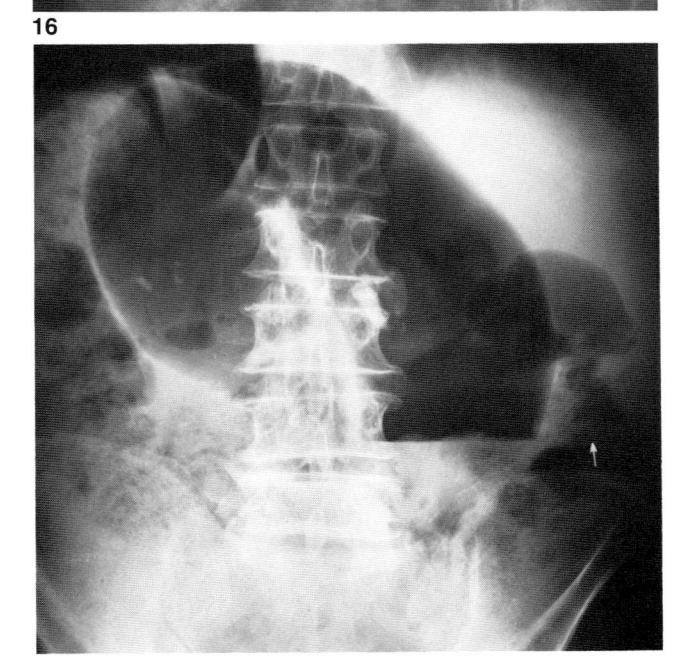

Table 2 (Cont.) Large Bowel Distension

Disease	Radiographic Findings	Comments
Cecal volvulus (Fig. 18)	Severely distended, kidney- or bean-shaped cecum projects upwards and may be in the epigastrium or left upper quadrant. One large air–fluid level is present in the cecum, the rest of the colon contains little or no gas or feces. The small bowel is distended.	The second most common colonic volvulus (15 to 44%). Torsion of cecum is only possible when it has a mesentery. Volvulus usually occurs in a clockwise direction.
Intestinal knot syndrome	Dilated sigmoid loop as in sigmoid volvulus. The remainder of the large bowel contains a variable amount of gas and fluid. Obstructed and twisted ileal loops are usually seen on the left side of the abdomen (reversed positions of sigmoid and ileal loops).	Twisting of the terminal ileum around the sigmoid colon that in turn has rotated on its own axis to create a volvulus is a relatively common (approximately 9%) presentation. Both ileum and sigmoid must have a long mesentery. When severe obstruction of the small bowel is present together with a typical sigmoid volvulus, an intestinal knot should be suspected. It requires prompt surgical intervention.
Volvulus of the transverse colon	Dilatation of the proximal large bowel, elevation of the distended hepatic flexure under the right hemidiaphragm. Small-bowel distension. The point of twist may be seen at the level of the proximal transverse colon.	A rare type of colonic volvulus (1% or less). It occurs only when the transverse colon is very redundant and the flexures approach each other.
Fecal impaction (Fig. 19)	Mottled radiolucencies of fecal debris, dilatation of colon above the fecal mass. Common locations of impaction are rectum (60%), sigmoid (15%), cecum (10%).	Fecal impaction may be secondary to loss of defecation reflex (old age, psychosis), loss of peristalsis (spinal cord injury, tertiary syphilis), or an anal lesion causing pain (hemorrhoid, fissure, fistula). Anatomic causes include carcinoma, diverticulitis, and Hirschsprung's disease. Rare causes include impacted gallstone, bezoar, foreign body, and enterolith.
Adhesions, hernias, extraintestinal masses (Fig. 20) *Obstruction with open lumen*	Signs of partial or complete (simple) large bowel obstruction.	
Jejunoileal bypass (for morbid obesity)	*Colonic pseudo-obstruction:* colonic distension with normal bowel outline. Air–fluid levels both in large and small bowel. Gas may be present also in the bowel wall.	Dilatation of the large bowel to a diameter of more than 7 cm is present in 50% of patients. Increase of the small-bowel diameter and increased thickness of the valvulae conniventes are almost regularly seen.
Megacolon (idiopathic, acquired, psychogenic) **Chronic constipation**	The entire colon down to the lower rectum is dilated and filled with fecal material and gas.	In *congenital megacolon* (Hirschsprung's disease) and *Chagas' disease* (South American trypanosomiasis) dilatation of the rectum is usually absent. A neurogenically dilated colon may complicate *diabetes mellitus*. Chronic constipation and megacolon is a common feature in *parkinsonism*.

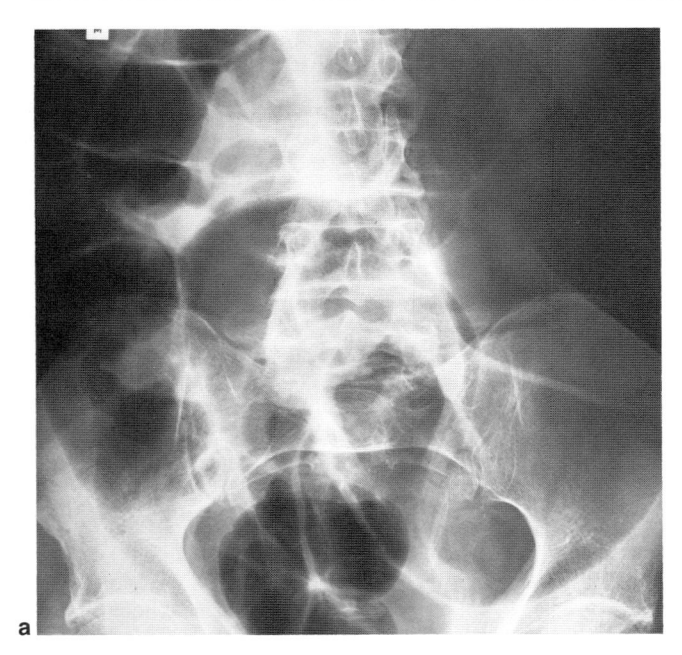

Figure **18a, b**   **a** Supine and **b** upright. **Cecal volvulus.** Massively dilated cecum projects into the left epigastrium and contains an air–fluid level. The proximal colon and the distal small bowel are moderately distended. The hepatic flexure is displaced between the diaphragm and the liver **(Chilaiditi syndrome).**

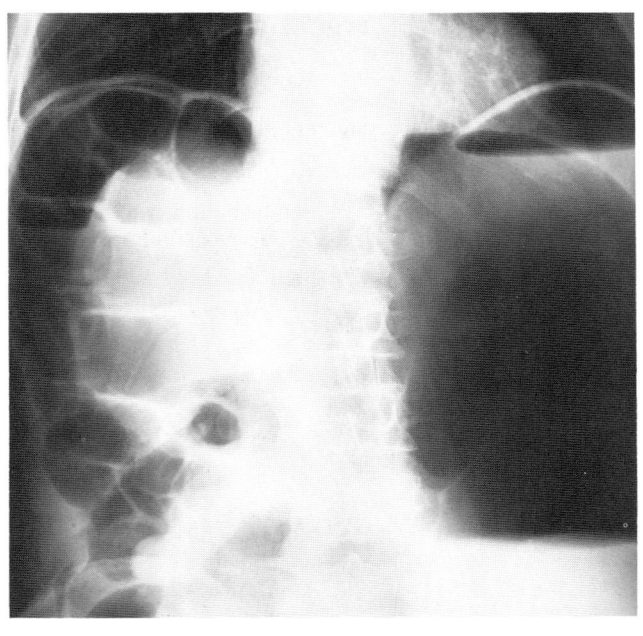

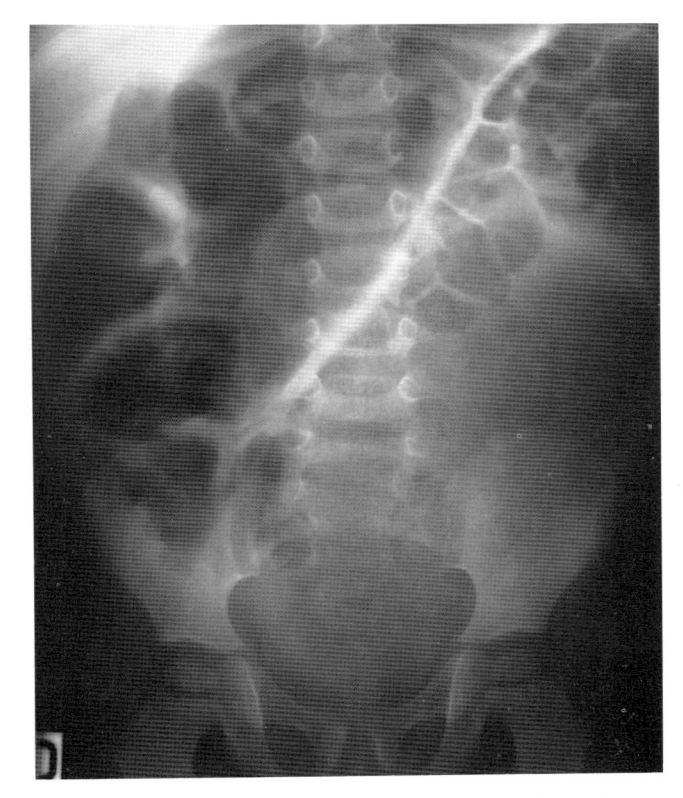

Figure **19 Fecal impaction.** Fecal material distends the rectum and colon. Dilatation of the colon proximal to the impaction. A three-year-old boy with **Hirschsprung's disease.**

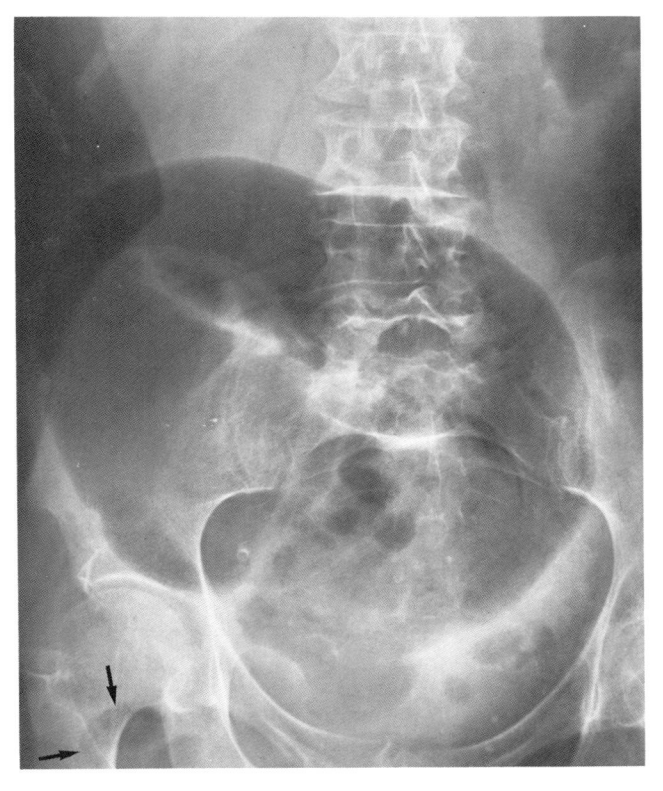

Figure **20 Incarceration of the transverse colon** in a right femoral hernia. There is subtle radiolucency over the right femoral neck representing the incarcerated segment (arrows). The dilated large bowel loop above it mimics volvulus of the sigmoid colon.

Table 2 (Cont.) Large Bowel Distension

Disease	Radiographic Findings	Comments
Paralytic (adynamic) ileus, generalized peritonitis (Fig. 21)	Dilatation of both large and small bowel with air–fluid levels in both. There is no stepladder arrangement of small bowel loops and no significant interval change in the gas pattern between examinations.	For various causes of paralytic ileus see Chapter 4, page 83. Colonic dilatation tends to be prominent in peritonitis.
Colonic pseudo-obstruction (Colonic ileus, Ogilvie's syndrome)	Predominantly colonic dilatation with little or no dilatation of the small bowel.	Common causes of colonic ileus include: *acute appendicitis* (see below), *acute cholecystitis, acute pancreatitis, congestive heart failure, idiopathic, low serum potassium concentration, low spinal and cauda equina lesions, inferior mesenteric thrombosis* (see below), *morphine overdosage, peritonitis, pelvic postsurgical states, renal failure, urinary calculus.*
Appendicitis	Moderate dilatation of cecum with an air–fluid level. Atonic distal ileum with fluid levels. Appendicolithiasis. Fluid in the pericecal area. Gas in irregularly distended appendix. Mass (abscess) indenting the cecum.	Dilatation of cecum and terminal ileum with fluid levels, and haziness due to fluid collections, is designated as appendiceal ileus and is highly suggestive of acute appendicitis. Recognition of an appendiceal stone is the single most important finding.
Ischemic colitis	Slight to moderate distension of involved bowel segment(s). Thumbprinting, produced by submucosal hemorrhage. Transverse ridging, produced by multiple parallel lucent bands crossing the involved segment of colon. Thickened and blunted mucosal folds. Loss of haustral patterns.	In superior mesenteric artery occlusion these changes are seen in small bowel and proximal colon. In inferior mesenteric artery occlusion, these changes occur in the distal colon. Intramural gas, gas in portal veins, and megacolon are rare complications of ischemia. Occlusion of the superior mesenteric vein produces thick bowel wall and a narrow, gas-filled lumen. Localized ischemic colitis may occur in small vessel sclerosis, cardiac disease, collagen diseases, and after surgery and cause minimal plain film changes.
Toxic megacolon (Fig. 22)	Extensive unchanging colonic distension, most severe in the transverse colon, which has a diameter of 6 cm or more. Air–fluid levels are present especially in the distal transverse colon. Normal haustral pattern and redundancy are absent. Soft-tissue defects may protrude into the lumen and represent sloughing mucosa or pseudopolyps. Submucosal radiolucent lines may parallel the colonic wall.	Severe dilatation of the colon associated with colitis, most commonly in ulcerative colitis (2 to 3% of ulcerative colitis patients), usually early in the course of the disease. For other causes of toxic megacolon, see Table **3**, page 16. In children, Hirschsprung's disease with exudative enteropathy may produce a similar appearance.
Typhlitis	Enlarging soft-tissue density in the right flank due to a dilated and atonic fluid-filled right colon. Small bowel dilatation may be present.	A complication of end-stage *leukemia* or *aplastic anemia* in children, caused by severe hemorrhagic necrosis of the cecum or surrounding bowel, without perforation.

Abnormal Gas Pattern 15

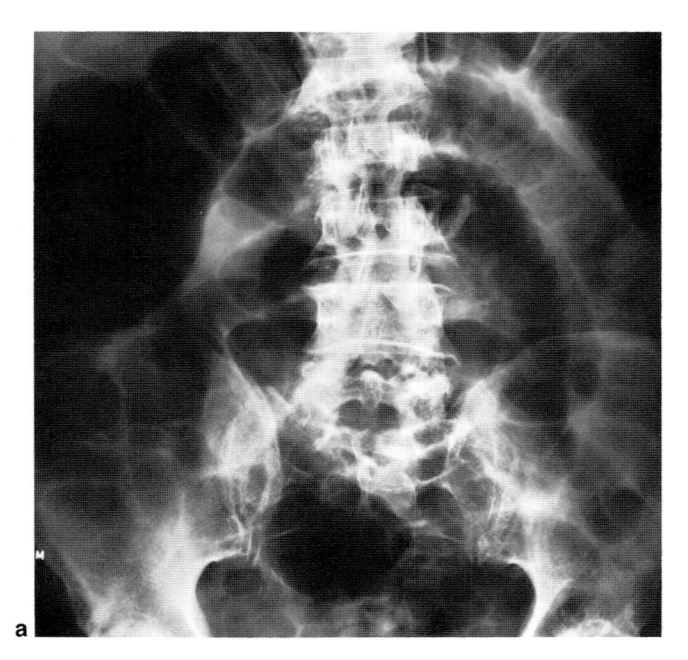

Figure **21a, b** **a** Supine and **b** upright. **Paralytic ileus.** Both the small and large bowel are dilated and contain air–fluid levels.

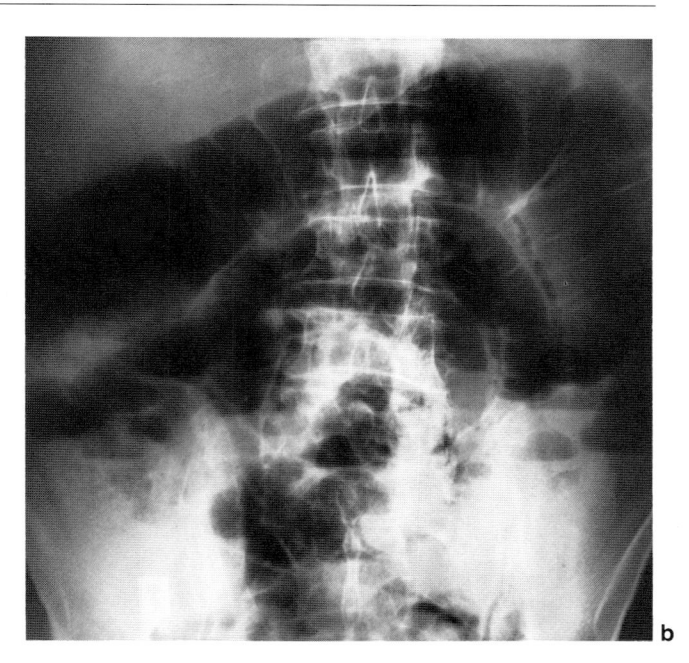

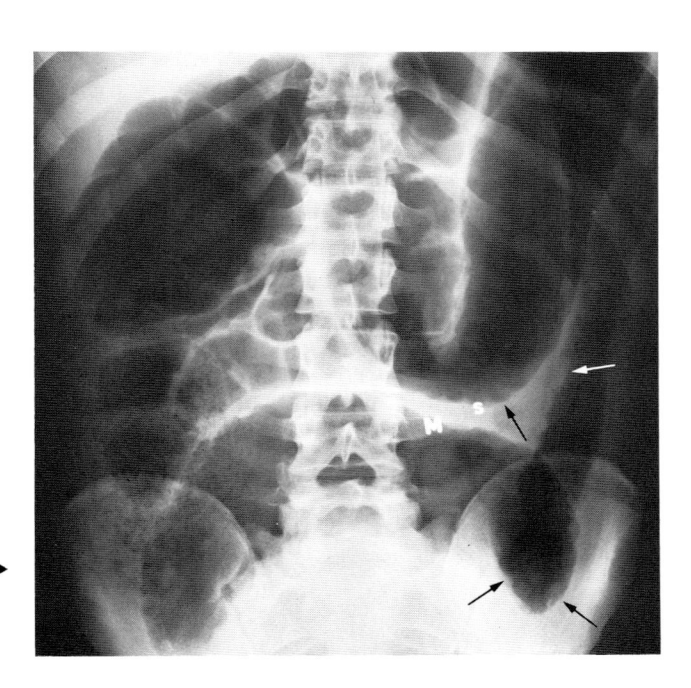

Figure **22** **Toxic megacolon** (colitis ulcerosa). Colonic distension, most severe in the transverse colon. Normal haustral pattern is lost. Soft-tissue densities (pseudopolyps, arrows) project into the lumen in the left colon.

Table 3 Abnormal Gas Pattern in a Neonate

Disease	Radiographic Findings	Comments
Esophageal atresia without fistula	Gasless abdomen. A blind gaseous pouch in the neck.	In approximately 10% of cases of esophageal atresia there is no fistula between distal segment and trachea. Associated anomalies are common.
Duodenal atresia or stenosis **Annular pancreas** (Fig. 23, 24)	"Double bubble", air–fluid levels in the dilated stomach and dilated first part of the duodenum. Gas in distal small bowel is either absent (atresia) or diminished (stenosis).	About 30% of duodenal atresias are associated with Down's syndrome. Other anomalies are frequent. Annular pancreas in infants is associated with duodenal stenosis in about 50%.
Atresia or stenosis of the ileum or jejunum	Multiple distended bowel loops with fluid levels. The most distal loop may be grossly dilated and mimic colonic obstruction. Jejunal atresia has fewer dilated loops. Loops may be completely fluid-filled.	Ileal atresia or stenosis is the most common type of intestinal atresia (50%) and may be multiple. Contrast enema will show a microcolon and possibly an associated malrotation. *Colonic atresia* is indistinguishable from ileal atresia on plain films.
Imperforate anus **Rectal atresia** (Fig. 25)	Pattern of low colonic occlusion: Gaseous distension of the colon and small intestine with fluid levels. Gas in the urinary bladder indicates a high lesion with an enterovesical fistula. The inverted lateral view will show the level of obstruction.	Associated malformation and fistulas are frequent. Fistulas may prevent bowel obstruction.
Malrotation **Peritoneal bands** **Midgut volvulus**	Dilated stomach and duodenum with air–fluid levels. Duodenal obstruction lower than in duodenal atresia or annular pancreas. Small amounts of gas may be seen in the distal intestine.	The rotation of the midgut loop has been arrested, e.g., cecum lies anterior to the duodenum and is fixed by bands that obstruct the third portion of duodenum (*Ladd–Waugh syndrome*) and there is tendency to midgut volvulus. Dilated small bowel indicates obstruction of the superior mesenteric vein and devitalized bowel.
Pyloric stenosis (Fig. 26)	Distended stomach with air–fluid level. Relative paucity of gas in the intestines. Hyperperistalsis may be seen.	Barium meal or ultrasound examination are diagnostic.

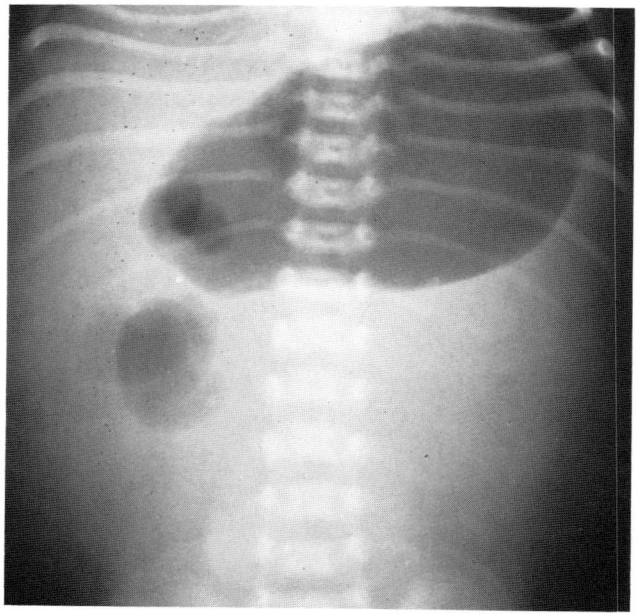

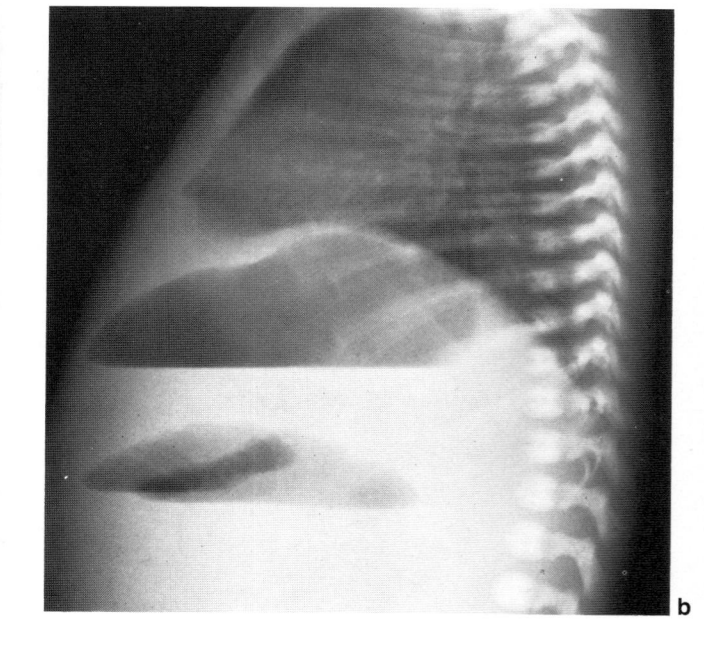

Figure **23a, b Duodenal atresia.** A characteristic "double bubble" gas pattern of the abdomen.

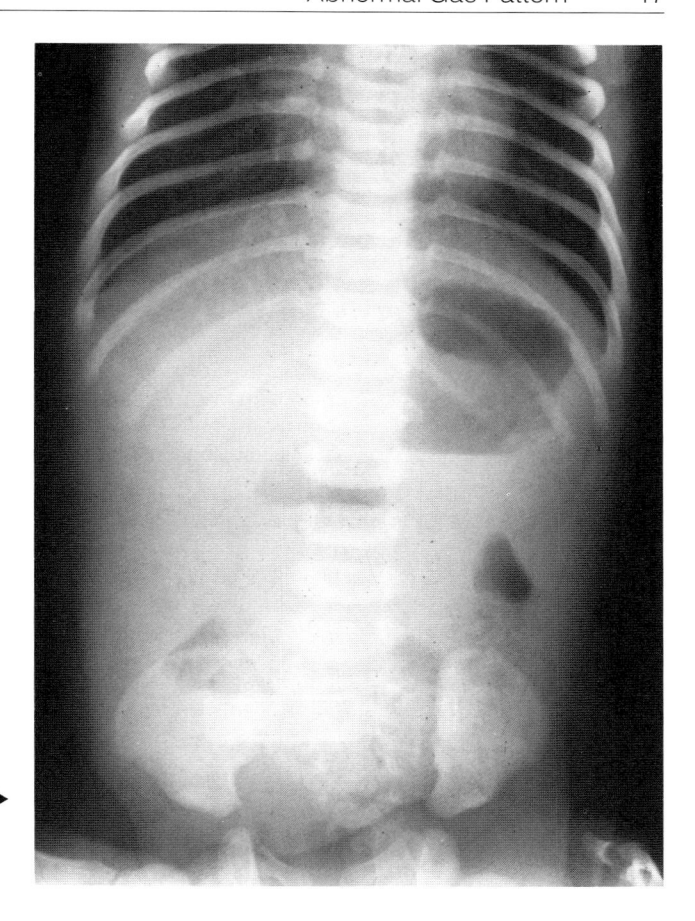

Figure 24 **Partial duodenal obstruction** (annular pancreas) associated with Down's syndrome. Relatively gasless abdomen, air–fluid levels in the stomach and duodenum. Flared iliac wings.

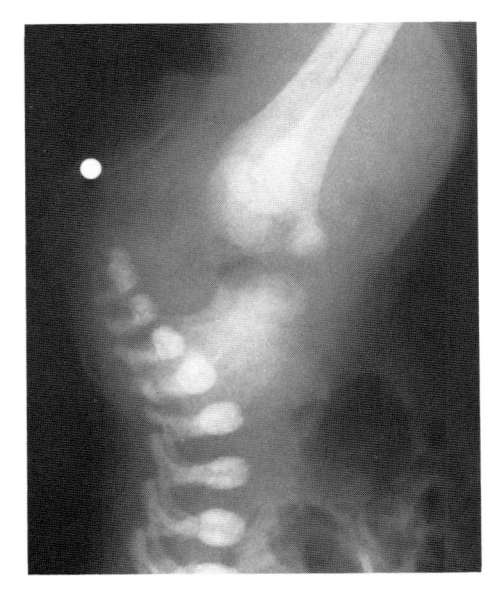

Figure 25 **Rectal atresia.** Inverted lateral view demonstrates a long segment on nonpatent bowel.

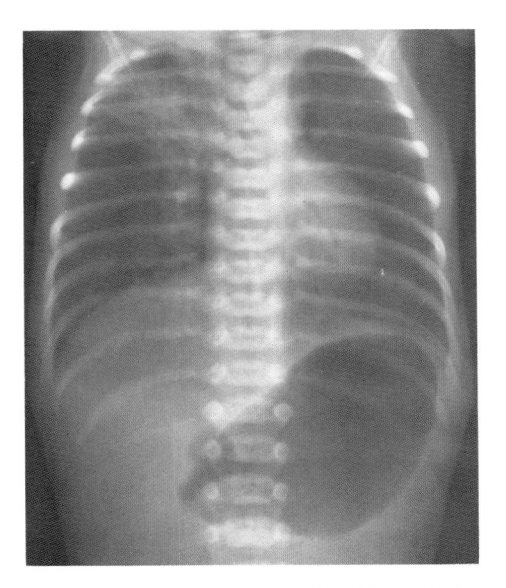

Figure 26 **Pyloric stenosis.** Distended stomach, gasless abdomen.

Table 3 (Cont.)   **Abnormal Gas Pattern in a Neonate**

Disease	Radiographic Findings	Comments
Diaphragmatic hernia of Bochdalek (Fig. 27)	Loops of bowel containing air are herniated usually into the left hemithorax. The mediastinum is displaced and the abdomen is relatively airless.	If the herniated bowel is obstructed, air–fluid levels and bowel distension are present.
Intramural duplication cyst of the terminal ileum	Multiple distended bowel loops with fluid levels. (Nonspecific intestinal obstruction).	Duplications may grow large enough to be palpable. When large enough, any duplication may cause intestinal obstruction.
Meconium plug syndrome	Moderate dilatation of both small bowel and colon with eventual fluid levels. Water soluble contrast enema will reveal the plug and normal-sized colon and dislodge the plug.	Normally meconium is passed during the first 12 to 24 hours of life. The pattern may mimic Hirschsprung's disease (aganglionosis).
Hirschsprung's disease (congenital intestinal aganglionosis)	A pattern of distal large bowel obstruction: Dilated bowel with multiple fluid levels. If only a short segment is involved, the distended sigmoid may resemble sigmoid volvulus. Inverted lateral film may show the narrowed rectum outlined with air, and an "egg on end" appearance of the distended abdomen. Barium enema will identify the length of the aganglionic (narrow) segment.	Congenital absence of ganglia in the submucosal and myenteric plexuses of the distal part of the colon. The disease is limited to the rectosigmoid in 80%. May cause urgent symptoms (obstruction or diarrhea) in the neonate. Enterocolitis occurs in 50% of infants suffering from aganglionosis.
Meconium ileus (Fig. 28)	Multiple dilated loops of bowel that vary greatly in size. Absence of fluid–levels is pathognomonic. Masses of granular meconium are often visualized.	The terminal ileum is obstructed by masses of abnormal meconium. An early manifestation of *cystic fibrosis*. Masses of meconium may be seen also in *Hirschsprung's disease* and in *anorectal malformations*.
Meconium peritonitis (Fig. 40, p. 27)	Intra-abdominal, extraluminal calcifications. Multiple distended bowel loops with fluid levels (due to the underlying intestinal obstruction). Loculated pneumoperitoneum.	Intrauterine perforation of the bowel due to any obstructing lesion (atresia, meconium ileus, volvulus, Meckel's diverticulum, internal hernia, or bands) or without any obvious cause. If perforation is not sealed at birth, a secondary septic peritonitis develops.
Functional obstruction	Dense, amorphous intraluminal masses in the bowel, frequently surrounded by a halo of gas. Fluid levels are scarce.	Impaired intestinal motility without an obvious cause. Occurs particularly in premature infants. Pellets of inspissated milk collect in the colon and terminal ileum.
Necrotizing enterocolitis (ischemic bowel disease) (Fig. 29)	Either decrease of the amount of intestinal gas or gaseous distension of the bowel with possible air–fluid levels. Gas in the bowel wall is characteristic. It is seen as fine bubbles or radiolucent lines in the wall of the small and/or large bowel.	Enterocolitis occurs predominantly in premature infants due to various causes of perinatal stress. A pneumoperitoneum indicates a perforation unless ventilatory assistance was used, whereas gas in the portal veins indicates a probable fatal outcome. Bowel strictures may develop as complications.

Abnormal Gas Pattern 19

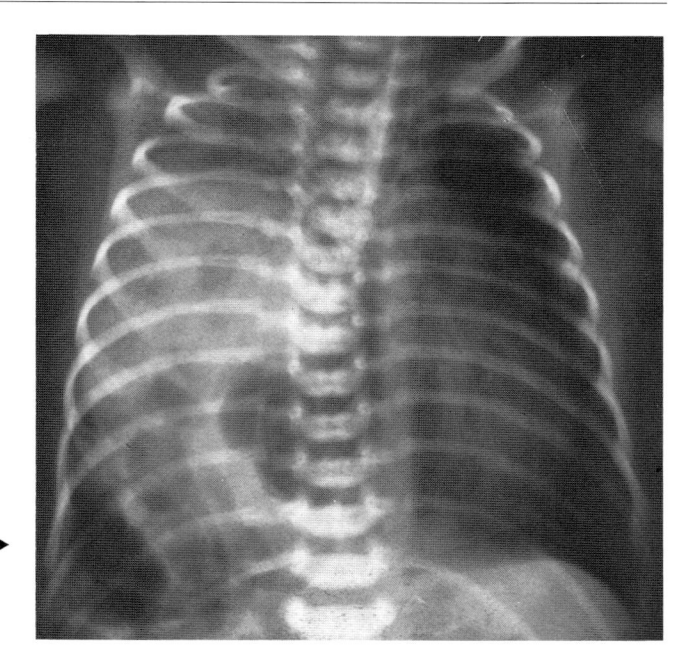

Figure **27 Diaphragmatic hernia of Bochdalek** containing the right liver lobe, cecum, ascending colon and parts of the ileum. The right hemithorax is opaque with bowel gas lucencies. The mediastinum is displaced toward the left.

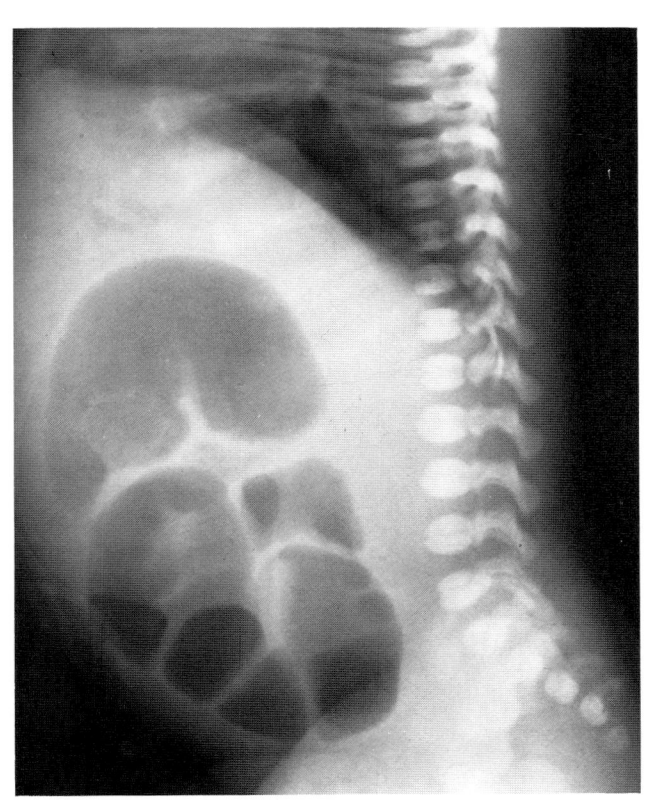

Figure **28 Meconium ileus.** Dilated bowel loops without air–fluid levels in a radiograph with a horizontal roentgen beam is a pathognomonic finding.

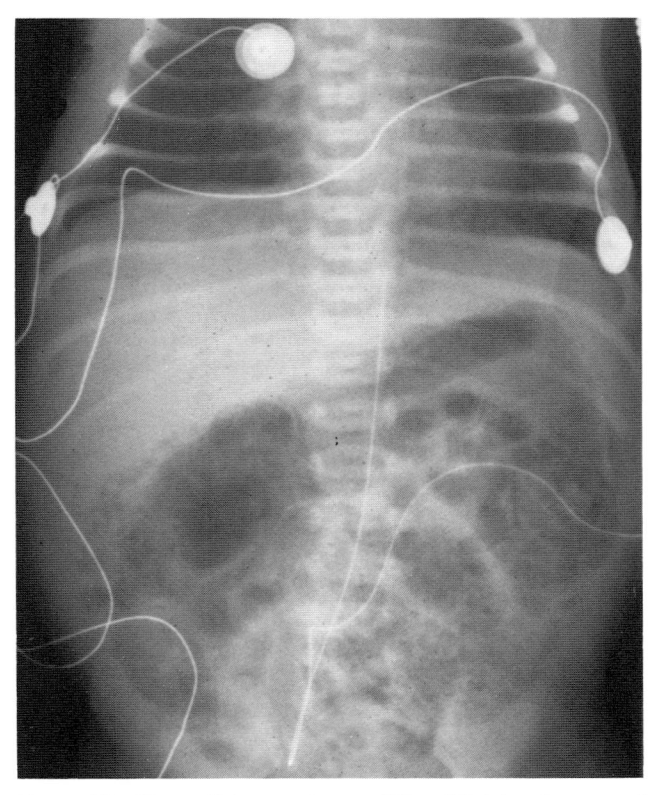

Figure **29 Necrotizing enterocolitis.** Slightly decreased amount of intestinal gas with gas in the bowel wall evident as small lucent straks and bubbles.

Table 3 (Cont.) Abnormal Gas Pattern in a Neonate

Disease	Radiographic Findings	Comments
A. Pneumoperitoneum		
Obstructed inguinal hernia	A pattern of small-bowel obstruction.	Usually of the indirect type, more common on the left.
Gastroenteritis	Dilated bowel loops and air–fluid levels simulate low colonic obstruction.	With excessive vomiting, the amount of gas will diminish.
Severe dehydration **Inability to swallow** **Peritoneal fluid**	Decreased amount of intestinal gas is a common observation in these conditions.	Secondary to: Severe gastroenteritis with vomiting Brain damage Respirator distress Obstruction of the lower urinary tract (urethral valve) Vitamin K deficiency
Pneumoperitoneum (secondary to perforated viscus, assisted respiration or postoperative leak (Fig. 30)	Free air in the abdomen with absence of the normal distended stomach suggests perforation of the stomach. Loculated pneumoperitoneum may occur in meconium peritonitis.	Perforation of the stomach is the most common cause and usually spontaneous. Small intestinal perforations are usually associated with obstructing lesions. Colonic perforations occur in necrotizing enterocolitis, Hirschsprung's disease, or strangulating volvulus. Postoperative gas in a newborn abdomen without leak is rare.

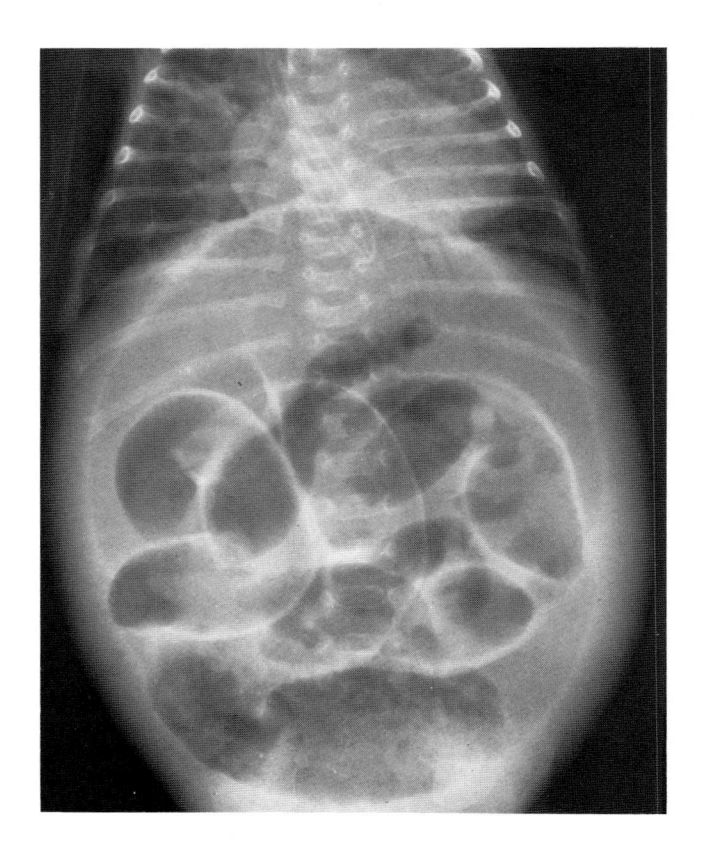

Figure **30** **Pneumoperitoneum after perforation of the cecum.** A large collection of gas is seen in the peritoneal cavity and the bowel loops are distended, indicating bowel paralysis. This infant also had patent ductus arteriosus.

Table 4   Extraluminal Gas Collections in the Abdomen or Pelvis

Disease	Radiographic Findings	Comments
Postoperative (laparotomy, abdominal drainage tubes, peritoneal dialysis)	Gas in the uppermost part of the peritoneal cavity without air–fluid level. Best visualized under the right hemidiaphragm in upright position and in the right-side-up decubitus position between the liver and the right lateral peritoneum. Gas may be present up to 24 days after operation; it usually disappears within 3 to 6 days.	Radiograph should be taken 5 to 10 min after placing the patient to the appropriate position. Postoperative gas is present more often in asthenic patients (80%) than in obese ones (25%), and in greater quantities after upper abdominal or pelvic surgery. Peritonitis has no influence on the disappearance of the gas. A leak should be suspected if gas is present after 3 days in an obese patient or in a child. Colonic interposition between the liver and the diaphragm (Chilaiditi syndrome) may be mistaken for intraperitoneal gas.
Perforated viscus (Figs. 31, 32)	Free intraperitoneal gas usually with clinical and radiographic signs (peritoneal fluid, paralytic ileus, pain-induced scoliosis) of peritonitis. Gas may also appear as a triangular subhepatic collection overlying the right kidney.	The most common causes are: *perforated peptic ulcer* and *perforated colonic diverticulum,* especially in renal transplant patients, rarely abdominal *trauma, perforated appendicitis* or ruptured *pneumatosis cystoides intestinalis.* Free intraperitoneal gas is present in 67% of perforated ulcers. Colonic perforation tends to produce large gas collections.
Resuscitation, anesthesia or endoscopic instrumentation	Small amount of intraperitoneal gas with or without gastric dilatation or pneumomediastinum.	Gas leaks from the mediastinum or thinned dilated segment of the intestine without perforation and peritonitis.
Spontaneous pneumoperitoneum without peritonitis (idiopathic)	Free intraperitoneal gas in the absence of disease, suggestive history, or symptoms.	The most common cause is suction of air through the female genital tract. A *forme fruste* perforation of a peptic ulcer should be considered.

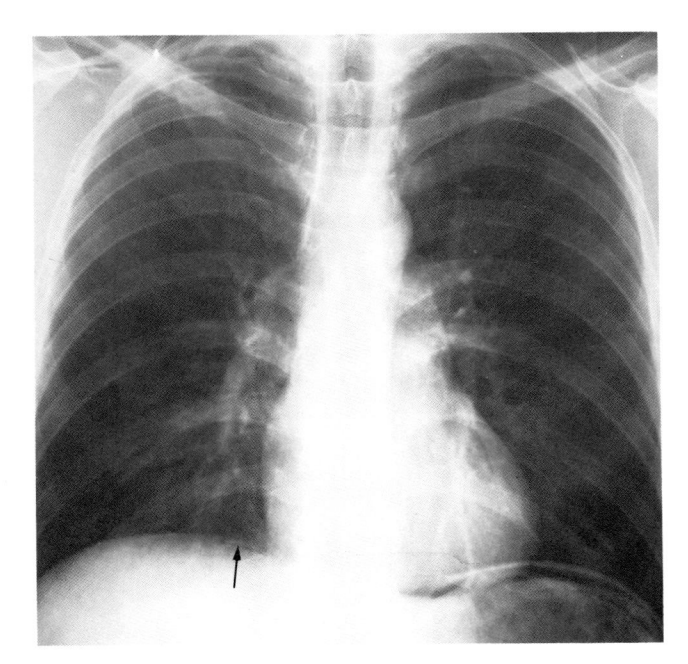

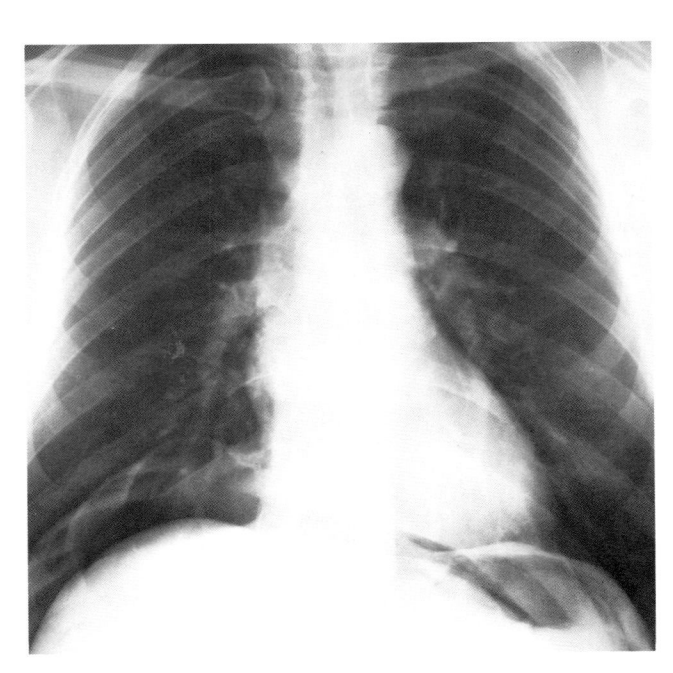

Figure 31   **Free intraperitoneal gas** under both hemidiaphragm. Perforated duodenal ulcer.

Figure 32   **Large free intraperitoneal gas** collections. Perforated colon, a complication secondary to ulcerative colitis.

Table 4 (Cont.) **Extraluminal Gas Collections in the Abdomen or Pelvis**

Disease	Radiographic Findings	Comments
B. Gas in the Bowel Wall		
Pneumatosis cystoides intestinalis (Fig. 33)	Round extrinsic and intrinsic gas containing cysts in the bowel wall, usually best seen in the colon.	Caused by air spread from the mediastinum or associated with ulcerative disease, acute or chronic distension, or ischemic necrosis of the bowel mucosa. May be postoperative or idiopathic.
Necrosis of the intestine	A lucent line of gas in the diseased segment of intestine.	Necrosis of the intestinal wall may be a complication of vascular occlusion, toxic megacolon, necrotizing enterocolitis or an adjacent abscess.
Intramural leakage after injury (Fig. 34)	Small intramural gas collections adjacent to an intramural perforation of a peptic ulcer or surgical injury (anastomosis).	A rare complication of localized mucosal injury resulting in transmural gas leakage. Very rarely such an incident is secondary to *diabetic infection* or *cystic fibrosis*.
C. Gas in the Bilary Tree		
Abnormal communication (postoperative reflux, cholecystoenteric fistula) (Fig. 35)	Lucent lines of gas density overlying the liver with or without gaseous lucency of the gallbladder. The gas is usually near the porta hepatis and in extrahepatic bile ducts. DD: Gas in the portal veins.	The most common cause of intrabiliary gas is a surgical procedure (choledochoduodenostomy, cholecystoenterostomy, sphincterotomy). Without previous surgery, perforation of a gallstone into the intestine is the usual cause, sometimes complicated by a gallstone ileus. Carcinoma is a rare cause of a fistula.
Emphysematous cholecystitis (Fig. 36)	Gas in the lumen and/or wall of an enlarged gallbladder with a possible air–bile level. Gas may be present in the bile ducts. DD: Subhepatic or liver abscess, gas in the duodenal bulb.	Blockage of the cystic duct and subsequent overgrowth of gas producing organisms, usually *Clostridium welchii* and *Escherichia coli*. Occurs usually in elderly men with *diabetes*.
D. Gas in the Portal Veins		
Bowel necrosis	Linear streaks of intrahepatic portal venous gas extending toward the periphery of the liver in a severely ill patient. DD: Gas in the biliary tree.	Usually associated with *mesenteric infarction* or *necrotizing enterocolitis*. Gas may be seen in the bowel wall. Rarely it may be seen in severe bowel dilatation or inflammatory bowel disease and emphysematous or corrosive gastritis.
Umbilical vein catheterization	As above.	Accidental, secondary to diagnostic or therapeutic catheterization of a neonate.

Abnormal Gas Pattern 23

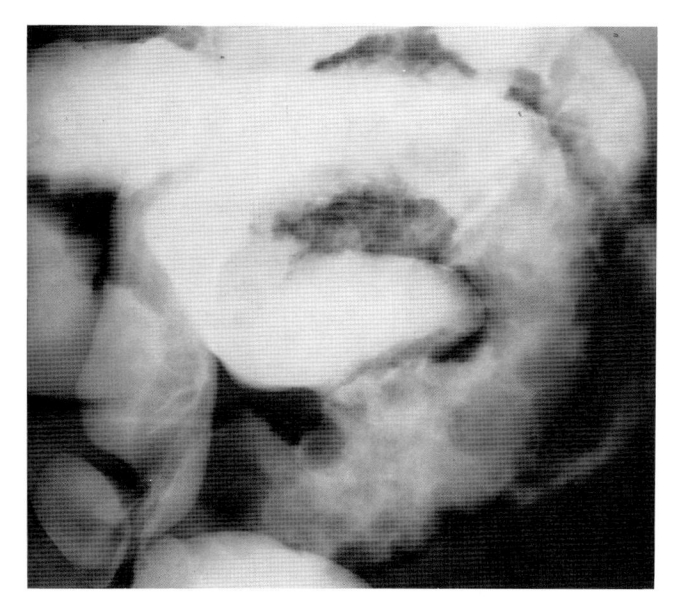

Figure 33 **Pneumatosis cystoides intestinalis.** Gas-containing cysts in the wall of the colon.

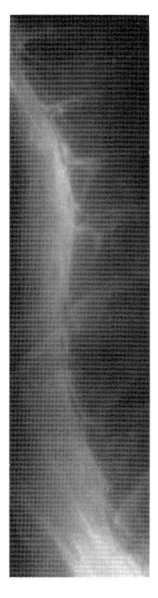

Figure 34 **Intramural gas** in the colonic wall is seen as a thin stripe, which follows the haustral pattern. A postoperative condition.

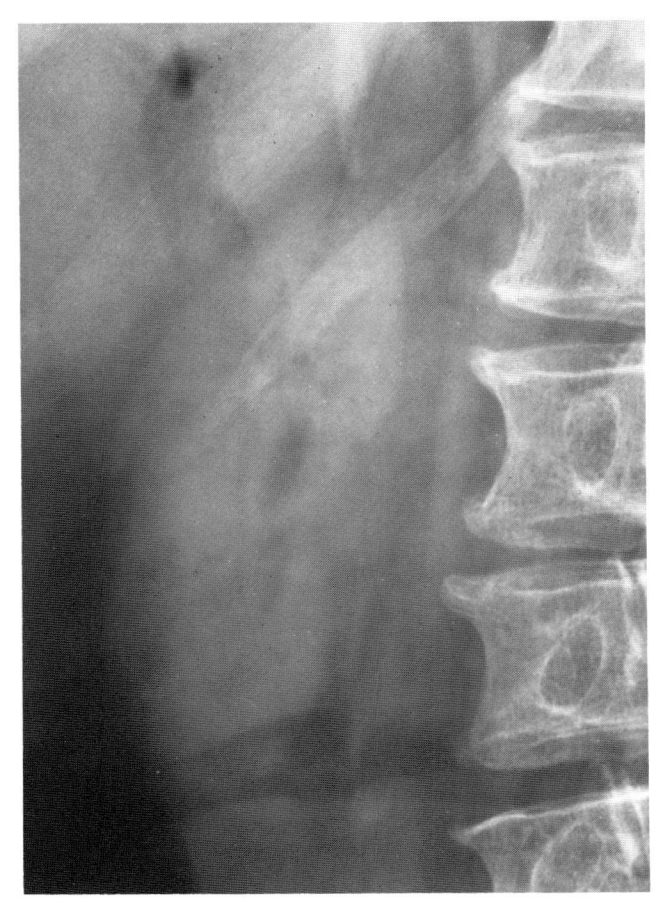

Figure 35 **Gas in the biliary tree** in a patient with a cholecystoenteric fistula (perforation of a gallstone into the duodenum).

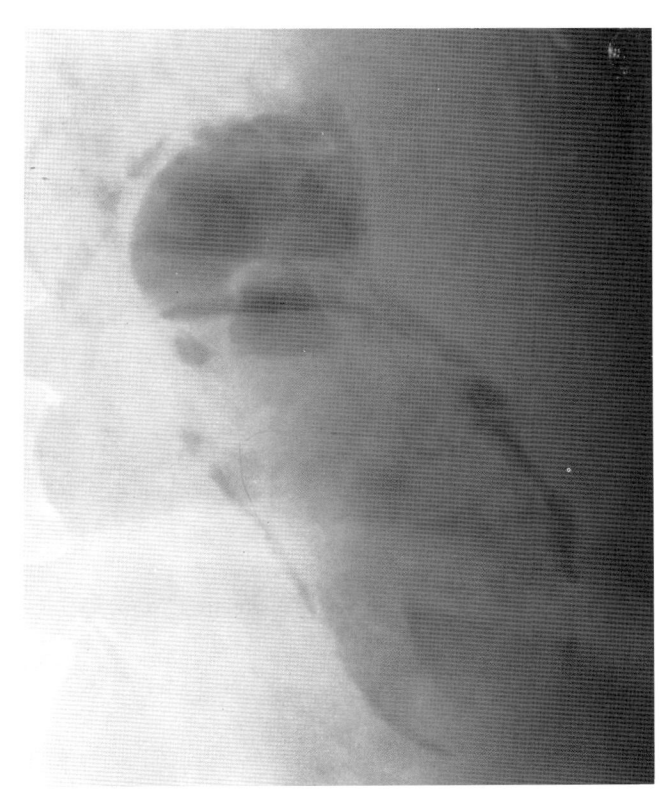

Figure 36 **Emphysematous cholecystitis.** Gas is seen both in the wall and in the lumen of an enlarged gallbladder. An air–bile level is also present. Thin stripes of gas extend to the bile ducts.

Table 4 (Cont.) Extraluminal Gas Collections in the Abdomen or Pelvis

Disease	Radiographic Findings	Comments
E. Diffuse Retroperitoneal Gas		
Rupture or perforation of the descending duodenum (Fig. 37)	Gas extends medially beyond the lateral border of the right psoas muscle toward the spine in the anterior pararenal space.	Perforation of duodenum into the extraperitoneal space is usually caused by blunt trauma. The appearance of symptoms may be delayed. There may be accompanying traumatic pancreatitis. Penetrating postbulbar ulcer is a rare cause. Right perirenal gas occurs in only one-third of cases of retroperitoneal duodenal rupture.
Extraperitoneal perforation of the colon or appendix (Fig. 38)	Mottled gaseous lucencies overlap the psoas muscle on the right, approach the spine, and do not obscure the flank stripe laterally.	In children, a relatively common cause is extraperitoneal appendicitis associated with an abscess. In adults, it may be a complication of colonoscopy, perforated carcinoma, diverticulitis of the right colon, or secondary to granulomatous ileocolitis. Abscess formation is common in these conditions.
Retroperitoneal sigmoid perforation	Extraperitoneal gas progresses up the left side, extending medially over the psoas muscle. Extension into the posterior compartment dominates the radiologic findings.	If the sigmoid perforation occurs between the leaves of the mesocolon, the extraperitoneal gas may rise bilaterally within the anterior pararenal spaces. Perforation may be due to diverticulosis or endoscopy.
Rectal perforation	Bilateral spread of extraperitoneal gas parallel to the lateral contour of the psoas muscles outlining the suprarenal and subdiaphragmatic structures.	Usually due to trauma or iatrogenic (leakage of a postoperative anastomosis or after endoscopy and biopsy).
Retroperitoneal gas from pneumomediastinum (Fig. 39)	Gaseous lucencies extend preferentially within the flank fat into the posterior pararenal space.	Extraperitoneal gas within the posterior pararenal space may dissect into the immediate subdiaphragmatic tissue planes. It can be differentiated from free peritoneal air, since it parallels a lower plane of the diaphragmatic curvature with a crescenting outline, may be medial or lateral to the apex of the peritoneal cavity, and appears to increase on expiration and decrease on inspiration.
External penetrating trauma	The localization of mottled gaseous lucencies depends on the site of trauma.	

Abnormal Gas Pattern 25

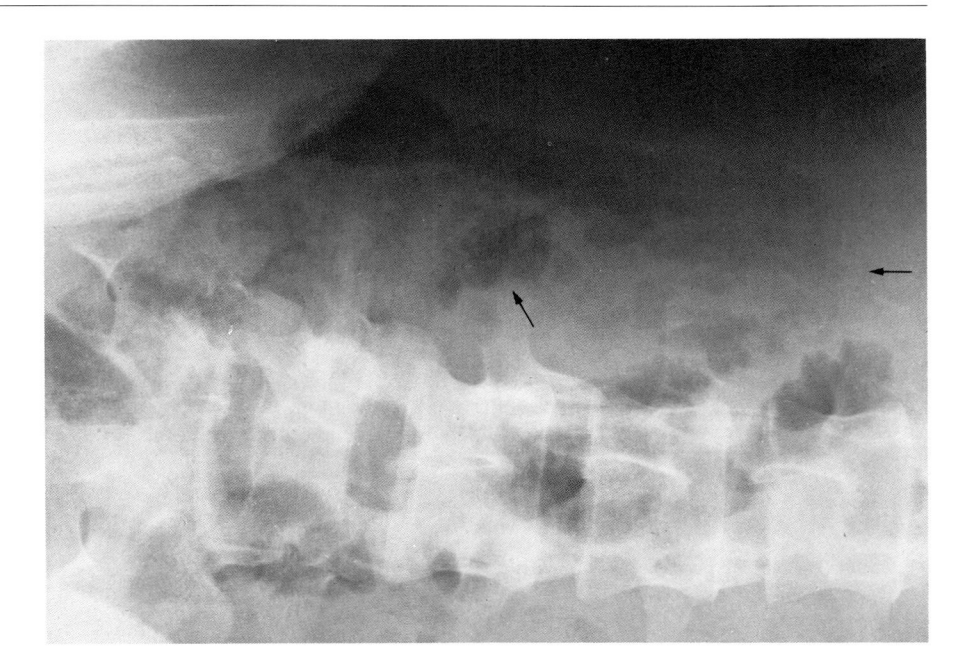

Figure 37 **Traumatic rupture of the duodenum.** Mottled gaseous lucencies are seen in the retroperitoneal space (arrows). They do not coalesce. (A left lateral decubitus projection).

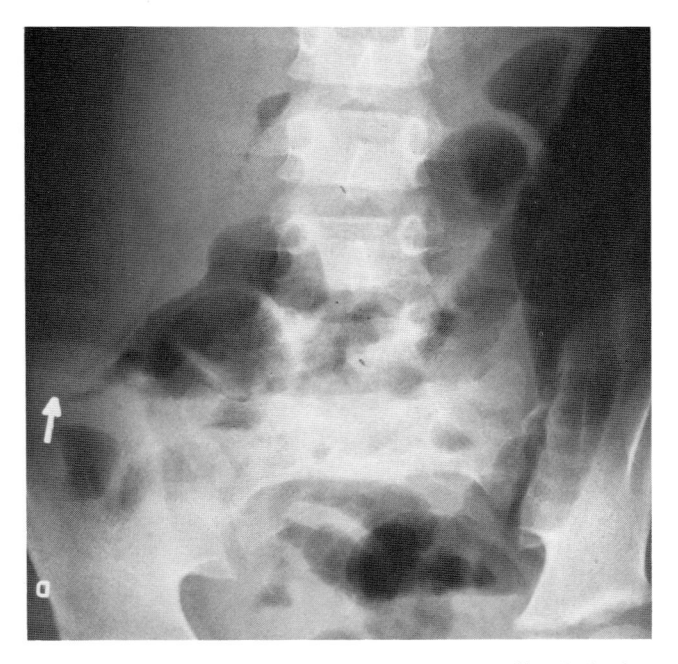

Figure 38 **Perforation of retrocecal appendix.** A "string of pearls" collection of gas rises along the lateral border of the psoas muscle indicating retroperitoneal location of the gas (arrow).

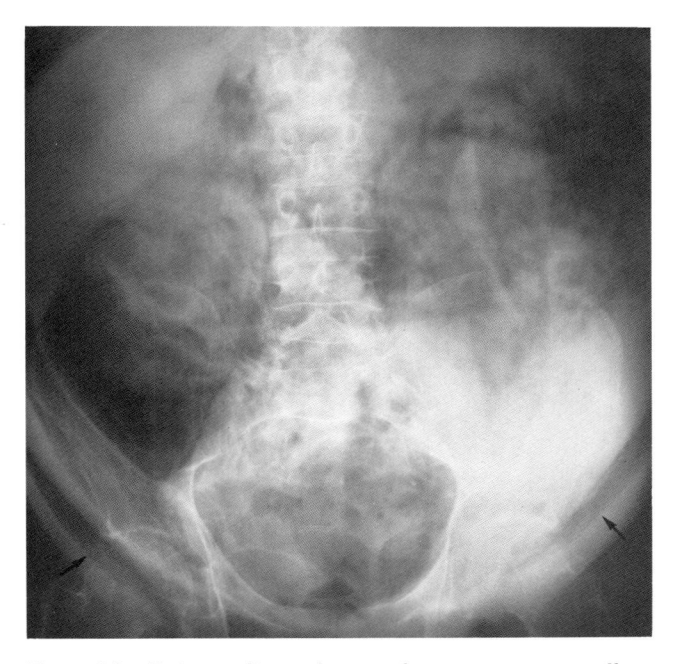

Figure 39 **Retroperitoneal gas from pneumomediastinum.** The pneumomediastinum resulted from respirator treatment for an asthmatic attack. Gaseous lucencies extend within the flank fat (arrows).

Table 4 (Cont.) Extraluminal Gas Collections in the Abdomen or Pelvis

Disease	Radiographic Findings	Comments
F. Extraluminal Pelvic Gas Collection(s)		
Pelvic abscess	Extraluminal gas and/or air–fluid level. Extrinsic distortion of the dome of the urinary bladder. Displacement of the sigmoid colon, usually posteriorly or superiorly.	Usually associated with peritonitis, after pelvic surgery, genital infection, or colonic diverticulitis.
Pneumatosis cystoides intestinalis	Gas within the wall of the colon.	See section B of this Table (p. 22).
Emphysematous cystitis (Fig. 40)	Gas bubbles in the wall of the urinary bladder with or without gas in the lumen. DD: Large fecal impaction with multiple trapped gas bubbles.	Usually associated with diabetes, urinary stasis, or bladder outlet obstruction with urinary infection.
Vesicocolic fistula	Gas in the urinary bladder without gas in the bladder wall.	May be congenital or secondary to colonic diverticulitis or malignancy.
Primary pneumaturia	Gas within the urinary bladder in the absence of fistula, instrumentation or other predisposing factors (e.g., fungus ball).	
Emphysematous vaginitis	Focal collection of gas bubbles, varying in diameter from a few millimeters up to 3 cm, Confined to the upper two thirds of the vagina and/or cervix. DD: Normal rectal gas, gas gangrene of the uterus, emphysematous cystitis.	A self-limited, benign condition, most common in pregnant women. Usually asymptomatic except for vaginal discharge. Associated with *Trichomonas vaginalis* or *Hemophilus vaginalis* infection.
Uterine gas gangrene	A large mass (uterus) in the pelvis containing mottled radiolucencies. Gas is present in the uterine wall and often in the cavity and in the fetus if present. Paralytic ileus and retroperitoneal abdominal gas may be present.	A *Clostridium perfringens* infection which is usually secondary to abortive manipulation of a pregnant uterus. *An infected uterine fibroid* is a rare cause of gaseous lucencies in the uterus. Gas in the abdominal wall (postoperatively) may mimic uterine gas collection.
G. Gas within an Abscess (Intraperitoneal or Extraperitoneal Localized Gas Collection with or without Air–fluid Level)		
Subphrenic abscess (Fig. 41)	Air–fluid level or mottled gas lucencies intermixed with necrotic material. Elevation and restricted motion of the hemidiaphragm. Pleural effusion (sympathetic). If left-sided, may separate the fundus of the stomach from the diaphragm.	Usually a complication of intra-abdominal surgery. May be secondary to *perforated appendix, peptic ulcer, diverticulitis,* or *cholecystitis.* Left-sided subphrenic abscess usually complicates splenectomy, gastric surgery, left colonic surgery, or hiatal hernia repair. Right-sided subphrenic abscess may follow biliary, gastric, duodenal, or right colonic surgery.
Perirenal abscess (Fig. 42)	Extraluminal gas around a kidney and in the retroperitoneal space. Loss of definition of the lower renal outline. Displacement and sometimes axial rotation of the kidney. The lower pole is displaced medially, upward and anteriorly. Loss of the upper segment of the psoas muscle margins. Fixation of the kidney. Restriction of the diaphragmatic motility and scoliosis may be present.	Usually secondary to renal infection *(pyelonephritis, tuberculosis, carbuncle)* and *perforation* of the renal capsule. Often associated with diabetes. Pus collection may displace adjacent bowel. *Osteomyelitis* of the spine may rarely create an abscess in the posterior pararenal space. A *urinoma* does not contain gas, pushes the lower pole up and laterally, is associated with hydronephrosis, and obscures the lower psoas shadow.
Renal abscess (subcapsular)	Visualization of the displaced renal capsule or fascia. Flattening or compression of the kidney.	In the absence of gas, a subcapsular hematoma may look identical.
Liver abscess	Gas may occasionally be present in a liver abscess either due to a gas-forming organism or due to connection to biliary tree. The liver may be enlarged and ascites or pleural effusion may be present.	Can be caused by pyogenic organisms or amebic infestation in severely ill patients. Plain film findings are nonspecific in the absence of gas.

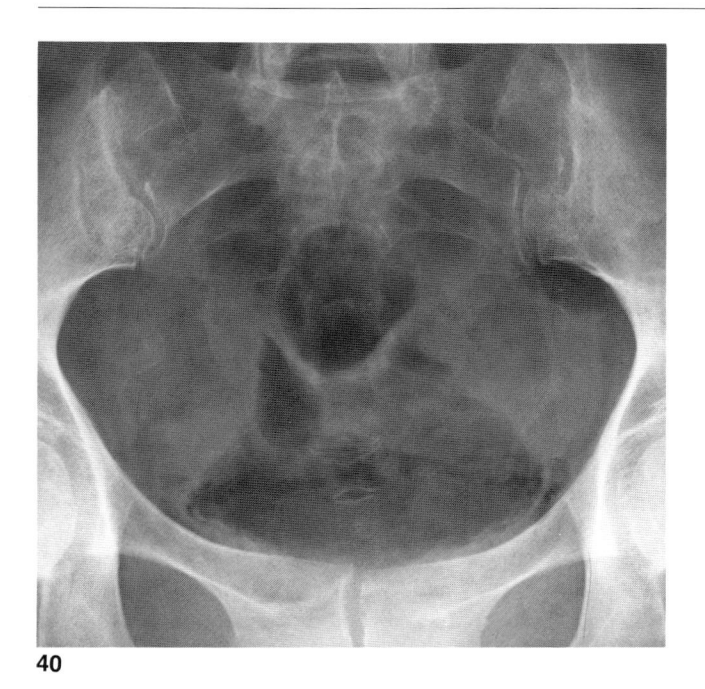

Figure **40 Emphysematous cystitis** in a diabetic. Gas is seen both in the wall and in the lumen of the urinary bladder.

Figure **41a, b Right subphrenic abscess.** An air–fluid level below the right hemidiaphragm (arrow) that projects further away from the lung than free air. Elevation of the hemidiaphragm is associated.

Figure **42 Left perirenal abscess.** Extraluminal gas on the medial side of the laterally displaced left kidney.

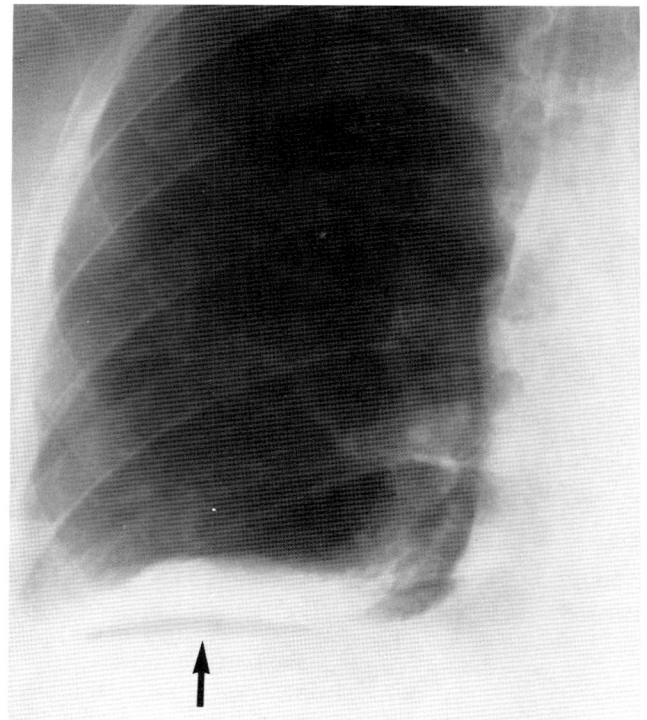

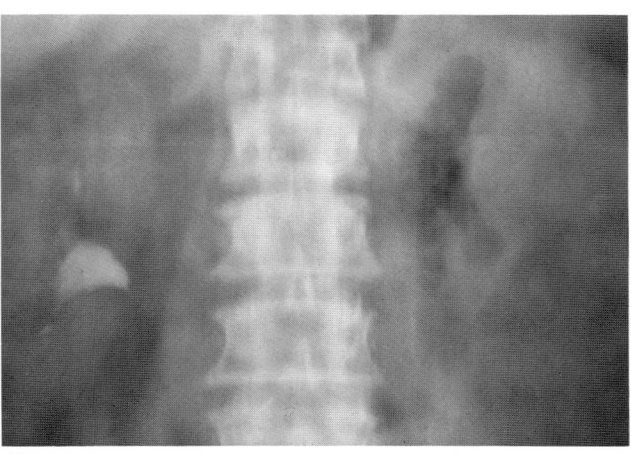

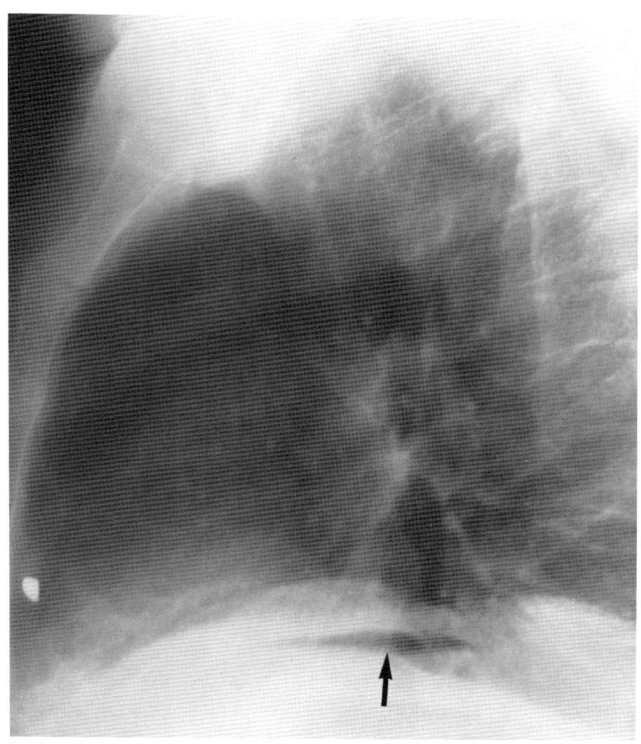

Table 4 (Cont.) Extraluminal Gas Collections in the Abdomen or Pelvis

Disease	Radiographic Findings	Comments
Pancreatic abscess	Peritoneal fat necrosis produces a pathognomonic mottled pattern of normal fat intermingled with areas of water density, best appreciated, on CT scans. True gas lucencies may be seen, too. Spread from the head of the pancreas tends to be downward and to the right. Emphysematous or fulminating pancreatitis may spread bilaterally downward in the anterior pararenal space with gas and mottled fat necrosis overlying the psoas muscles.	Pancreatic abscess may dissect within fascial planes to the posterior pararenal space, push the kidney and colon forward, and obliterate psoas muscle and flank stripe.
Lesser sac abscess (Fig. 43, 44)	A gas–fluid level in the left upper abdomen extending slightly over the midline but not reaching the diaphragm. The stomach is displaced anteriorly and the colon inferiorly.	Gas collection in the lesser sac may be due to bowel perforation or a hernia through the foramen of Winslow. A necrotic tumor containing an air–fluid level may mimic an abscess.
Intraperitoneal abscess (Fig. 45)	Depending on location: *Right paracolic abscess:* Gas shadow and a mass effect lateral to the ascending colon below the hepatic flexure. *Subhepatic abscess:* Displacement of the proximal transverse colon, lateral wall of the duodenum; loss of visualization of the hepatic angle and of the right kidney, depending on anteroposterior position of the abscess. *Gastrohepatic recess abscess:* Posterior and left displacement of the stomach. *Gastrosplenic recess abscess:* Medial and posterior displacement of the stomach. *Renosplenic recess abscess:* Medial and anterior displacement of the stomach.	A supramesocolic abscess may appear similar to a lesser sac abscess on upright films, but is situated in the midline beneath the central tendon of the diaphragm.
Periappendicular abscess	An extrinsic defect of the cecum, with possible displacement of the terminal ileum and multiple gas densities overlying the psoas muscle.	

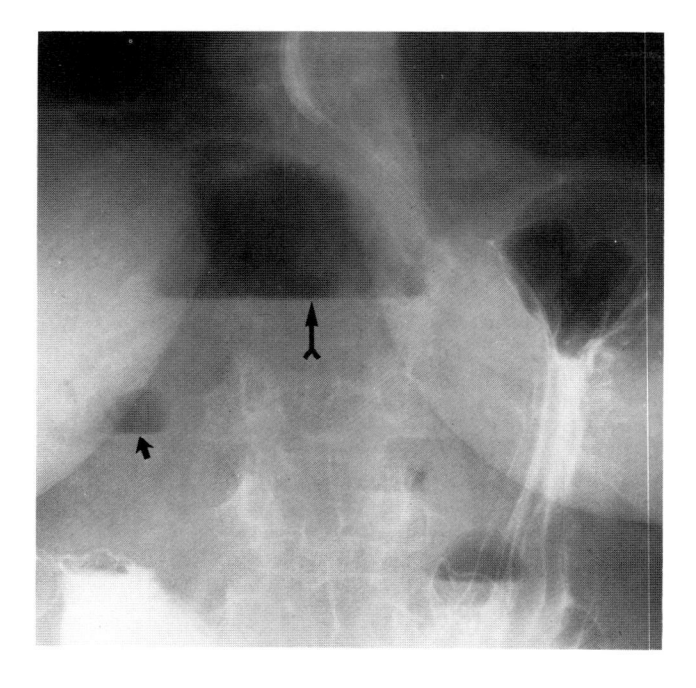

Figure **43 Lesser sac abscess** (arrow) and cholecystoduodenal fistula (short arrow) in the same patient. A large gas–fluid level is seen in the midline, just below the level of the diaphragm, representing the lesser sac abscess. The smaller gas–fluid level is located in the gallbladder.

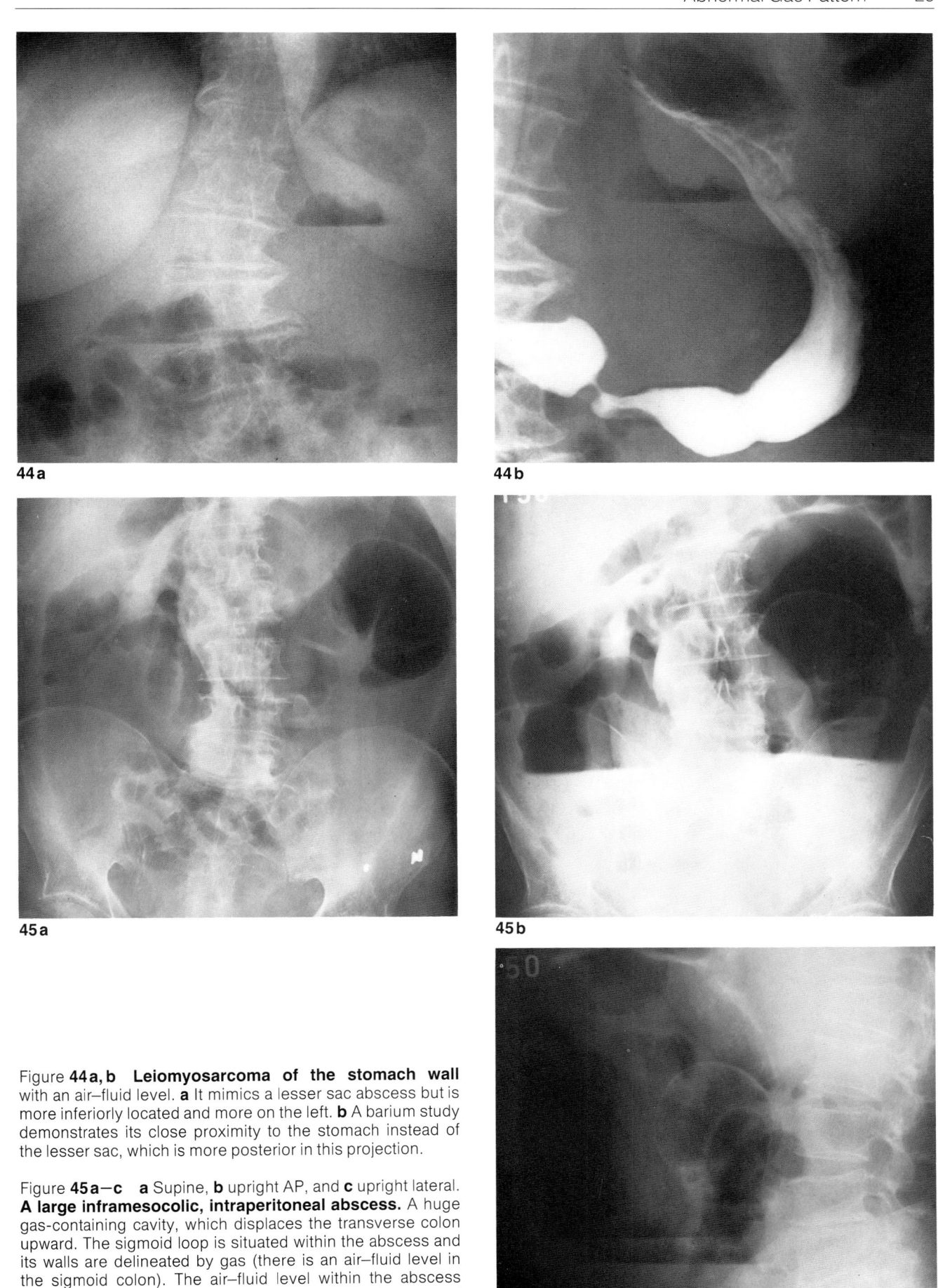

Figure **44a, b Leiomyosarcoma of the stomach wall** with an air–fluid level. **a** It mimics a lesser sac abscess but is more inferiorly located and more on the left. **b** A barium study demonstrates its close proximity to the stomach instead of the lesser sac, which is more posterior in this projection.

Figure **45a–c**   **a** Supine, **b** upright AP, and **c** upright lateral. **A large inframesocolic, intraperitoneal abscess.** A huge gas-containing cavity, which displaces the transverse colon upward. The sigmoid loop is situated within the abscess and its walls are delineated by gas (there is an air–fluid level in the sigmoid colon). The air–fluid level within the abscess does not extend throughout the entire abscess because of loculations within the abscess.

Chapter 2 Abdominal Calcifications

As elsewhere in the body, abdominal calcifications may be *dystrophic,* resulting from precipitation of calcium salts in necrotic tissue (e.g., pancreatitis, renal cortical necrosis) or may result from *chemical interaction* (e.g., hypercalcemia, diet). Some calcifications develop without known underlying pathology (e.g., prostatic calculi).

The majority of calcifications on the abdominal films are of little clinical significance, but some indicate areas of pathology or allow even a precise histologic diagnosis. Some calcifications can be classified on the basis of their radiographic appearance (location, number, size, shape, distribution, or density). The following calcifications may be of significance in the assesment of an acute abdomen:
- Calcifications of the biliary tract
- Calcified aneurysm of the abdominal aorta or of the hepatic or splenic artery
- Appendicoliths – indicative of appendicitis
- Calcification of an appendiceal mucocele, ringlike or amorphous
- Ribbon-like calcifications in Meckel's diverticulum
- Pancreatic calculi
- Ureteral calculus
- Calcium deposits in a dermoid cyst

Oblique or lateral projections are of value in differentiating abdominal wall calcifications from calcifications within the intraperitoneal or retroperitoneal space. Calculi less than 1 mm in diameter are not recognizable on plain films.

Intramuscular injections of quinine, calcium gluconate, or calcium penicillin can result in calcifications, usually in the gluteal region. Bismuth injections have a higher density (Fig. 1). Injection sites are usually bilateral. They are easy to differentiate from intra-abdominal calcifications.

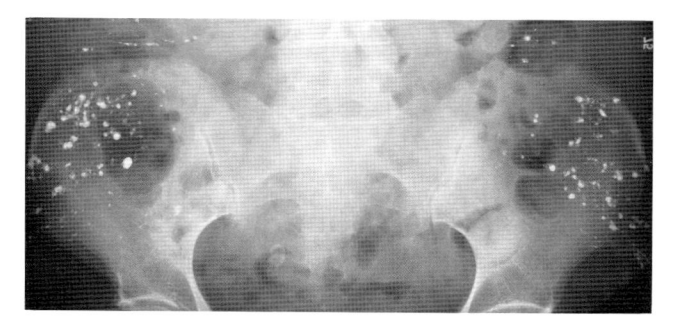

Figure 1 **Bilateral metal (bismuth) deposits** in needle tracks, a residue of injections given for the treatment of lues. Note the high density of the deposits in comparison with bone.

Table 1 Differential Diagnosis of Abdominal Calcifications

Site and Pattern of Calcification	Common Causes	Radiographic Findings and Comments
Calcification in the liver **A. Disseminated**	Histoplasmosis, tuberculosis	Small (up to 3 cm), multiple, dense, scattered throughout the liver. If calcifications of the spleen and lung are associated, the pattern is virtually diagnostic of histoplasmosis.
	Brucellosis	Snowflake, fluffy calcifications. Similar lesions may be seen in the spleen.
	Tongue worm *(Armillifer armillatus)*	*Typical comma-shaped or semilunar calcifications occur in the liver, lungs, pleura, peritoneum, and spleen.*
	Metastatic mucinous carcinoma (of the colon or rectum, less frequently ovary, breast, stomach)	*Finely granular calcifications have a diameter of 2 to 4 mm and a poppy-seed appearance.*
	Metastases from other primary tumors (adrenal, bronchogenic, melanoma, mesothelioma, neuroblastoma, osteogenic sarcoma, pancreatic, renal, testicular, thyroid)	*Calcification of metastases in these tumors is much rarer than in mucinous carcinomas. They also tend to be larger and denser. Growth indicates malignancy.*
B. Cystic	Hydatid cysts *(Echinococcus granulosus)* (Fig. **2a**)	Oval or circular calcifications are characteristic. Arc-like daughter cyst calcifications within the mother cyst may occur also. Usually asymptomatic.
	Alveolar hydatid disease *(Echinococcus multilocularis)*	Multiple small (2 to 4 mm) cysts with calcified walls lie within large areas of amorphous calcification; are seen in 70%. Symptomatic, may be fulminant, even fatal.
	Liver cyst (nonparasitic) (Fig. **2b**)	Calcification of the cyst wall is rare.

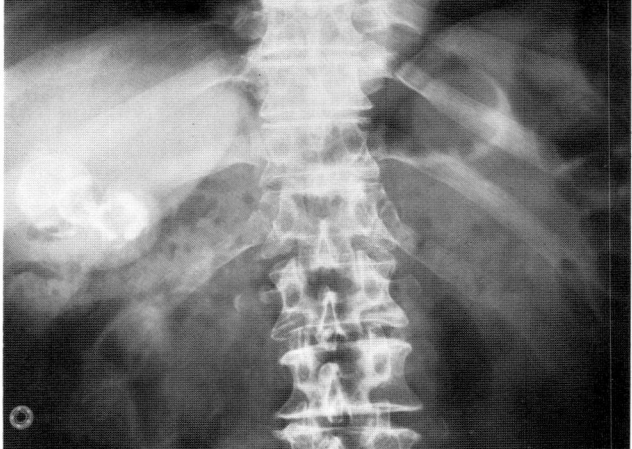

Figure **2a** Calcified hydatid cysts in the liver.

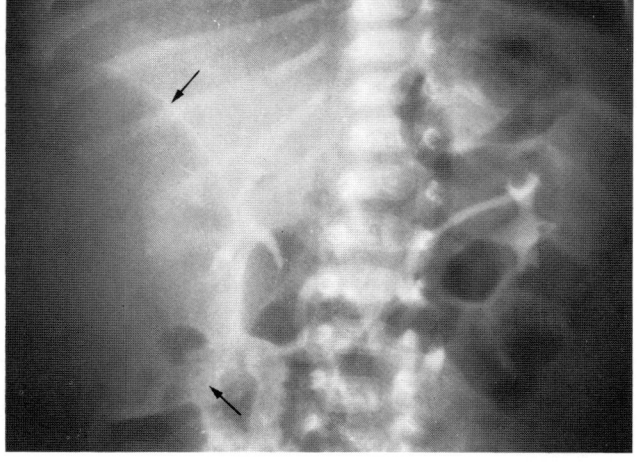

Figure **2b** Calcified cystic hematoma in the liver. A faintly calcified rim (arrows) is seen in this infant.

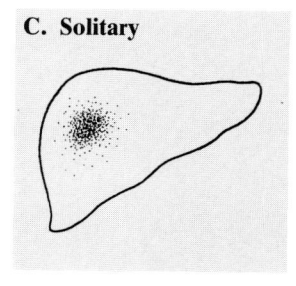

C. Solitary	Healed liver abscess (pyogenic or amebic)	Dense, mottled calcification, usually solitary. Calcification of an amebic abscess is often associated with secondary infection.
	Coccidioidomycosis Gumma (tertiary syphilis)	These are rare causes of hepatic parenchymal calcification.
	Guinea worm *(Dracunculus medinensis)*	Calcified large worms are more commonly seen in extremities, rarely in the liver.
	Filariasis	Coiled calcified densities are rarely seen in the liver, more commonly in soft tissues.

Table 1 (Cont.) **Differential Diagnosis of Abdominal Calcifications**

Site and Pattern of Calcification	Common Causes	Radiographic Findings and Comments
	Toxoplasmosis Cysticercosis Ascariasis Clonorchiasis	Liver calcification in these conditions is unusual.
	Cavernous hemangioma	A sunburst pattern of calcified spicules may be seen. Most hemangiomas are not calcified. Unlike hemangiomas of soft tissue elsewhere, calcified phleboliths are uncommon in hepatic hemangiomas.
	Primary carcinoma of the liver	Dystrophic calcification of necrotic tumor tissue may occur, especially in children; seen as flecks or spherical calculi resembling cholelithiasis.
	Hematoma	Traumatic liver hematoma may later calcify.
D. Vascular	Calcified thrombus of the portal vein	A linear density crossing the vertebral column. Rare, usually associated with cirrhosis and portal hypertension.
	Hepatic artery aneurysm	A cracked eggshell appearance typical of aneurysm is rare in the hepatic artery, much more common in the splenic artery. May mimic a calcified cyst.
E. Gallstones	(See biliary calcification, p. 36.)	
F. Capsular	May occur in alcoholic cirrhosis, pyogenic infection, meconium peritonitis, or pseudomyxoma peritonei.	
G. Generalized increase of liver density	May be secondary to hemochromatosis, hemosiderosis, cirrhotic contraction, Thorotrast injection or lipiodol (Ethiodol) embolisation of the liver after lymphography.	

Table 1 (Cont.) Differential Diagnosis of Abdominal Calcifications

Site and Pattern of Calcification	Common Causes	Radiographic Findings and Comments
Calcification in the spleen		
A. Disseminated	Phleboliths	Multiple small, round calcific nodules throughout the spleen.
	Granulomatous disease (histoplasmosis, tuberculosis, brucellosis) (Fig. 3)	Histoplasmosis is the most common cause in endemic areas. Similar lesions are often present throughout the lungs, occasionally in the liver. Calcifications in brucellosis are larger than in histoplasmosis or tuberculosis, about 1 to 3 cm in diameter. They consist of flocculent central calcifications and a surrounding calcific rim. Brucellosis may still be active when calcifications occur.
B. Cystic	Echinococcal cysts (Fig. 4)	Hydatid cysts are often multiple and heavily calcified in contrast to other cysts.
	Hematoma	A splenic hematoma may occasionally become cystic and calcify.
	Congenital cyst Dermoid Epidermoid	These lesions very rarely calcify.
C. Capsular and/or parenchymal calcification	Splenic infarct (Fig. 5)	Single or, rarely, multiple. Infrequently calcifies as a triangular density, with apex toward the center of the organ.
	Hematoma Abscess (pyogenic or tuberculous)	Plaques of calcification of the splenic capsule may occur secondary to an abscess, although calcification of splenic abscesses is rare.
D. Vascular	Calcified splenic artery (Fig. 3)	A common finding without clinical importance. Tortuous, corkscrew appearance of the linear calcification is characteristic.
	Splenic artery aneurysm	Circular or bizarre calcification with diameter larger than the normal artery.
E. Generalized increase of splenic density	Sickle-cell anemia	Produced by fine miliary calcifications and iron deposits.
	Hemochromatosis	Iron deposition. May also occur in excessive dietary intake of iron or in thalassemia, Fanconi's anemia, or rarely after multiple transfusions.
	Thorotrast deposits	Thorium dioxide particles are stored in the reticuloendothelial system. A history of Thorotrast angiography may be obtained. This contrast medium has not been used since the early 1950s.
Calcification in the pancreas		
A. Disseminated	Alcoholic pancreatitis Gallstone pancreatitis (Fig. 6)	Alcoholic pancreatitis is the most common cause of pancreatic lithiasis. Numerous irregular, small concretions are widely scattered within the pancreatic ducts throughout the gland. Present in 20–40% of patients with chronic alcoholic pancreatitis. The incidence of calcification in gallstone pancreatitis is only 2%, but the radiographic appearance is similar.

Table 1 (Cont.) Differential Diagnosis of Abdominal Calcifications

Site and Pattern of Calcification	Common Causes	Radiographic Findings and Comments
	Hyperparathyroidism	Due to pancreatitis, which develops in up to 20% of patients with hyperparathyroidism. Often associated with renal calcifications.
	Hereditary pancreatitis	Rounded, often relatively large pancreatic calcifications which are already present in childhood.
	Cystic fibrosis	Fine granular calcifications of the pancreas in a pediatric patient.
	Kwashiorkor (protein malnutrition)	Typical calcifications of chronic pancreatitis in a young patient.
	Cavernous lymphangioma	A very rare tumor that may contain multiple phleboliths.

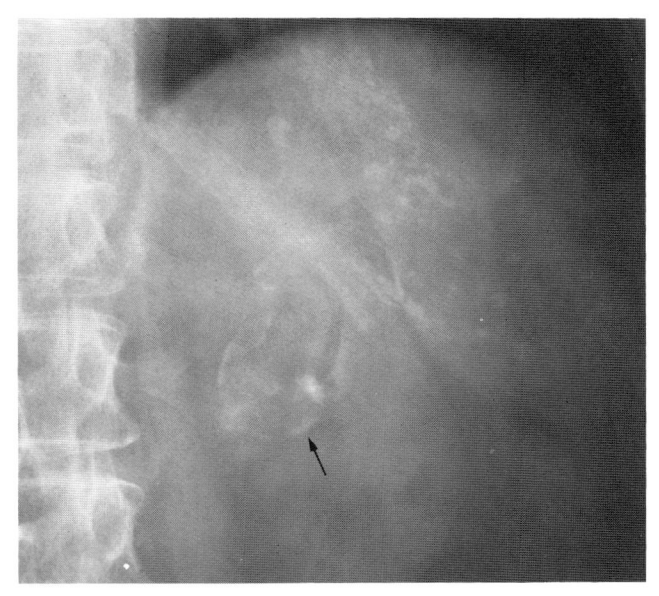

Figure 3 **Tuberculosis.** Disseminated granulomatous calcifications in the spleen. Calcification of the splenic artery is associated (arrow).

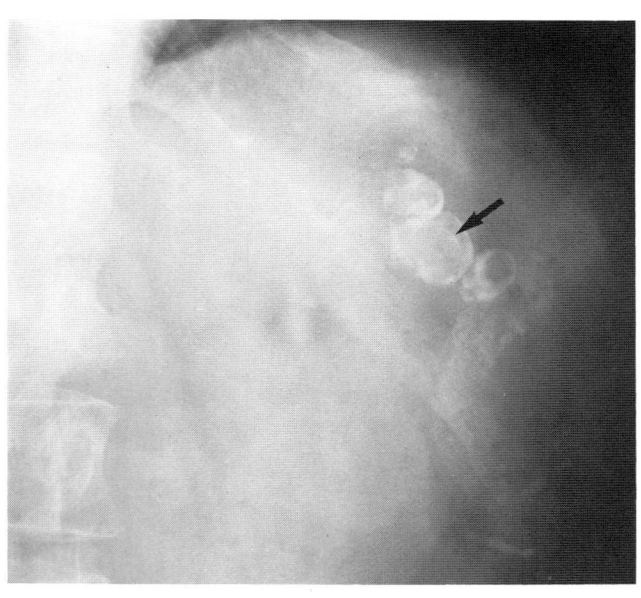

Figure 4 **Echinococcal cysts of the spleen.** Arc-like calcifications (arrow) within the calcified mother cysts represent calcified daughter cysts.

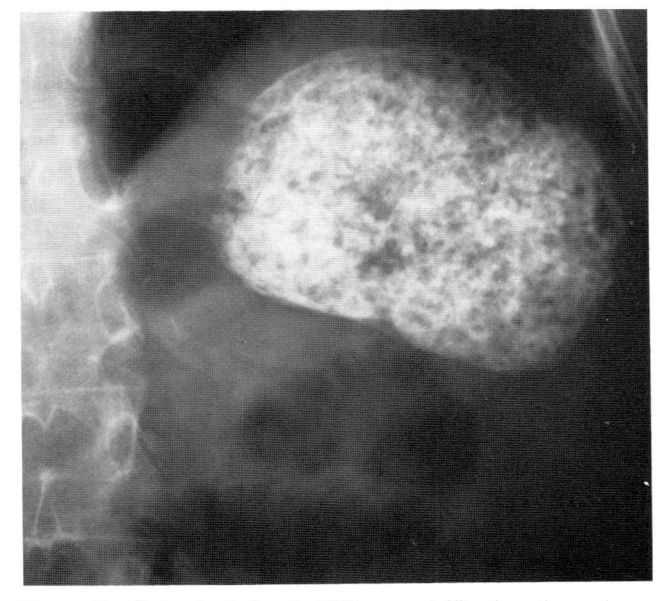

Figure 5 **Splenic infarct.** Diffuse calcification throughout the entire spleen after infarction.

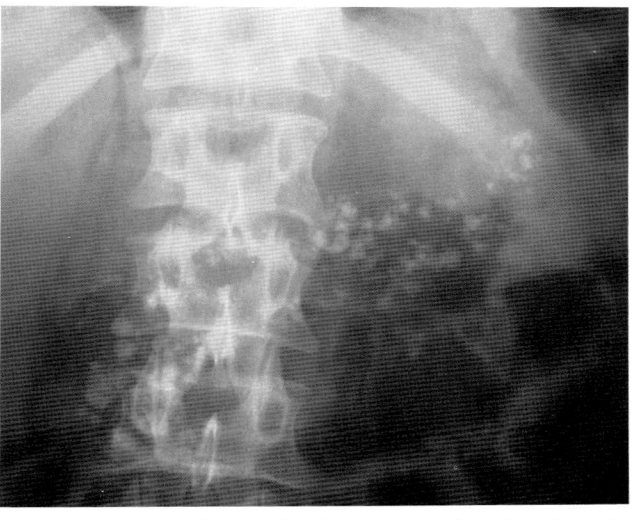

Figure 6 Pancreatic calcifications secondary to **chronic pancreatitis.** (Courtesy of Dr. Leena Kivisaari, Helsinki University Central Hospital.)

Abdomen

Table 1 (Cont.) Differential Diagnosis of Abdominal Calcifications

Site and Pattern of Calcification	Common Causes	Radiographic Findings and Comments
B. Cystic	Pancreatic pseudocyst	A rim of calcification occasionally outlines the wall of the pseudocyst. Pancreatic lithiasis is usually associated.
C. Solitary	Cystadenoma Cystadenocarcinoma	10% of these tumors contain radiographic calcification. Sunburst pattern of calcification is pathognomonic if present. Adenocarcinomas do not calcify.
	Hematoma	Intraparenchymal hemorrhage due to trauma, infarction, or a bleeding intraparenchymal aneurysm.
Calcifications in the biliary tract		
A. Calculous	Gallstone(s) (Fig. 7)	20% of gallstones are radiopaque. They tend to have a dense outer rim of calcium salts. Renal calculus or an appendicolith in a long retrocecal appendix may project into the right upper quadrant, but can be differentiated on oblique films. Calculi in the bile duct may be difficult to appreciate and to differentiate from renal stones.
B. Cystic	Porcelain gallbladder	Extensive mural calcification of the gallbladder in chronic cholecystitis. There is a high incidence of gallbladder carcinoma, requiring prophylactic cholecystectomy.
C. Homogenous	Milk of calcium bile	High biliary concentrations of calcium carbonate secondary to chronic cholecystitis and obstruction of the cystic duct. Simulates a contrast-filled normal gallbladder.
D. Punctate	Mucinous adenocarcinoma of the gallbladder	A rare cause of localized fine granular calcification in the gallbladder.

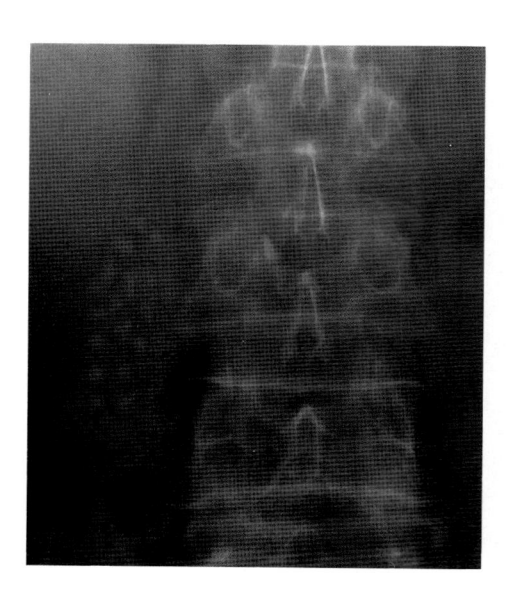

Figure 7 **Multiple radiopaque gallstones.**

Table 1 (Cont.) Differential Diagnosis of Abdominal Calcifications

Site and Pattern of Calcification	Common Causes	Radiographic Findings and Comments
Calcification in the alimentary tract		
A. Calculous	Appendicoliths (Fig. 8)	A round, laminated enterolith, usually located in the right lower quadrant. Demonstration of an appendicolith in a patient with fever, leukocytosis and right lower quadrant pain is highly suggestive of acute appendicitis, likely a gangrenous one. May mimic gallstone or ureteral stone.
	Meckel's stone	An occasionally faceted enterolith is seen in Meckel's diverticulum, located low midline or in the right lower quadrant. May be complicated by inflammation, hemorrhage, or perforation.
	Rectal stone	Low midline enterolith with possible rectal symptoms or even fecal impaction.
	Diverticular stone	An enterolith within a colonic diverticulum.
B. Cystic	Calcified mucocele of the appendix	A large crescent-shaped or circular calcification in the right lower quadrant. May displace the cecum.
	Calcified appendix epiploica.	An infarcted appendix epiploica is seen as a cystic calcification adjacent to the gas-filled colon, most commonly in the ascending portion. May become detached and mobile.
	Mesenteric or peritoneal cysts	Especially chylous and hydatid cysts of the mesentery tend to have calcific walls.

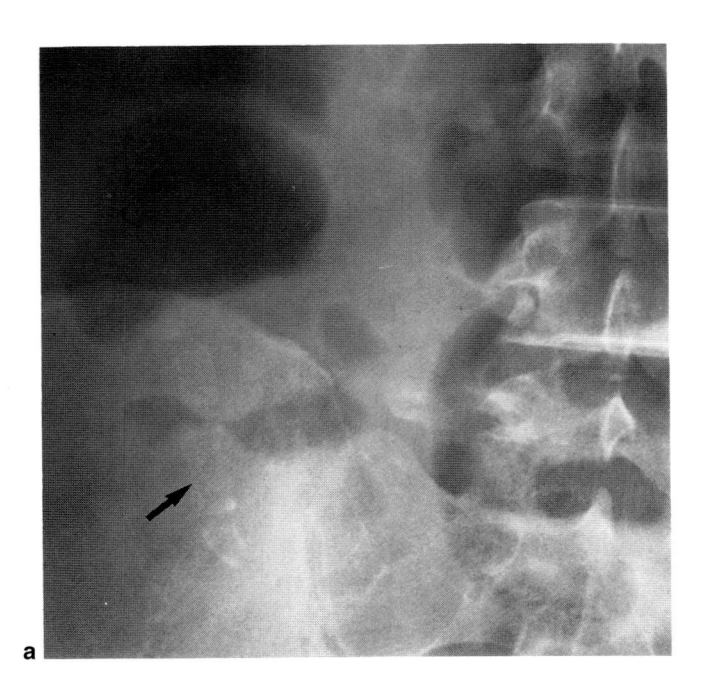

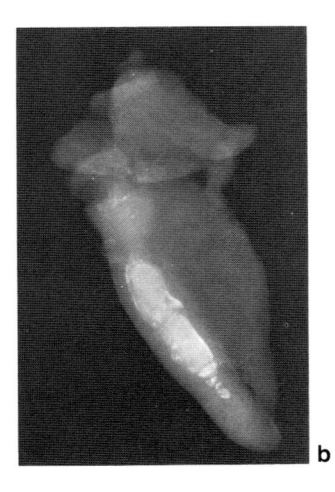

Figure **8a, b** **Appendicolith. a** A tubular calcification of the right lower quadrant on a supine film (arrow). **b** Roentgenogram of the surgical specimen.

Table 1 (Cont.)   **Differential Diagnosis of Abdominal Calcifications**

Site and Pattern of Calcification	Common Causes	Radiographic Findings and Comments
C. Parenchymal	Mucinous adenocarcinoma of the stomach or colon	Small, mottled, or punctate calcifications of mucinous carcinoma occur predominantly in patients under 40.
	Leiomyoma Leiomyosarcoma	Calcium deposits occur in 4% of leiomyomas of the stomach, and even less commonly in the remaining gastrointestinal tract. A very large lesion suggests leiomyosarcoma.
	Mesenteric lipoma Omental fat necrosis	Rare causes of calcification in the alimentary tract.
D. Ingested material	Trapped nonopaque foreign bodies.	They tend to have a ring-like appearance due to peripheral deposition of calcium.
Calcification in the kidney		

A. Nephrolithiasis (Figs. 9, 10)	Often idiopathic but commonly associated with:
	Chronic urinary infection
	Hyperparathyroidism
	Loss of calcium from bones due to immobilization, menopause, senility, or metabolic reasons
	Stasis of urine due to obstruction or neurogenic bladder
	Calcium phosphate stones are uniformly dense. They occur commonly in:
	   Idiopathic hypercalciuria
	   Idiopathic hyperuricosuria
	   Hypercalcemic conditions
	   Distal renal tubular acidosis
	Calcium oxalate stones are very dense. They occur in:
	   Intestinal malabsorption, bypass, Crohn's disease
	   Primary hyperoxaluria
	Struvite (magnesium ammonium phosphate) stones are moderately opaque, often staghorn stones and occur often in:
	   Persistent urinary tract infection
	   Neurogenic bladder
	Cystine stones (slightly opaque) occur in:
	   Cystinuria, seen in children and young adults, may form staghorns
	Uric acid stones are nonopaque. They occur often in:
	   Gout
	   Diet high in purines
	   Rapid cell destruction (e.g., treatment of lymphoma)
		90% of urinary calculi are sufficiently opaque to be seen on the plain film. Expiration and inspiration films help in correct localization of the calcification. Urate and matrix stones are radiolucent. Staghorn calculi form a cast of the pelvocaliceal system and tend to be relatively radiolucent.

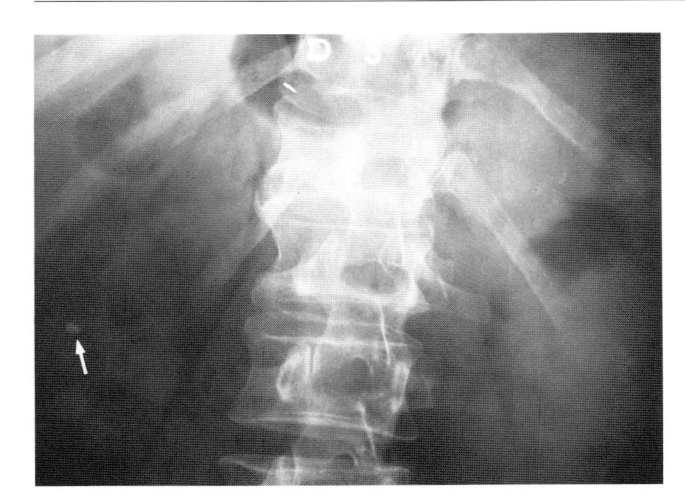

Figure 9 **Caliceal stone.** The intrarenal location is shown with oblique projection.

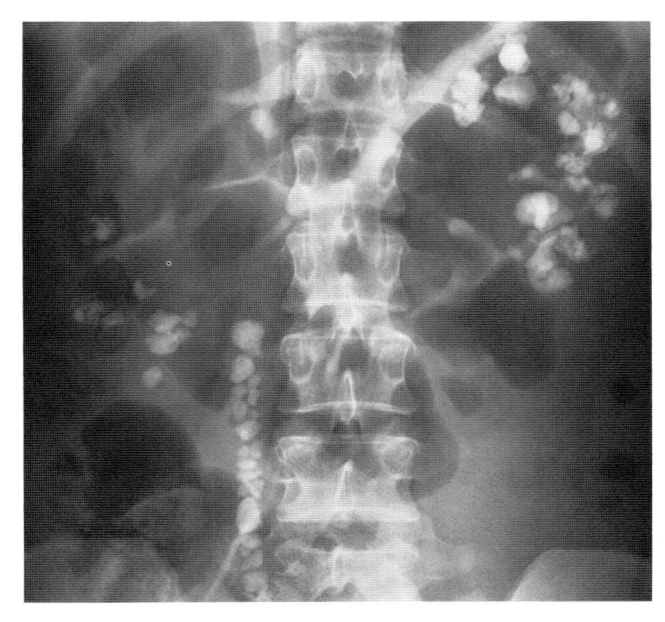

Figure 10 **Renal tubular acidosis.** Extensive nephro-ureterolithiasis and renal parenchymal calcifications are seen.

Table 1 (Cont.)   **Differential Diagnosis of Abdominal Calcifications**

Site and Pattern of Calcification	Common Causes	Radiographic Findings and Comments
B. Predominantly pyramidal nephrocalcinosis	Medullary sponge kidney (Fig. 11)	Small calcifications within cystic dilatations of the distal collecting tubules, bilateral in 75%, may involve a single pyramid only.
	Hyperparathyroidism (Fig. 12)	Small nodular or streaky calcifications in renal pyramids are seen in about 25%. Often associated with stones and bone abnormalities.
	Renal tubular acidosis: Primary (idiopathic) or associated with systemic diseases: Ehlers–Danlos syndrome, sickle-cell anemia, thyroiditis, primary hyperparathyroidism, vitamin D intoxication, idiopathic hypercalciuria, medullary sponge kidneys, toxic nephropathy, chronic pyelonephritis secondary to urolithiasis, and hyperoxaluria. (Figs. 10, 13)	Inability of the distal portion of the nephron to effectively secrete hydrogen ions to lower urinary pH. Nephrolithiasis and nephrocalcinosis occur in the majority of cases of primary renal tubular acidosis. Staghorn calculi are common.
	Skeletal demineralization secondary to: Carcinoma metastatic to bone Paraneoplastic hypercalcemia Severe osteoporosis Cushing's disease Steroid therapy Paget's disease	Metastatic bone destruction is common, but rarely causes nephrocalcinosis. Paraneoplastic hypercalcemia occurs especially in lung and kidney carcinomas. Immobilization may cause acute demineralization with hypercalcemia and nephrocalcinosis.
	Increased intestinal absorption of calcium in: Sarcoidosis Hypervitaminosis D Milk-alkali syndrome	There is increased intestinal sensitivity to vitamin D in sarcoidosis resulting in increased absorption of calcium. Increased tubular load of calcium and phosphate causes nephrocalcinosis.
	Hyperoxaluria (Fig. 14) Primary Secondary to inflammatory bowel disease, intestinal bypass, or pancreatic insufficiency	Primary hyperoxaluria is a rare congenital disease in which urinary calculi and nephrocalcinosis occur early in childhood. Secondary hyperoxaluria results from increased intestinal absorption of oxalate, most commonly seen in Crohn's disease.
	Renal papillary necrosis secondary to: Analgesic abuse (e.g., phenacetin) Diabetes mellitus Obstructive uropathy Pyelonephritis Sickle-cell anemia	A triangular radiolucency surrounded by a dense ring shadow is a characteristic radiographic finding. The pattern may vary and mimic renal tuberculosis or medullary sponge kidney. A detached papilla may form a renal stone. Uroepithelial carcinoma occurs with an increased incidence in analgesic nephropathy.
C. Predominantly medullary	Renal tuberculosis (Fig. 15)	May produce single or multiple flecks of nephrocalcinosis, gross amorphous and irregular calcifications, or massive calcification of the whole kidney (autonephrectomy). There is a history of pulmonary tuberculosis years earlier in most cases.
	Chronic pyelonephritis	Radiographically demonstrable calcifications are rare unless associated with papillary necrosis.

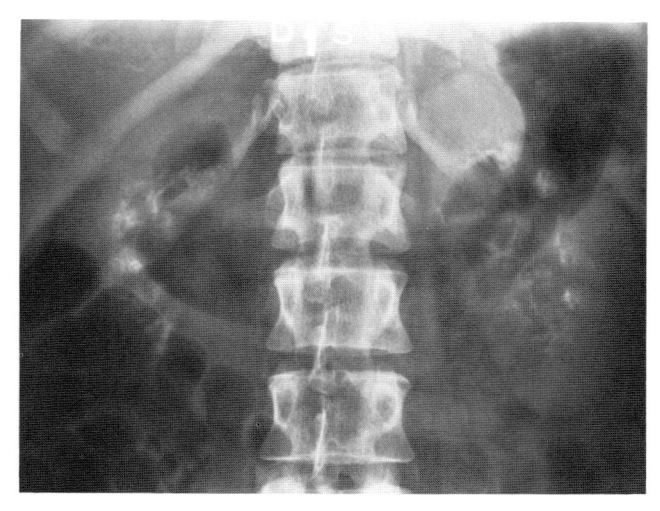

Figure 11 **Medullary sponge kidney.** Small calcifications within cystic dilatations of the distal collecting tubules are seen bilaterally.

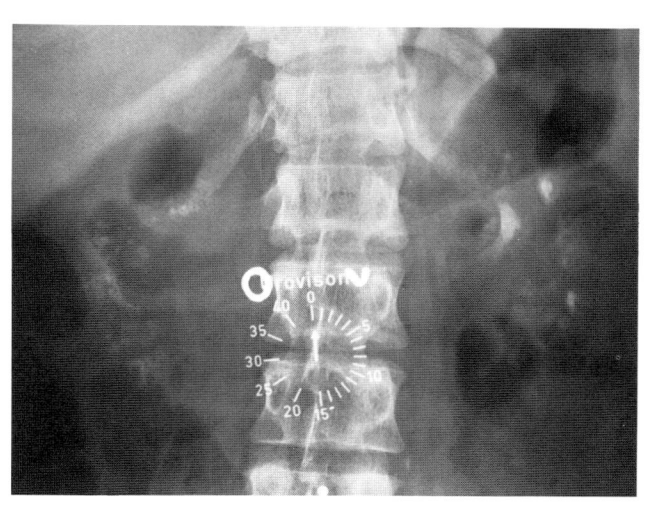

Figure 12 **Hyperparathyroidism.** Small nodular calcifications are seen throughout the renal pyramids bilaterally.

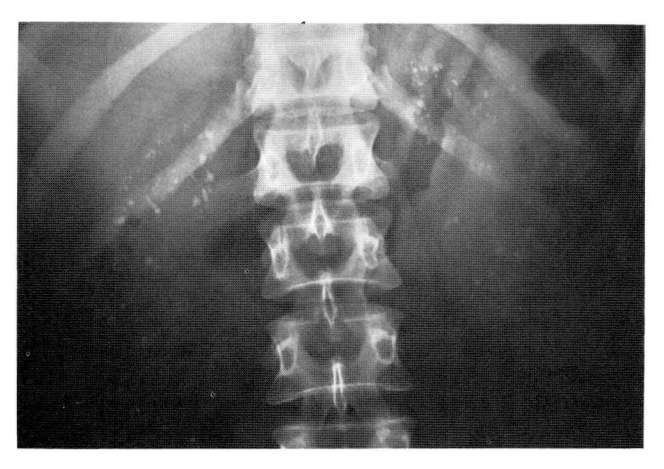

Figure 13 **Renal tubular acidosis.** Multiple small calcifications throughout the medullary portion of the renal parenchyma are seen.

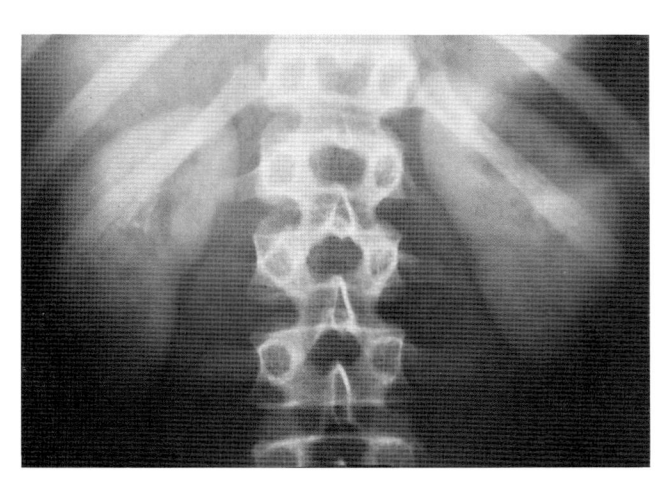

Figure 14 **Hyperoxaluria.** Both kidneys are abnormally dense. The renal cortices are homogeneously dense and the pyramids contain dense calcific flecks.

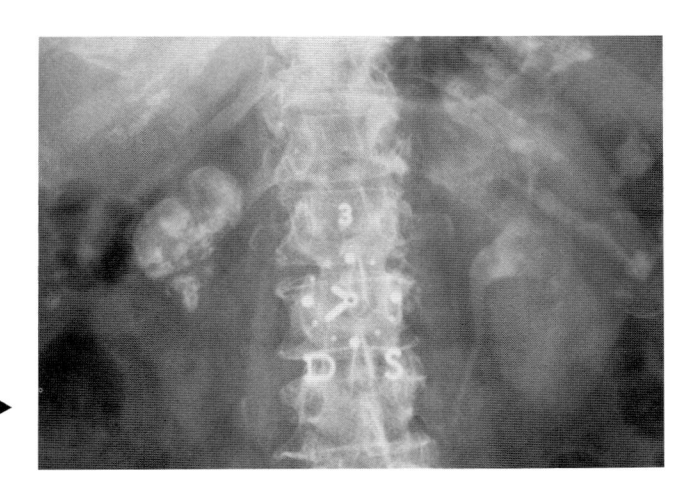

Figure 15 **Renal tuberculosis** with massive parenchymal ▶ calcification of the shrunken right kidney. No excretion of contrast medium on the right side.

Table 1 (Cont.) Differential Diagnosis of Abdominal Calcifications

Site and Pattern of Calcification	Common Causes	Radiographic Findings and Comments

D. Disseminated cortical calcification of kidneys	Acute cortical necrosis secondary to:
	  Shock
	  Toxic substances
	  Acute tubular necrosis
	  Acute pyelonephritis
		Punctate or linear calcifications of the cortex occur within one month of the onset.

	Hyperoxaluria	Calcifications may involve predominantly cortex. See above.
	Hereditary nephritis (Alport's syndrome)	Recurrent microscopic hematuria, slowly progressive renal failure, and later often deafness. May be a disorder of basement membrane synthesis. Fully expressed only in males (X-linked penetrance) who usually die before the fifth decade.
	Chronic glomerulonephritis Dialysis therapy Polycystic disease Sickle-cell disease Fabry's disease Nail-patella syndrome (osteo-onychodysplasia)	These are rare causes of renal cortical calcification. *Fabry's disease,* or *angiokeratoma corporis diffusum universale* (accumulation of ceramide hexoside), is radiologically characterized by cardiomegaly with congestive heart failure and poor renal function.
	Calcified subcapsular hematoma	Linear calcification around the kidney, often associated with hypertension.
E. Focal parenchymal calcification of the kidney	Tuberculosis (Fig. **16**)	May appear as a single nodular or irregular calcification (see above).
	Adenocarcinoma (Fig. **17**)	About 10% of renal adenocarcinomas calcify. If a renal mass contains calcium in a nonperipheral location, it is very likely malignant. Even a curvilinear cystic peripheral calcification of a mass does not exclude malignancy.
	Nephroblastoma (Wilms' tumor) (Fig. **18**)	Cystic, streaky, or amorphous calcification of the tumor is uncommon, but may occur in older children and adults with nephroblastoma.
	Xanthogranulomatous pyelonephritis (Fig. **19**)	Simulates carcinoma, but inflammatory masses may be multiple and diffusely calcified. A large pelvic calculus is present in the majority of cases, causing pelvocaliceal obstruction.

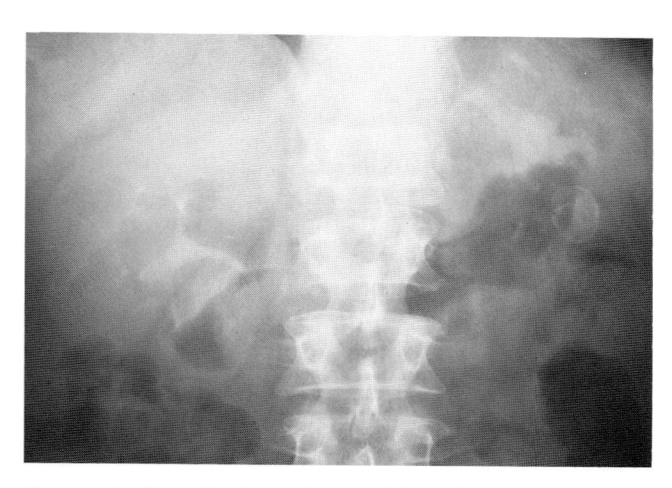

Figure 16 **Renal tuberculosis** of the left kidney with focal calcification. The calcification appears cystic but internal calcifications are also present.

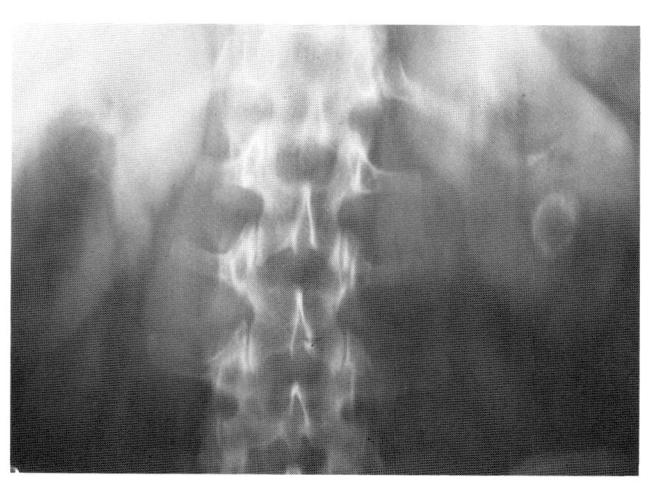

Figure 17 **Adenocarcinoma** of the left kidney with calcification – a thick-walled, somewhat cystic calcification with irregular internal calcific deposits.

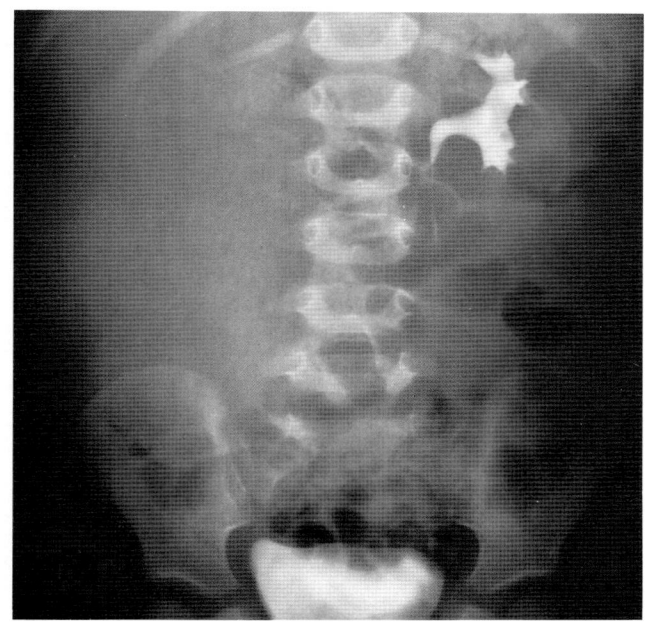

Figure 18 **A large Wilms' tumor** in the right kidney of a three-year-old boy, seen as an enlarged, nonexcreting kidney containing flecks of calcification.

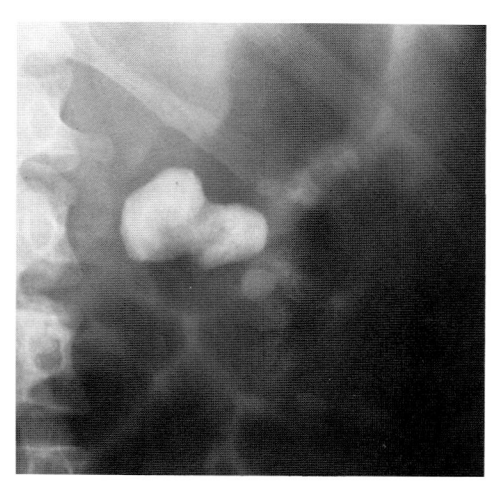

Figure 19 **Xanthogranulomatous pyelonephritis.** Scout film shows pelvic stones and parenchymal calcifications.

Table 1 (Cont.) Differential Diagnosis of Abdominal Calcifications

Site and Pattern of Calcification	Common Causes	Radiographic Findings and Comments
F. Cystic (curvilinear) renal calcification	Simple renal cyst (Fig. 20)	A thin curvilinear calcification can be demonstrated in 3%.
	Adenocarcinoma (Fig. 21)	20% of thin curvilinear calcifications are due to a calcified fibrous pseudocapsule of a renal adenocarcinoma.
	Polycystic or multicystic disease (Fig. 22)	Curvilinear calcifications similar to that of a simple cyst may occur.
	Echinococcal cyst	The majority are calcified. Complete circumferential ring of calcium is characteristic but not always present.
	Organized perirenal hematoma (Fig. 23) Old perirenal abscess	May appear as large cyst-like calcifications.
	Nephroblastoma (Wilms' tumor)	May appear cystic due to peripheral calcification.
	Renal artery aneurysm	A cracked eggshell-like circular calcification at the renal hilus is seen in about one third of renal artery aneurysms.
	Renal milk of calcium DD: Residual Pantopaque from prior cyst puncture	Calcium-containing sediment in a cyst, caliceal diverticulum, or obstructed renal pelvis. Mimics calculus in supine films. In upright position calcific material gravitates to the bottom of the cyst.
Ureteral calcification	Ureteral calculus: Mostly idiopathic but the following conditions predispose: Decreased mobility Pre-existing ureteral obstruction Metabolic diseases (see nephrocalcinosis Pre-existing infection Postoperative ureteral stump DD: phleboliths (round located laterally, and below the interspinous line)	Characteristically irregular, often oval, lodged at three levels: Ureteropelvic junction (large calculi) Pelvic brim Ureterovesical junction (small calculi) Stones less than 4 mm will eventually pass spontaneously in over 80%. 4–6 mm stones will be passed spontaneously in 50%, but often cause renal obstruction. Stones larger than 6 mm rarely pass spontaneously and have a high incidence of serious complications.
	Schistosomiasis	Tubular calcification of the distal ureter occurs in about 15% of patients.
	Tuberculosis (Fig. 24)	Ureter calcifies less frequently than the kidney and its appearance is variable. Ipsilateral renal calcification is often present.
Adrenal and retroperitoneal calcification		
A. Triangular	Neonatal adrenal hemorrhage	Occurs in infants born to mothers with diabetes and/or with an abnormal obstetric history. The periphery of the adrenal calcifies a few weeks after hemorrhage. Can be an incidental finding.
	Adrenal tuberculosis (Addison's disease)	In about one-fourth of patients discrete, stippled densities outline the entire adrenal. Calcification can also be confluent and dense.

Abdominal Calcifications

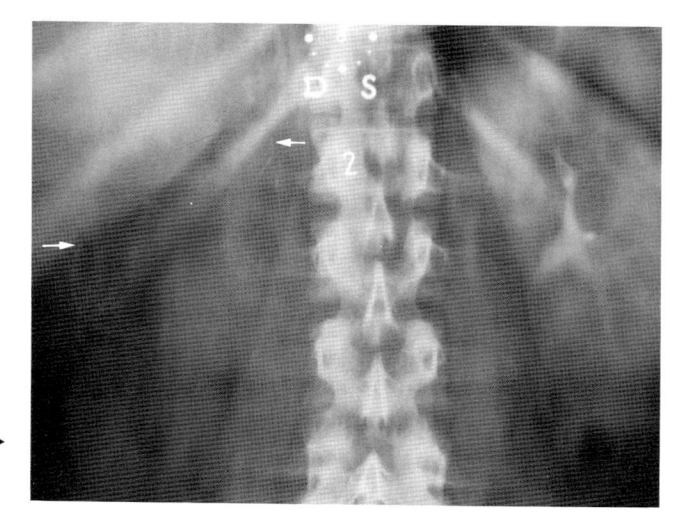

Figure 20 **Two calcified simple renal cysts** in the right ▶ kidney (arrows). A tomographic section is shown for better visualization.

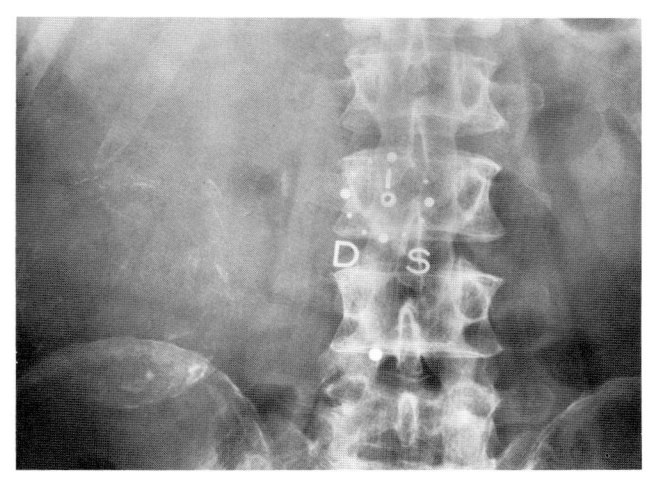

Figure 21 **Adenocarcinoma of the kidney.** Curvilinear calcification (with possible internal calcifications) in a large tumor of the lower pole of the right kidney.

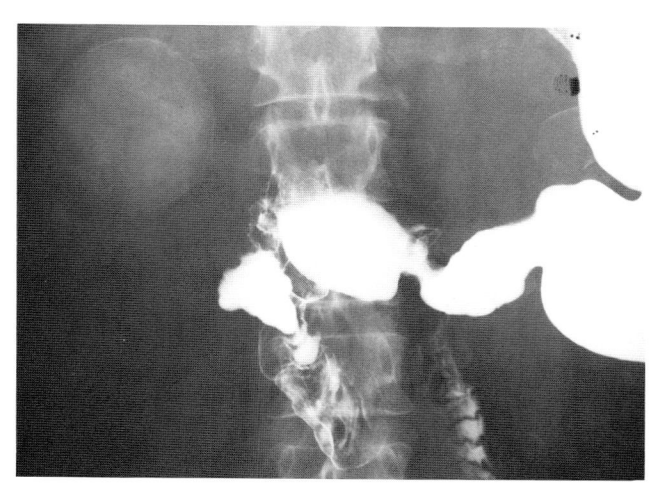

Figure 22 **Polycystic kidneys** with renal failure and calcification of the cyst walls bilaterally.

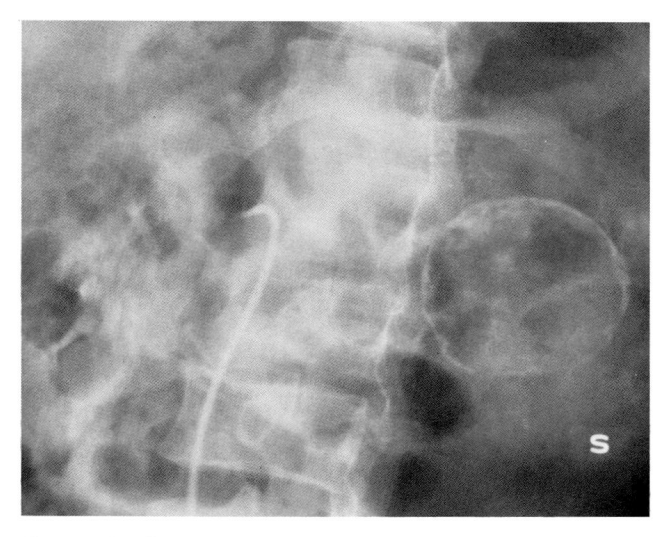

Figure 23 **Calcification of an organized perirenal hematoma** on the left.

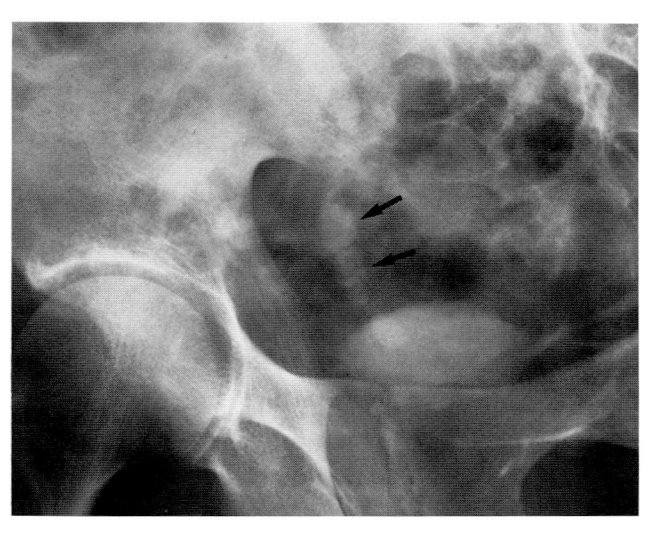

Figure 24 **Tuberculosis of the right distal ureter** with characteristic ribbon-like calcifications (arrows).

Table 1 (Cont.) Differential Diagnosis of Abdominal Calcifications

Site and Pattern of Calcification	Common Causes	Radiographic Findings and Comments

B. Cystic (curvilinear)	Adrenal cyst:
	  Lymphatic
	  Necrotic pseudocyst (Fig. 25)
	  Cystic adenoma
	  Echinococcal
	  Old hemorrhage (Fig. 26)
		A thin rim of curvilinear calcification above the kidney.

C. Mottled mass calcification	Adrenal cortical carcinoma Pheochromocytoma (rare) Adrenal cortical adenoma (rare) Adrenal choristoma (a small mass of bone marrow and fat) (very rare)	Scattered flecks of calcification throughout the mass.
	Neuroblastoma	Calcification that is fine granular or stippled, rarely massive, occurs in about 50% of neuroblastomas. It is the second most common malignancy in children (after Wilms' tumor).
	Retroperitoneal teratoma	Calcified spicules of cartilage or bone are seen near the midline of upper abdomen. Teeth inclusions may be identifiable.
	Retroperitoneal cavernous hemangioma (Fig. 27)	A large mass with multiple phleboliths.
	Other retroperitoneal tumors (Fig. 28)	Calcification is extremely rare.
	Calcified lymph node	1 to 1.5 cm dense calcification may move according to different body positions.
	Retroperitoneal hematoma Tuberculous psoas abscess	May present as a large calcification.
D. Longitudinal tubular calcification	Atherosclerosis	Sclerotic plaques of the aortic wall are common in the elderly. The aorta characteristically narrows toward the bifurcation. It may be curved and simulate an aneurysm.
	Abdominal aortic aneurysm (Fig. 29)	Walls of the aneurysm tend to calcify more than the normal aorta. Calcified plaques outline the aneurysm that most commonly occurs below the renal arteries. Oblique films can be used to avoid superimposition of the spine.

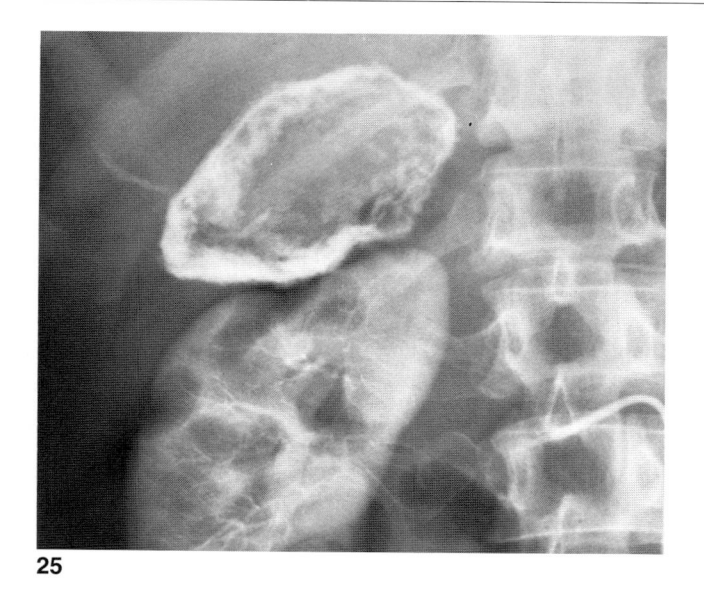

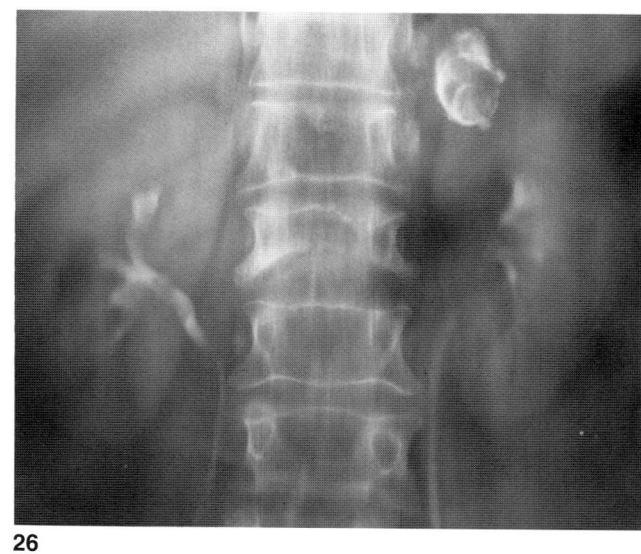

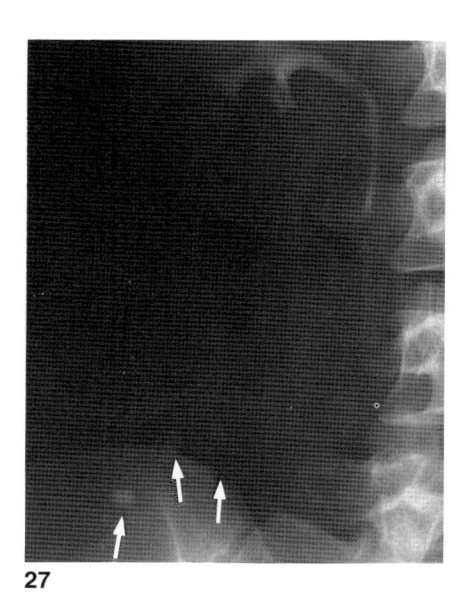

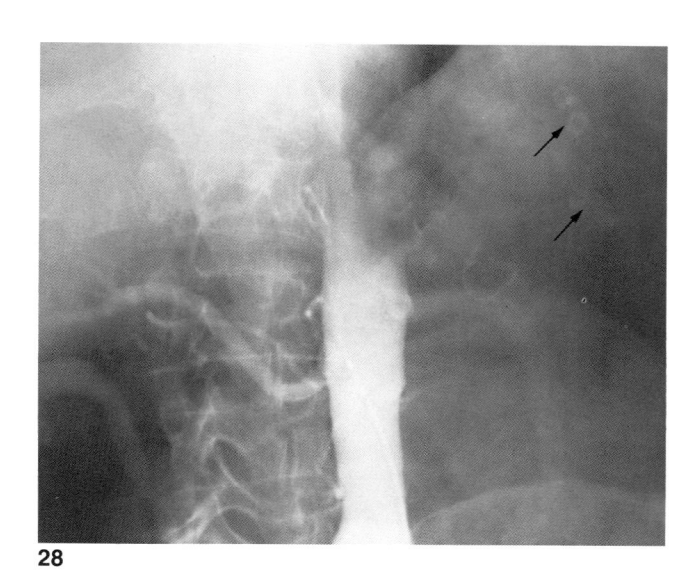

Figure 25 **Necrotic pseudocyst of the right adrenal.** A large cystic calcified mass, separate from the kidney, is seen.

Figure 26 **Calcified old adrenal hemorrhage** above the left kidney.

Figure 27 **Right retroperitoneal cavernous hemangioma,** containing 3 phleboliths. Due to their location they simulate appendicoliths.

Figure 28 **Retroperitoneal leiomyosarcoma.** Faint calcifications (arrows) are seen in this mass. The film was obtained during aortography.

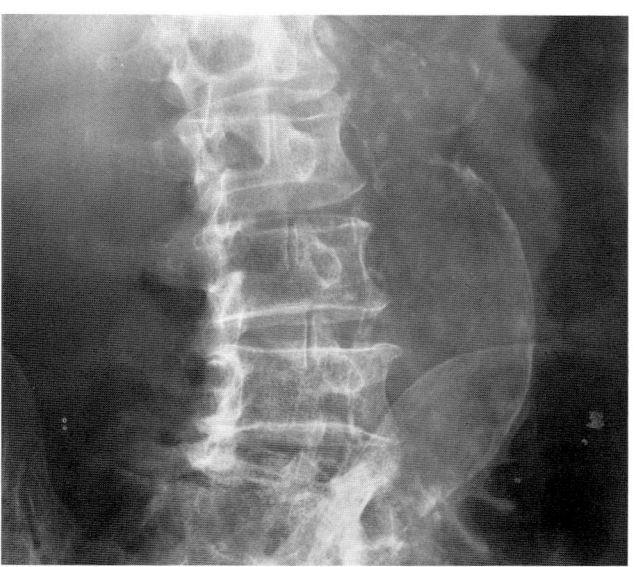

Figure 29 **Calcified abdominal aortic aneurysm.**

Table 1 (Cont.) Differential Diagnosis of Abdominal Calcifications

Site and Pattern of Calcification	Common Causes	Radiographic Findings and Comments
Pelvic calcification		
A. Tubular calcification	Arteriosclerosis	The aorta and the iliac arteries are frequently calcified and seen as irregular plaque-like densities. May be seen in young persons with diabetes.
	Vas deferens Associated conditions: Diabetes mellitus Tuberculosis Degenerative change (Fig. **30**)	Bilaterally symmetric tubular densities that run medially and caudally to enter the base of the prostate, somewhat mimicking a medium-sized arteriosclerotic artery. Vas deferens calcification due to chronic inflammation (tuberculosis, syphilis) is intraluminal and has an irregular pattern.
B. Calcified bladder wall	Schistosomiasis (Fig. **31**)	About 50% of patients with schistosomiasis of the bladder have visible calcifications of the bladder, most apparent at the base. A linear opaque shadow may surround a relatively normal-sized bladder. A disruption in the continuity of the homogenous line of calcification is suggestive of bladder carcinoma, a common complication.
	Tuberculous cystitis	A rare cause of bladder wall calcification. Usually a faint calcified rim is seen in a contracted bladder, associated with calcifications in a kidney and ureter.
	Encrusted cystitis: nonspecific infection post-irradiation	A very rare cause of calcification of the bladder wall.
C. Calculi	Bladder calculi (Fig. **32**) – migrated down the ureter – formed in the bladder secondary to obstruction or infection of the lower urinary tract or formed around a foreign body nidus	Usually circular or oval with variable internal structure. Small calculi may be confused with phleboliths in the vicinity of the bladder.
	Urethral calculi (Fig. **33**) – migrant or primary	Midline stones usually in the subpubic angle. In males they are associated with urethral stricture, in females with diverticula and infection.
	Urachal calculus	An oval or dumbbell-shaped opacity is located anteriorly and superimposed on the sacrum. On cystograms, the upper portion of the bladder is pear-shaped and points toward the stone.
	Phleboliths	Phlebolith is a calcified thrombus within a vein, present in most adults. Round, homogeneous or ringlike, most frequent in the lateral aspect of the pelvis. When seen in great quantity in a localized area, they are suggestive of a *hemangioma*.

Abdominal Calcifications 49

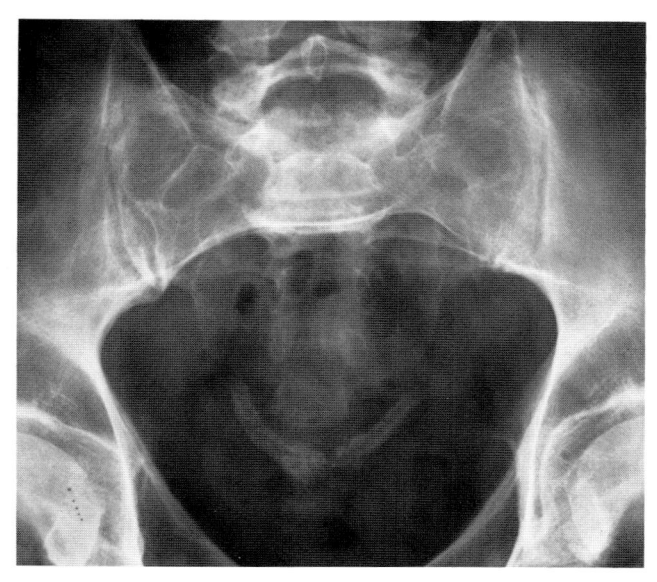

Figure 30 **Calcified vas deferens** in a 65-year-old patient, an incidental finding.

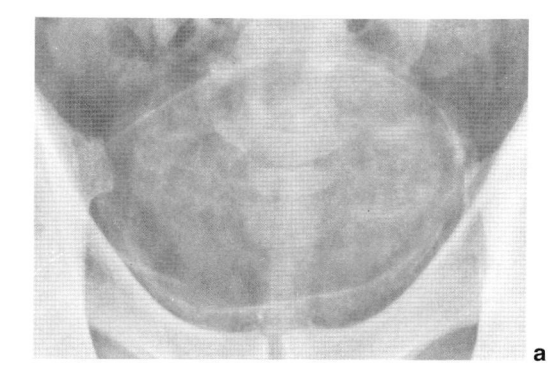

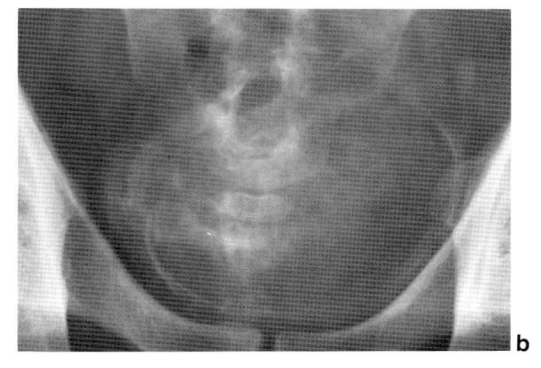

Figure 31a **Schistosomiasis** of the urinary bladder. A linear calcified ring represents the bladder wall. **b** The same patient, two years later. The disruption of the right wall of the bladder indicates bladder carcinoma.

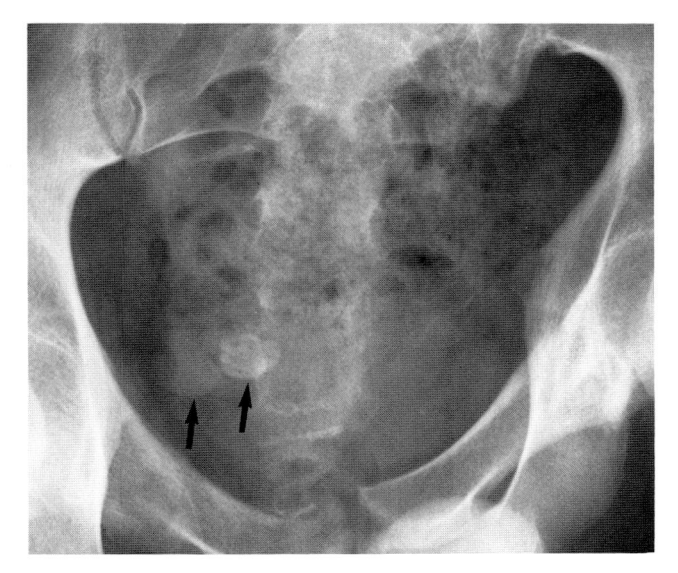

Figure 32 **Bladder calculi** (arrows) in a young male (age 22) with trauma, prolonged immobilization and urinary tract infection.

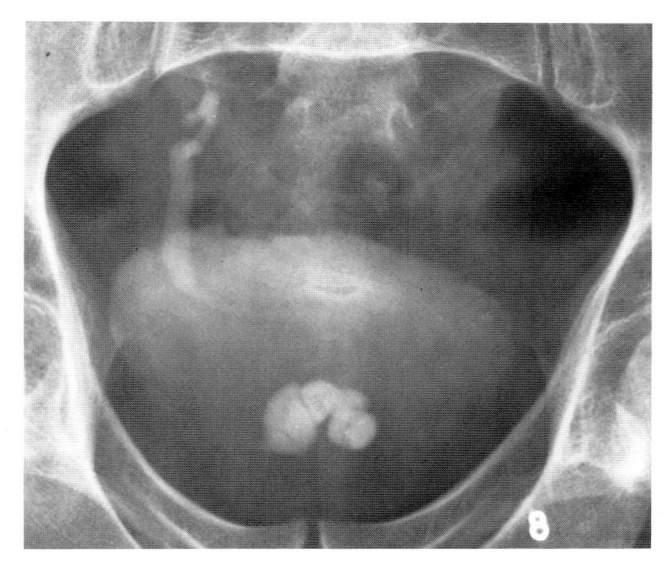

Figure 33 **Urethral calculi** in the proximal urethra. A male with gonorrheal urethral stricture.

Table 1 (Cont.) Differential Diagnosis of Abdominal Calcifications

Site and Pattern of Calcification	Common Causes	Radiographic Findings and Comments
D. Mass calcifications (stippled or conglomerate) in a female	Uterine fibroid (leiomyoma) (Fig. 34)	The most common calcified lesion of the female genital tract. A mottled or "mulberry" type of calcification is characteristic.
	Ovarian dermoid cyst (Fig. 35)	About half of them contain calcification, either partial or complete teeth or the cyst wall is calcified.
	Papillary cystadenoma or papillary cystadenocarcinoma of the ovary (Fig. 36)	Psammomatous calcifications of these tumors are scattered, and amorphous. They are easily missed on plain films. Implants in the peritoneal cavity may show similar calcifications, but may be mistaken for feces.
	Gonadoblastoma	Circumscribed mottled calcifications in the pelvis are frequent but the tumor is rare.
	Spontaneous amputation of the ovary	Probably the result of torsion and infarction of the adnexa. A small, coarsely stippled calcified mass in the pelvis moves with changing position.
	Pregnancy (Fig. 37)	Fetal bones may be seen
	Placental calcification	Occurs after the 32nd week of fetal life, has an average width of 15–20 cm and thickness of 3 cm. Calcification is greatest in the periphery.
	Lithopedion	Fetal skeletal parts are mixed with calcification. Can be intrauterine (old missed abortion) or extrauterine (previous ectopic pregnancy).
Mass calcifications (stippled or conglomerate) in a male	Prostatic calculi: Primary (idiopathic) Secondary to obstruction, stasis, or infection Postoperative (in prostatic fossa, rare)	Frequent in men after 40. Discrete 2 to 4 mm calcifications may be present throughout the prostate or have a horseshoe or ring arrangement. Depending on the size of the prostate they may be seen above, behind, or rarely beneath the symphysis pubis. The most common cause of secondary prostatic calculi is a urethral stricture. *Prostatic tuberculosis* may cause an identical pattern. Postoperative stones are usually large and most common after an open prostatectomy.
	Seminal vesicle calculi	Very rare, variable in diameter, single or multiple.

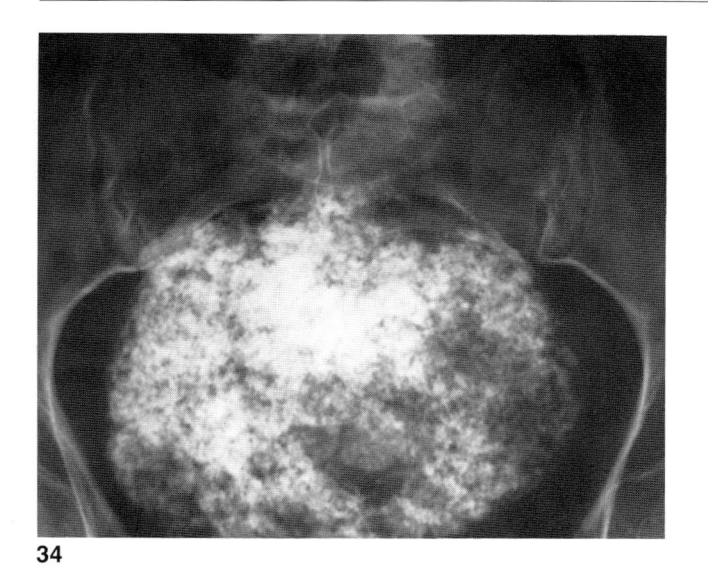

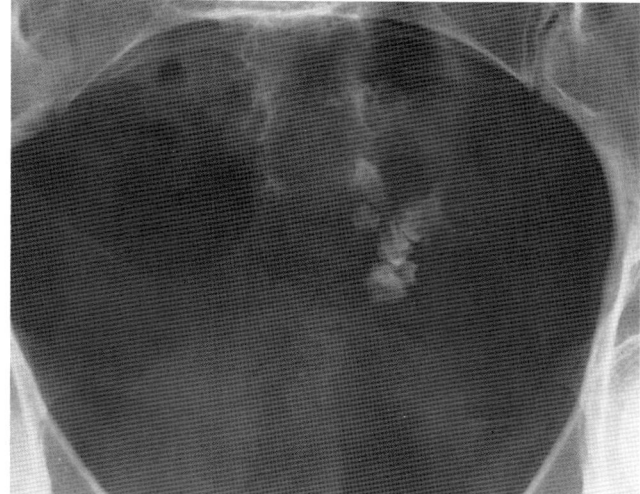

Abdominal Calcifications 51

Figure 34 **A large calcified uterine fibroid.**

Figure 35a, b a **Ovarian dermoid cyst** containing several teeth. **b** Ovarian dermoid with layered calcification.

Figure 36 **Papillary cystadenocarcinoma** of the right ovary detected as an incidental finding by observing the fine amorphous psammomatous calcifications (arrows).

Figure 37 **Normal pregnancy** showing fetal bones. A calcified uterine fibroid, displaced into the left upper quadrant (arrow) is seen as an incidental finding.

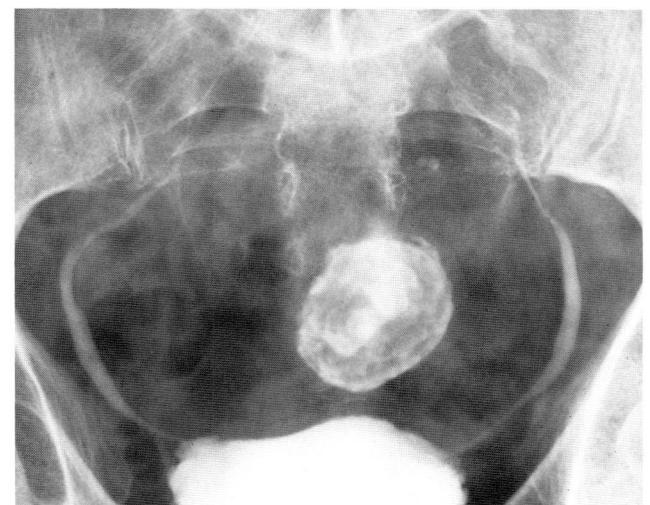

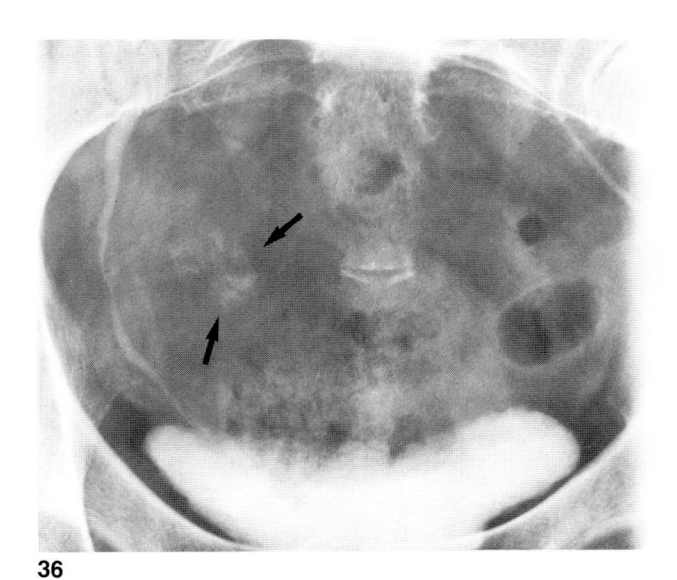

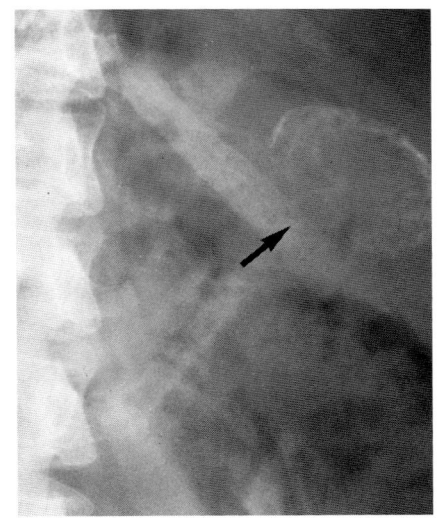

Table 1 (Cont.) Differential Diagnosis of Abdominal Calcifications

Site and Pattern of Calcification	Common Causes	Radiographic Findings and Comments

E. Mass calcifications (stippled or conglomerate) in both sexes	Bladder neoplasm:
	   Transitional cell carcinoma
	   Squamous cell carcinoma
	   Mesenchymal tumors (rarely)
		Calcification associated with a mass in the bladder usually indicates the presence of a bladder neoplasm. Tumor calcification can be punctate, coarse, or linear, and is often located on the surface of the tumor.

	Calcified lymph node	Represents old granulomatous infection and has a diameter of 1 to 1.5 cm. Calcification is usually coarser than in phleboliths or in calculi.
"String of pearls" calcification	Tuberculous salpingitis	May be bilateral in the female pelvis.
	Tuberculosis of vas deferens	Intraluminal calcifications may produce an irregular string of densities with a typical course.
Widespread abdominal calcification	Ovarian cystadenocarcinoma with abdominal metastases (Fig. 38)	Granular or sandlike psammomatous calcifications adjacent to the peritoneal fat stripe are characteristic.
	Pseudomyxoma peritonei (ruptured pseudomucinous cystadenoma of the ovary or mucocele of appendix)	Annular curvilinear calcifications may appear secondary to a foreign body reaction in the peritoneum.
	Undifferentiated abdominal malignancy	Variable forms of calcification may occur rarely.
	Tuberculous peritonitis (Fig. 39)	Mottled, widespread calcifications may simulate residual barium.
	Meconium peritonitis (Fig. 40)	Multiple small calcifications secondary to intrauterine perforation of the bowel.

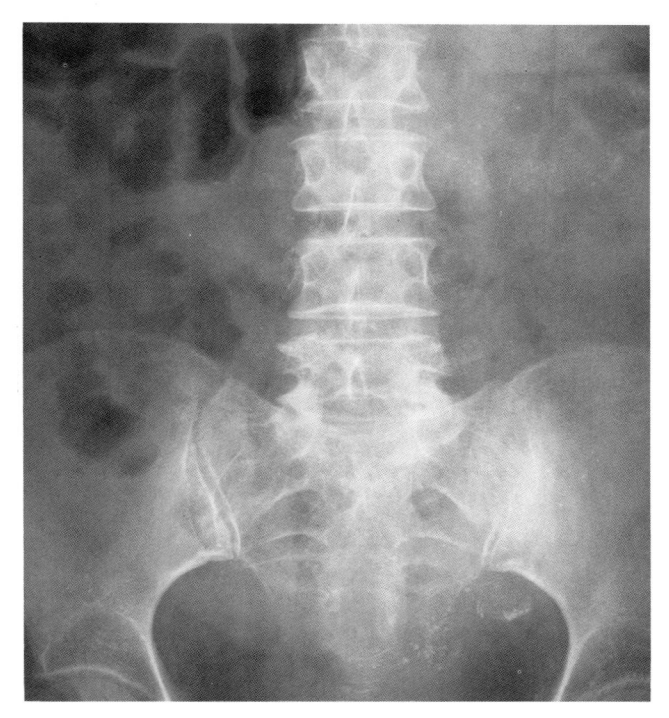

Figure 38 **Ovarian cystadenocarcinoma** with abdominal metastases. Faint granular psammomatous calcifications as demonstrated in the pelvis were seen throughout the peritoneal cavity.

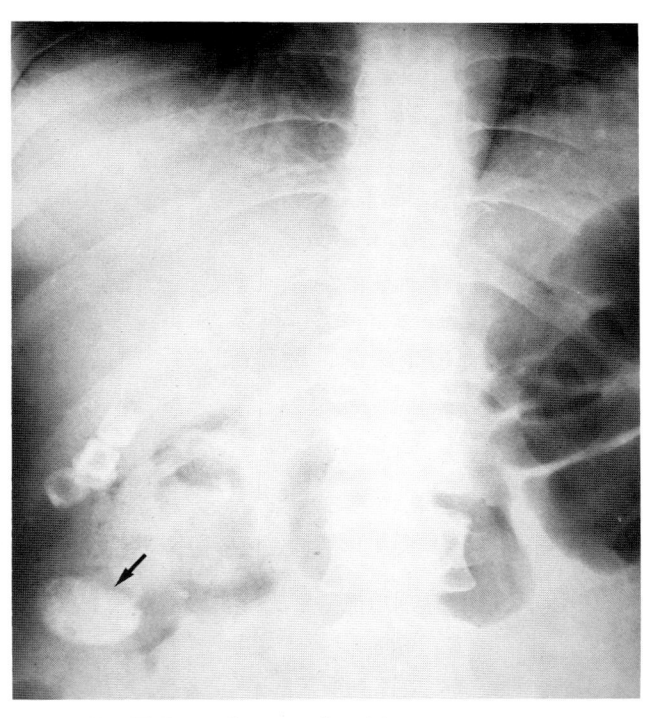

Figure 39 **Tuberculous peritonitis** (healed) with calcification (arrow). Gallstones are also seen on this film above the peritoneal calcification.

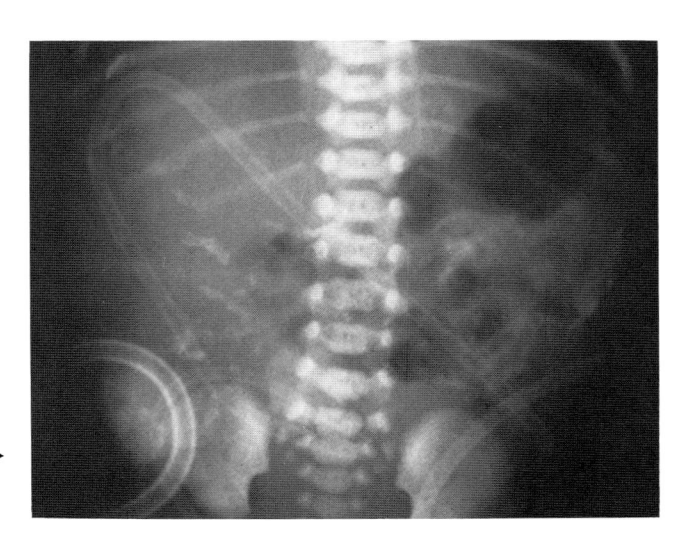

Figure 40 **Meconium peritonitis** with calcification secondary to ileal atresia. Widespread peritoneal calcifications are seen.

Chapter 3 Displacement of Abdominal Organs

Knowledge of the normal anatomic relationships and variants in the position of abdominal structures is essential to the detection and understanding of their displacement.

In general, the bowel, which has its own mesentery, will be prone to greater displacement than the visceral organs and bowel, which are tightly bound to the posterior wall of the abdominal cavity. Whereas the kidneys, liver, and spleen are visible on the plain film and even minor changes in their relatively constant positions are detected, a barium study may be required to disclose changes in the relative position of the intestinal loops both to each other and other organs.

The liver is relatively fixed in its position below the right hemidiaphragm. Normally the lower edge of the right lobe of the liver does not cross the right psoas margin or extend below the iliac crest. The anterior inferior edge is seen indirectly by its relationship to the hepatic flexure of the colon. The posterior aspect of the right lobe of the liver abuts the extraperitoneal adipose tissue and may be seen as a soft-tissue–fat interface. The area of the smaller left lobe of the liver is best evaluated radiologically as the space anterior to the stomach on lateral views during gastrointestinal series, since plain film identification is usually impossible, but it may occasionally displace the fundus of the stomach inferiorly.

The spleen normally lies in the left upper quadrant between the fundus of the stomach and the diaphragm in an oblique position. Rarely, it is horizontal, between the gastric fundus and the diaphragm, simulating a mass. Enlargement of the spleen tends to change the main axis of the spleen more vertically, but a vertically oriented spleen occurs without enlargement. The posteromedial border of the spleen is visualized by virtue of the extraperitoneal fat–spleen interface. The inferior tip of the spleen projects toward the splenic flexure of the colon.

The head of *the pancreas* is cradled by the descending duodenum, its body lies in the bed of the stomach, and the tail curves posteriorly to cross the left kidney and inserts within the splenic hilum. Depending on the position of the spleen, the pancreas is usually obliquely oriented (tail up), or rarely, horizontal. An insufficient amount of adjacent extraperitoneal fat prevents plain film visualization of the pancreas. The duodenojejunal junction serves as a useful demarcation between the body and tail of the pancreas. The longitudinal axis of the pancreas can be projected along a line from mid-descending duodenum to the splenic hilum.

The fundus of the *stomach* lies quite posteriorly in the left upper quadrant, whereas the distal body and antrum course anteriorly. The first and second portions of the duodenum are redirected posteriorly.

The root of the *small bowel* mesentery extends for a distance of about 15 cm from the region of the duodenojejunal junction to the cecocolic junction. Jejunal loops are commonly found in the left upper quadrant and ileal loops in the lower mid-abdomen and in the right lower quadrant. A common variant is nonrotation of the small bowel, wherein jejunal loops are in the right mid-abdomen.

The anatomic relationships of the *large intestine* are complex. The cecum may be completely extraperitoneal, but is often suspended intraperitoneally and seen as a more or less mobile cecum. This is particularly common in females. The ascending colon is extraperitoneal up to the anterior hepatic flexure and therefore fixed. The transverse colon is suspended anteriorly in the abdomen. From the splenic flexure the descending colon continues as a fixed extraperitoneal organ. A mesentery suspends the redundant sigmoid loops anteriorly off the level of the left sacroiliac joint. From the level of S2 to S4 the *rectum* continues subperitoneally.

In tall, thin females the stomach tends to be J-shaped and the transverse colon may curve into the lower abdomen or pelvis. In a short, stocky male the stomach is typically horizontally oriented in the upper abdomen with the duodenal bulb directed posteriorly, accompanied by a straight and high transverse colon that parallels the greater curvature of the stomach.

Renal outlines can be seen even on plain films because of perirenal fat. The left kidney is usually at the level of the 12th thoracic and 1st and 2nd lumbar vertebral bodies, 1–2 cm higher than the right kidney. The long axis of the kidneys diverges inferiorly and grossly parallels the psoas margins. The upper pole of the kidney is more posteriorly situated than the lower pole. Increased mobility of the kidney (commonly on the right) is demonstrated by comparing supine and upright films. In addition to the general downward displacement of the mobile kidney, axis rotation is common in the upright position with shortening of the kidney shadow.

The urinary bladder is fixed by the pelvic connective tissue and rarely shows major displacement (Fig. 1), but impressions from neighboring organs or tumors are common. In cystocele (prolapse of the bladder and the anterior vaginal wall into the vaginal cavity) and in certain instances of stress incontinence with rotational descent of the bladder neck, there is downward displacement of the bladder relative to the pelvic bones with or even without strain. Pregnancy or a huge pelvic tumor, usually of ovarian origin, may cause relative downward displacement of the bladder by completely flattening the dome of the urinary bladder, which normally is outlined by the subperitoneal fat and visible on plain films. Compression by a neighboring mass may also occur from the lateral and posterior aspects (colonic distension, pelvic or retroperitoneal tumor, abscess or hematoma, pelvic lipomatosis) or from below the bladder (prostatic enlargement).

Plain films, and even bowel-contrast examinations, are relatively insensitive in detecting any abnormal position of the parenchymal organs of the abdomen. Ultrasound, CT and MRI give more exact information on the organs' size and position. As far as the mobility of the parenchymal organs is concerned, ultrasound is usually the most convenient method of examination.

Conditions associated with abnormal position or displacement of the liver, spleen, kidneys, stomach, small bowel, and various segments of the large intestine are presented in Tables **1** through **7**. Displacement of the intestine is often associated with an abnormal gas pattern (see Chapter 1, p. 1).

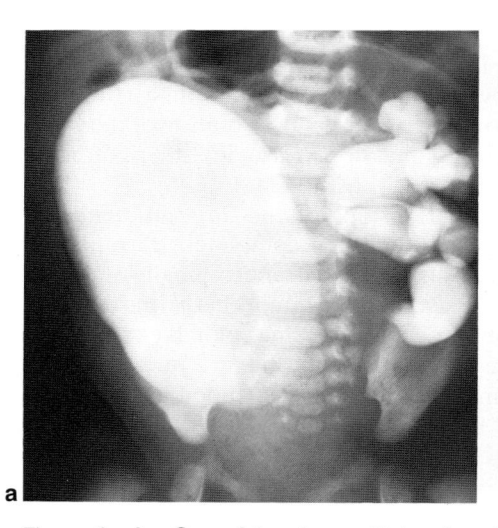

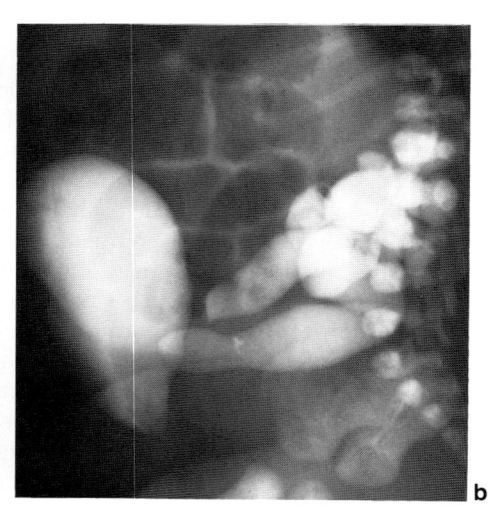

Figure **1a, b** **Sacral teratoma.** Extensive displacement of the bladder **a** upward and **b** anteriorly in an infant. There is also ureteral obstruction and bilateral hydronephrosis.

Table 1 Abnormal Position of the Liver

Presentation	Associated Conditions	Radiographic Findings and Comments
Left-sided liver	Situs inversus	Complete abdominal and thoracic mirror image.
	Abdominal heterotaxia	May be associated with asplenia, polysplenia, or anisosplenia and pulmonary isomerism.
Upward displacement	Eventration of the right hemidiaphragm	Localized or generalized elevation of the right hemidiaphragm. Restricted motion of the involved portion of the diaphragm. Elevation of the liver and hepatic flexure of the colon.
	Right pleuroperitoneal (foramen of Bochdalek) hernia	Opacification of the right hemithorax, displacement of mediastinum to the left, atelectasis of the right lung, elevation of the hepatic flexure of the colon. Free access of gas from a diagnostic pneumoperitoneum into the right hemithorax differentiates Bochdalek hernia from diaphragmatic eventration. Bochdalek hernia is much more common on the left side.
Downward displacement of the liver	Large pneumoperitoneum (Fig. 2)	The liver drops downward and gas replaces the subdiaphragmatic space.
	Colonic interposition between the right hemidiaphragm and the liver (Chilaiditi syndrome) Fig. 18, p. 13).	Caudal displacement of the liver depends on the degree of gaseous distension of the interposed colonic segment.
	Right subphrenic abscess	The distance from the dome of the diaphragm to the lower edge of the liver is increased mainly due to diaphragmatic elevation.

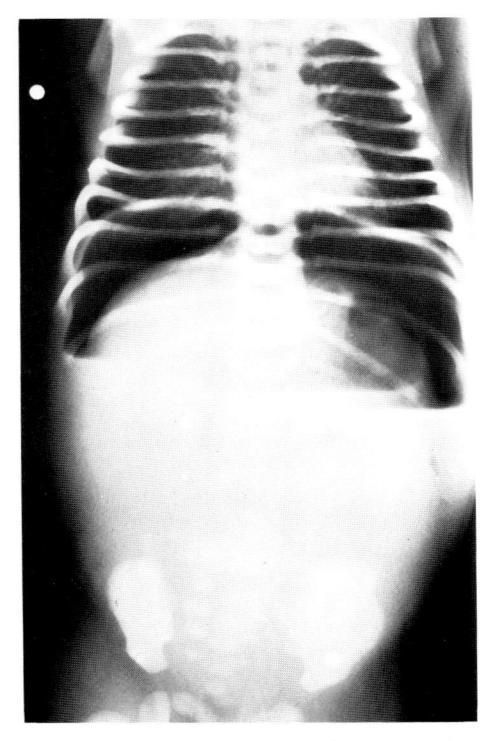

Figure 2 **Hydropneumoperitoneum.** Downward displacement of liver, stomach, and spleen in an infant with bowel rupture (duodenal atresia).

Table 2 Abnormal Position of the Spleen

Presentation	Associated Conditions	Radiographic Findings and Comments
Absent splenic shadow	Asplenia	A rare anomaly often associated with cardiovascular malformations, partial situs inversus (*abdominal heterotaxia*), persistence of dorsal mesenteries of the duodenum and colon, and symmetrical lobulations of the liver and lungs (*pulmonary isomerism*).
	Postsplenectomy	
Upward displacement	Congenital left pleuroperitoneal (foramen of Bochdalek) hernia	Intestinal loops, kidney, and spleen may be located in the left hemithorax.
Medial displacement	Medially located spleen	The spleen may lie between the tail of the pancreas and the anterior aspect of the left kidney and mimic a retroperitoneal mass, upper pole mass of the kidney, or pancreatic pseudocyst.
	"Wandering spleen"	A rare, usually asymptomatic deficiency or laxity of the ligamentous attachments of the spleen. May mimic an abdominal mass. Occurs most often in women of child-bearing age. The normal splenic shadow is absent. The spleen may be seen as a central abdominal or left flank mass displacing adjacent organs.
	"Upside-down" spleen	An anatomic variant without ligamentous laxity. The splenic hilum is directed superiorly or laterally. The convex splenic border adjacent to the left kidney may mimic a suprarenal mass.
	Accessory spleen	A spheric or ovoid structure up to 4 cm in diameter, can be mistaken for an adrenal, pancreatic, or retroperitoneal tumor. Can enlarge after splenectomy. Most commonly located in the splenic hilus.
Vertically oriented spleen (Figs. 3, 6)	Normal in an infant	
	Splenomegaly: The distance between the dome of the left diaphragm and the inferior pole of the spleen exceeds in an adult 16 cm or the height of T12 to L3, respectively. The spleen assumes a globular configuration.	The inferior splenic angle projects well below the left costal margin. Common causes of splenomegaly include: Lymphomas Leukemias Myelofibrosis Anemias Parasitic infections Portal hypertension Hematoma Right heart failure
	Mass between spleen and abdominal wall, e. g., hematoma.	The splenic shadow may be obscured by hematoma.

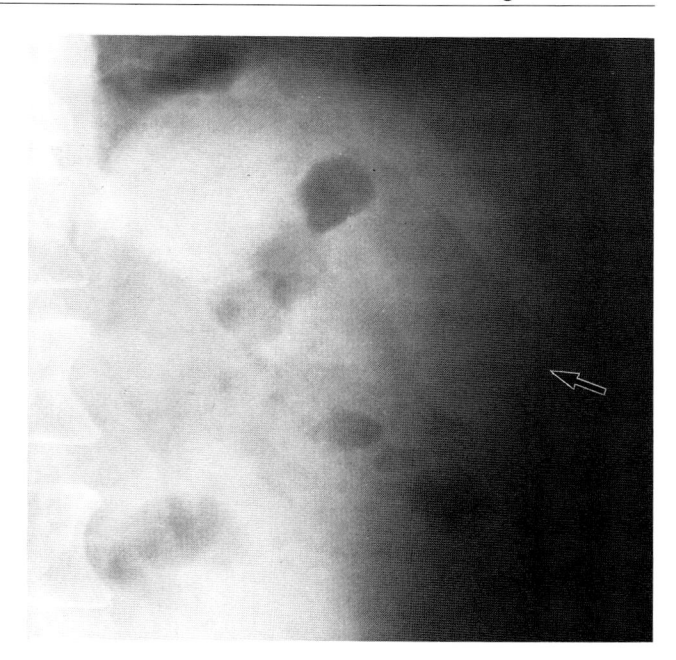

Figure 3 **Splenic rupture.** Medial displacement of the inferior end of the spleen (arrow) and the proximal descending colon by a hematoma.

Table 3 Abnormal Position of the Kidney

Presentation	Associated Conditions	Radiographic Findings and Comments
Downward displacement	Ptosis of the kidney (mobile kidney)	Downward displacement of usually the right kidney on erect films, often accompanied by rotation of the kidney. Most common in thin females.
(Fig. 4)	Renal ectopia DD: Renal agenesis, severe hypoplasia, or fusion malposition (Fig. 5)	A relatively common anomaly (approximately 1 : 1000), obvious in IVP. The kidney may be located in the pelvis (over 60%), above the iliac crest (over 20%), or at the level of iliac bone (about 10%). Intestine occupies the area of renal fossa on the side of ectopia. Absent renal shadow and extrinsic mass effect by the ectopic kidney in the pelvis are characteristic. There is an increased incidence of stones, infection and hydronephrosis. May complicate delivery. Other urogenital anomalies are commonly associated.
	Transplanted kidney	Kidney overlying ilium, often with surgical markers.
	Enlarged liver	Liver enlargement nearly always causes downward displacement of the right kidney.
(Fig. 6)	Enlarged spleen	Splenomegaly only infrequently causes downward displacement of the left kidney.

(Fig. 7)	Adrenal tumor:
	  Neuroblastoma (child under 2 ½ years)
	  Pheochromocytoma
	  Metastasis
	  Rarely a benign tumor
		A mass density above the kidney, displacing but not markedly distorting the kidney. Neuroblastoma is the second most common malignant neoplasm in children (after Wilms' tumor), and commonly calcifies. Pheochromocytomas may grow very large, whereas adrenal adenomas are usually too small to displace the ipsilateral kidney.

	Adrenal hemorrhage (neonate)	Adrenal hemorrhage may be large enough to displace the ipsilateral kidney.
	(Upper pole intrarenal mass)	A large intrarenal tumor may cause apparent downward displacement of the rest of the kidney. Severe distortion of the caliceal system is common.
Upward displacement	Congenital pleuroperitoneal hernia (Bochdalek hernia)	Usually a left-sided defect. The left kidney (together with the spleen and/or small bowel loops) may be seen in the left hemithorax.
	Small liver	In advanced cirrhosis with shrunken liver, the right kidney and duodenal bulb occupy an abnormally high position.

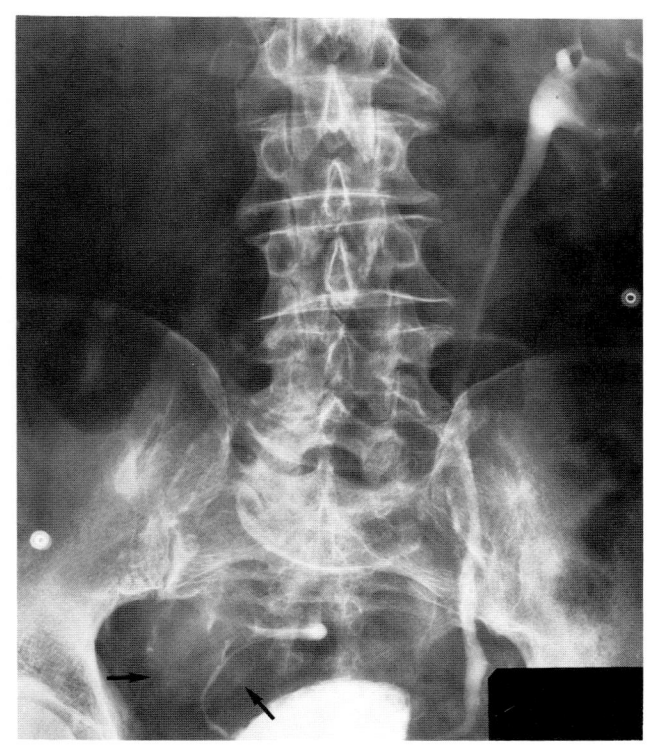

Figure 4 **Right pelvic kidney** without other abnormalities.

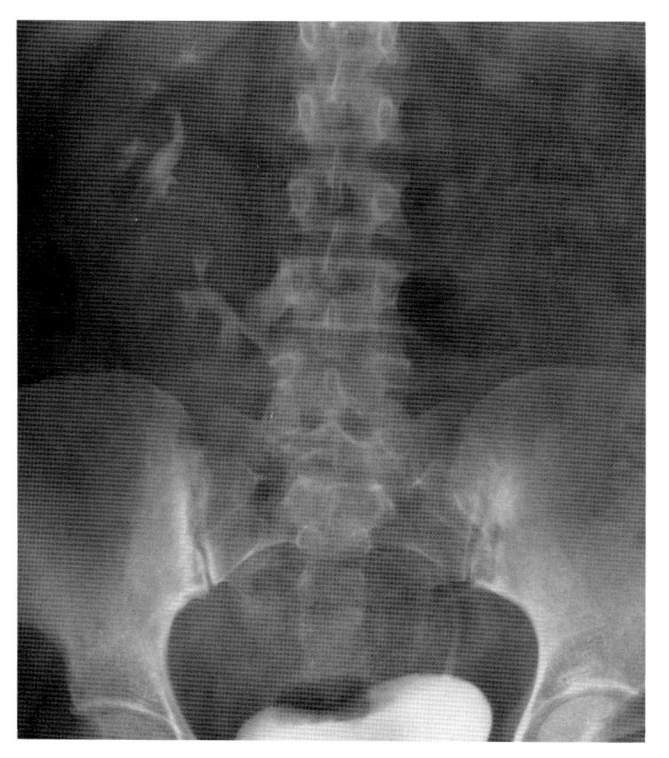

Figure 5 **Fusion malposition of the kidneys.** The left kidney is located below the right kidney, but its ureter is seen on the left side.

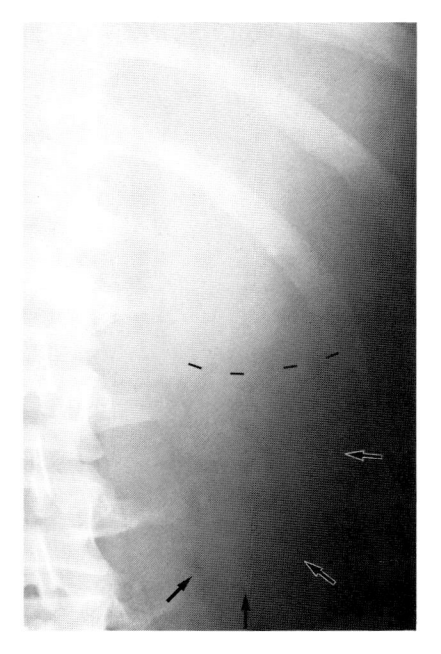

Figure 6 **Splenomegaly.** Vertically oriented large spleen displaces the left kidney down (arrows). The dashed line indicates the inferior splenic border.

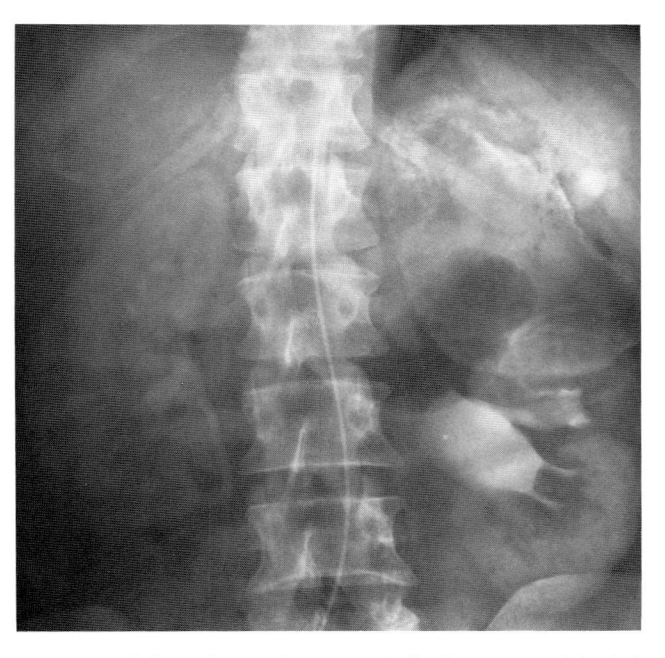

Figure 7 **Adrenal cyst.** Downward displacement of the left kidney by a large calcified adrenal cyst. There is also rotation of the kidney about its short axis.

Table 3 (Cont.) Abnormal Position of the Kidney

Presentation	Associated Conditions	Radiographic Findings and Comments
(Fig. 8)	Mass lesion below the lower pole	
Medial displacement (Fig. 9)	Horse-shoe kidney	Lower poles are joined by fibrous or renal tissue. The longitudinal axes of *both* kidneys are reversed with upper poles tilted away from the spine.
	Splenomegaly	Marked enlargement of the spleen may displace the left kidney medially.
	A lateral, extracapsular or sub-capsular mass (e.g., hematoma, lipoma)	
Lateral displacement (Figs. 10, 11)	Peripelvic expansion (cyst, tumor or abscess, or hydronephrosis) Lymphoma Metastatic lymph node enlargement, especially from gonadal tumors Retroperitoneal sarcoma Aneurysm of the aorta	Lateral displacement of the kidney or more commonly lateral rotation of upper or lower pole, associated with a close to midline extrarenal mass. May be bilateral or unilateral.
	Adrenal tumor Pancreatic tumor or pseudocyst (Liver tumor)	Unilateral upper pole lateral rotation or displacement of a kidney may occur.
Rotation about the short axis (Fig. 7)	Adrenal mass	The upper pole is displaced downward and the kidney is seen end on. Normal thickness of the renal parenchyma.
	Retroperitoneal tumor	The lower pole may rarely be pushed up by a retroperitoneal tumor and consequently the kidney is seen end on.
Rotation about the long axis (Fig. 9)	Horseshoe kidney Congenital malposition Peripelvic mass	The minor calices are seen end on or even medially. If bilateral, a horseshoe kidney should be suspected.

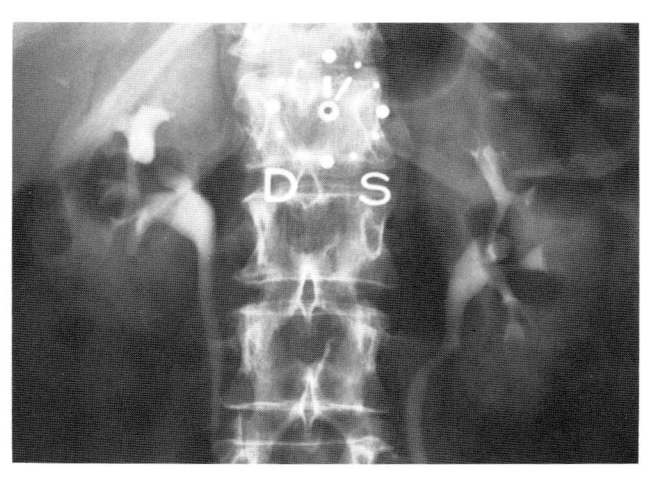

Figure 8 **Retroperitoneal cyst.** Upward displacement of the right kidney.

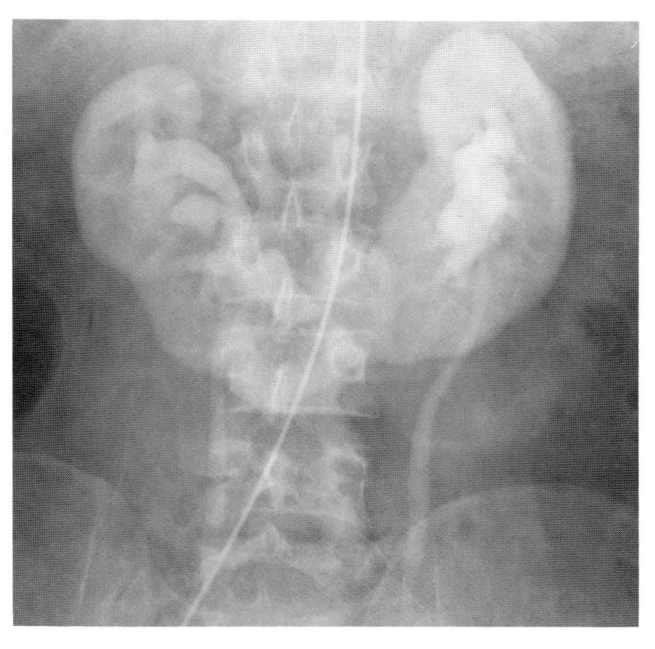

Figure 9 **Horseshoe kidney.** The lower poles are joined by renal tissue. The longitudinal axes are reversed from normal, and both halves are rotated so that the renal pelvis projects more anteriorly than in a normal kidney. Note also the characteristic lateral position of the left proximal ureter.

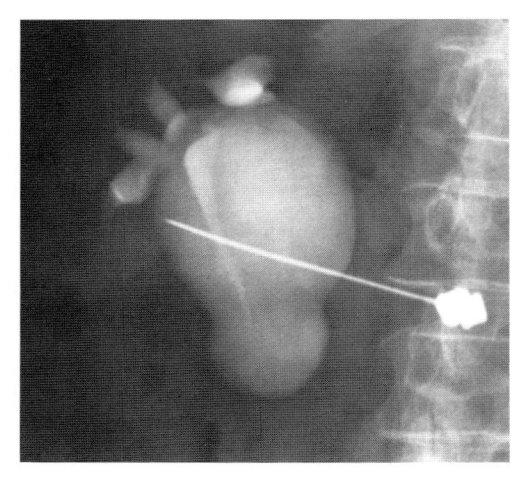

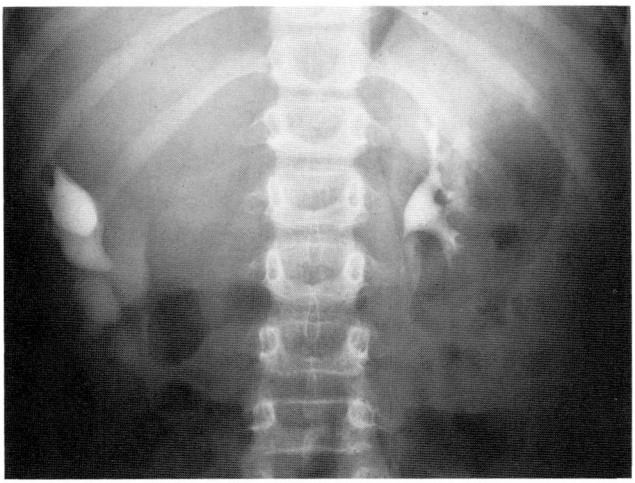

Figure 10 **Peripelvic cyst.** Lateral displacement of the right kidney. The cyst is filled with contrast medium.

Figure 11 **Renal adenocarcinoma.** Lateral displacement ▶ of the right kidney and obstruction of the ureter with hydronephrosis is also present.

64 Abdomen

Table 4 Abnormal Position of the Stomach

Presentation	Associated Conditions	Radiographic Findings and Comments
Upward displacement	Left diaphragmatic eventration or paralysis	Total eventration is more common on the left side. It may be differentiated fluoroscopically from paralysis by the absence of paradoxical movements.
(Fig. 12)	Hiatus hernia Paraesophageal hernia	If fixed, usually seen as a double density behind the heart on plain films. An air–fluid level is commonly present.
(Fig. 13)	Hernia through the hiatus of Morgagni	The hernia sac lies anteriorly and usually to the right of the heart. May occasionally contain either a small or large portion of stomach, but usually only omentum or large bowel.
(Figs. 14, 15)	Other diaphragmatic hernias (Bochdalek, traumatic, or intrapericardial)	Other organs (bowel, spleen, kidney) are herniated more often than the stomach.
Rotation (Fig. 16)	Posterior cascade stomach	Downward and posterior rotation of the gastric fundus. Emptying of the contents of the gastric fundus is therefore delayed in the upright position.
(Fig. 17)	Organoaxial volvulus	Rotation of the stomach upward around its long axis. May be associated with diaphragmatic hernia, eventration or paralysis of the diaphragm. May be asymptomatic if neither an outlet obstruction nor ischemia are associated.
(Fig. 12)	Mesenteroaxial volvulus	The stomach rotates about the long axis of the gastrohepatic omentum (right angles to the longitudinal axis of the stomach). Often associated with hiatus hernia. Symptomatic if associated with obstruction or ischemia.

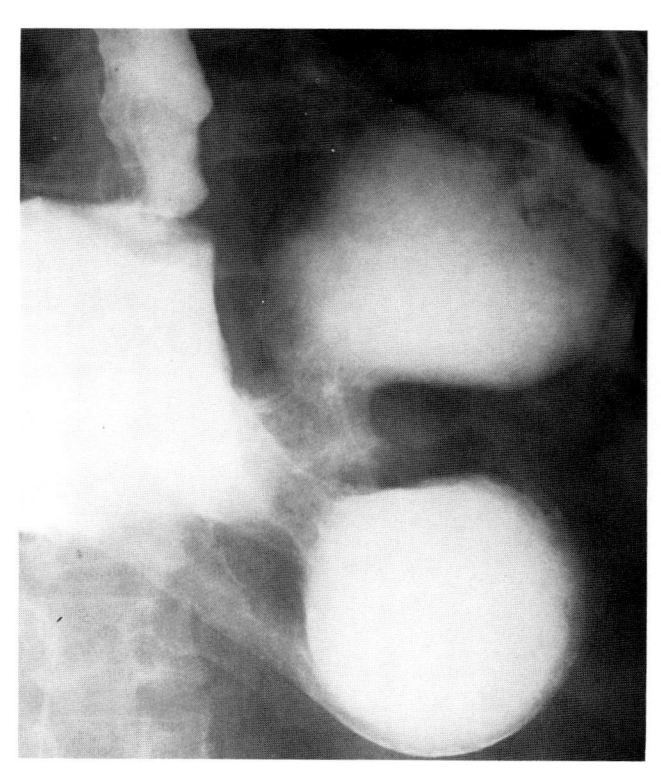

Figure **12** **A large paraesophageal hernia with mesenteroaxial volvulus of the stomach.** Part of the stomach is in the hernia sac.

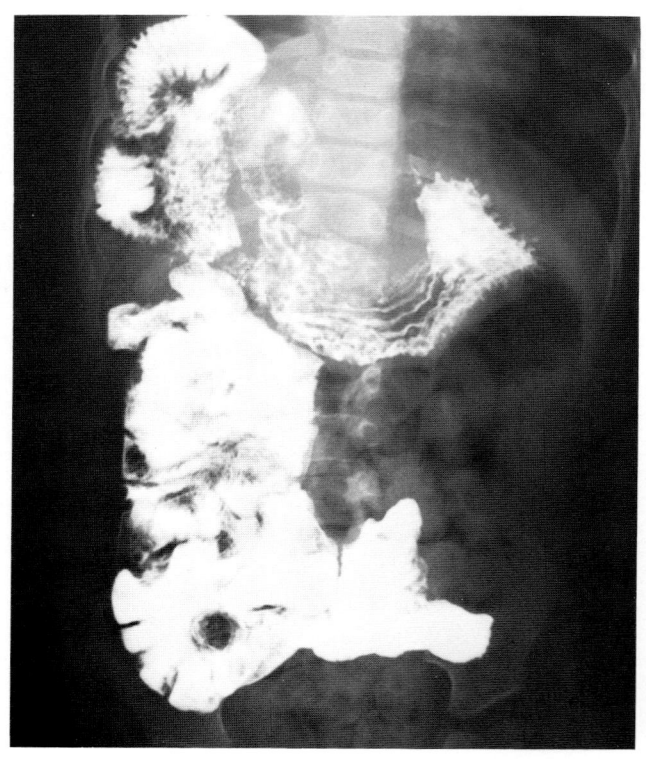

Figure **13** **Hernia of Morgagni.** Herniation of the distal stomach and the whole duodenum through the right hiatus of Morgagni. Malrotation of the small bowel is also present. Its appearance is complicated by herniation.

Displacement of Abdominal Organs 65

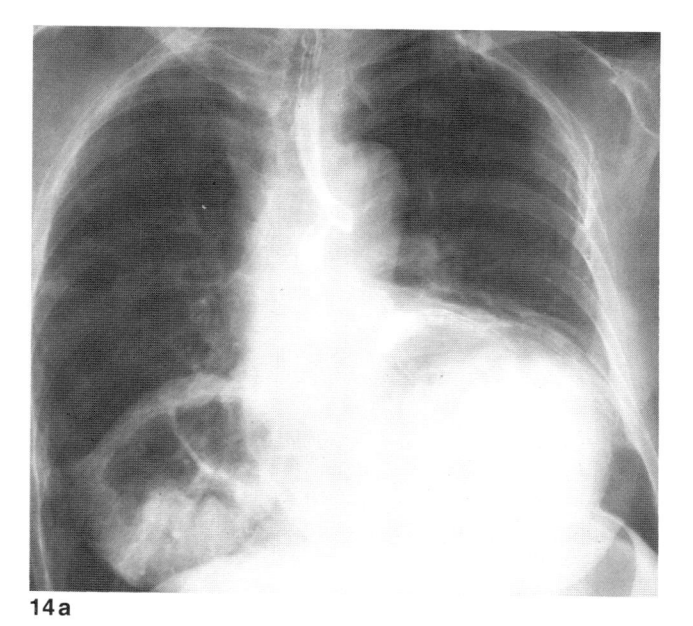

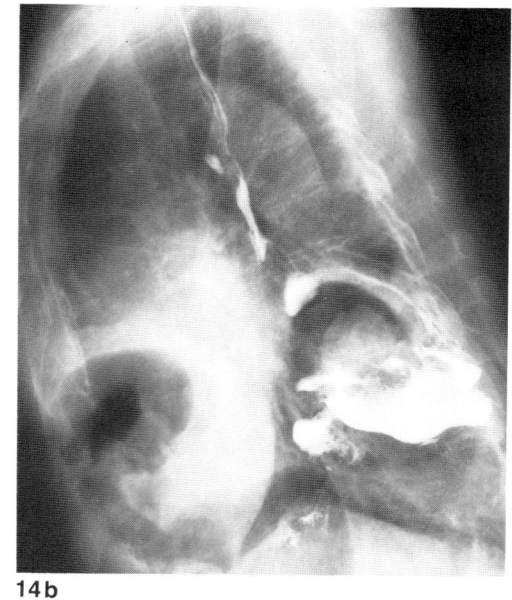

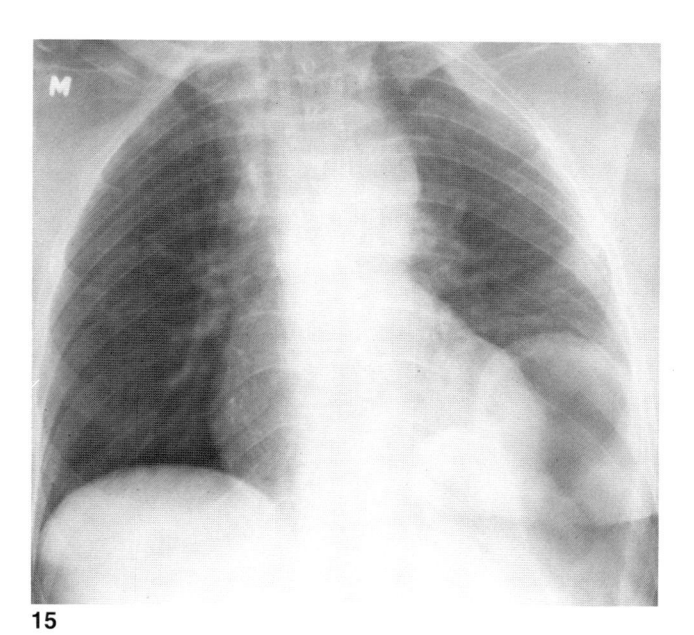

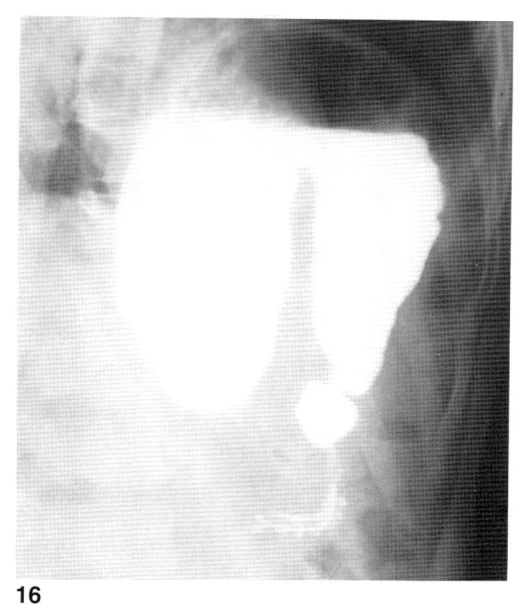

Figure **14a, b Morgagni hernia (right) and Bochdalek hernia (left)** in the same patient. The Morgagni hernia contains large bowel and the Bochdalek hernia contains stomach, delineated by barium sulfate.

Figure **15 Traumatic diaphragmatic defect** with herniated stomach. The gas-containing stomach projects above the left dome of the diaphragm.

Figure **16 Posterior cascade stomach.** The duodenum is also in an abnormal position.

Figure **17 Organoaxial volvulus** of the stomach without obstruction. The Stomach is rotated upward around its long axis.

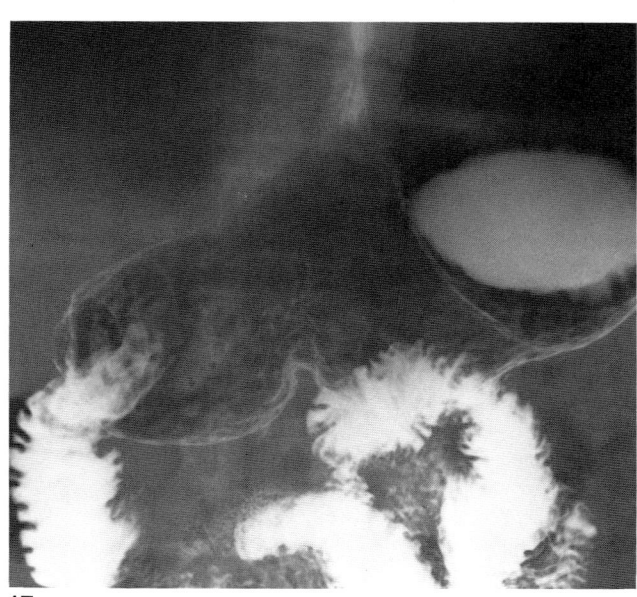

Table 4 (Cont.) Abnormal Position of the Stomach

Presentation	Associated Conditions	Radiographic Findings and Comments
Displacement by adjacent organs	Enlarged liver	Displacement to the left and posteriorly.
(Fig. 18)	Enlarged spleen	Displacement to the right and posteriorly.
(Fig. 19)	Enlarged left kidney or retroperitoneal tumor	Displacement to the right and anteriorly.
(Fig. 20)	Aorta (aneurysm or severe unfolding)	Displacement to the right and anteriorly.
	Pancreatic mass (especially pseudocyst)	May displace any part of the stomach, usually anteriorly and to the left.
	Lesser sac abscess or hernia	Anterior displacement of stomach. Air–fluid level(s) behind the stomach.
	Obesity, emphysema	In these patients, the stomach tends to be relatively anterior and the sagittal diameter of the upper abdomen is increased.

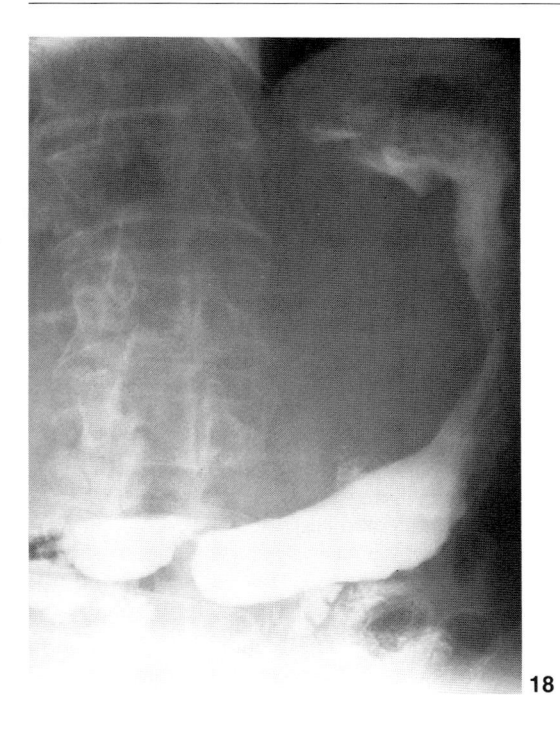

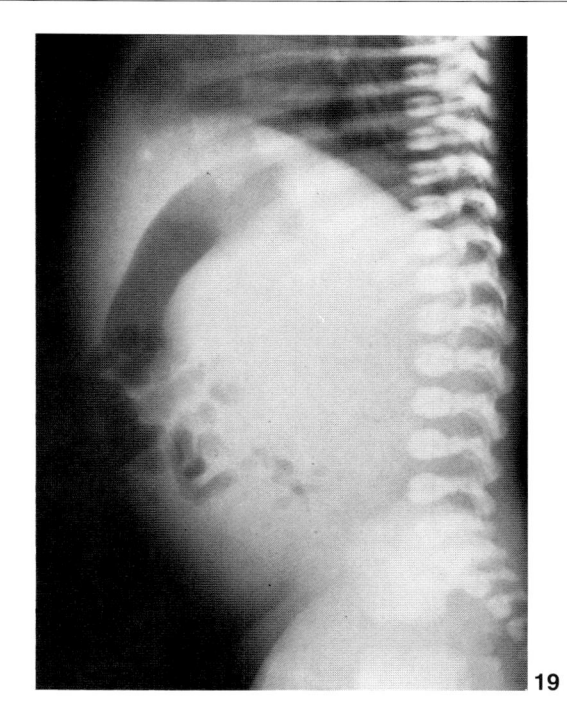

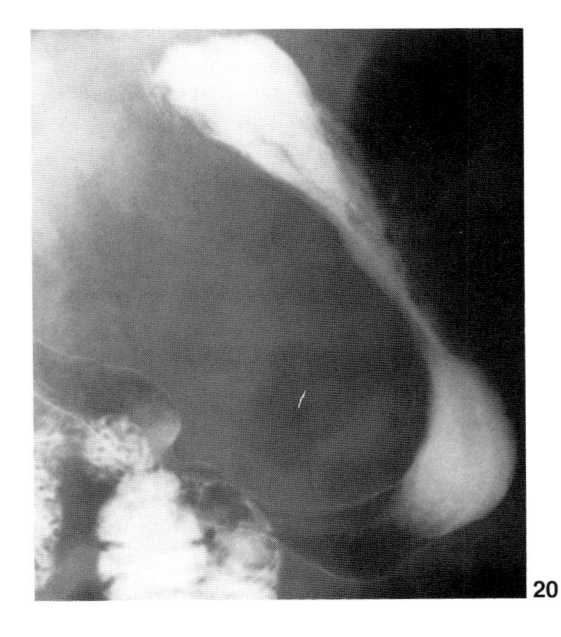

Figure 18 **Hepatomegaly.** Displacement of the stomach by an enlarged liver.

Figure 19 **Hydronephrosis.** Anterior displacement of the stomach by a hydronephrotic enlarged left kidney.

Figure 20 **Leiomyosarcoma.** Anterior displacement of body of the stomach by a gastric leiomyosarcoma mimicking a pancreatic mass. The gas-containing transverse colon is also anteriorly displaced.

Table 5 Duodenal Displacement

Presentation	Associated Conditions	Radiographic Findings and Comments
Widened duodenal sweep (Fig. 21)	Normal variant	An apparently large duodenal sweep is common in heavy patients with high, transverse stomach and vertical course of the descending duodenum.
	Acute pancreatitis	A smooth mass indenting the inner border of the duodenal sweep. "Inverted number 3" appearance of the inner margin, duodenal paresis, and edema of duodenal folds are common if the head of the pancreas is involved.
	Chronic pancreatitis	Flattening of the normal interfold crevices and straightening of the upper inner margin of the descending duodenum are secondary to fibrosis. Pancreatic calcifications may be seen.
	Pancreatic pseudocyst	Usually smooth mass impression on the inner border of the descending duodenum and often on the inferior or posterior wall of the stomach. The cyst wall and remaining pancreas may be calcified.
(Fig. 22)	Carcinoma of the head of the pancreas	Significant widening of the duodenal sweep is a late sign. Subtle indentations, double contour of the medial wall or an "inverted 3" sign may be present. Mucosal changes and mass impressions are usually indistinguishable from a benign pancreatic lesion. Can also represent direct extension of a tumor from an adjacent organ (stomach, colon, kidney, retroperitoneum), or lymph node enlargement. Cystic lymphangioma of the mesentery and dilated pancreaticoduodenal vessels (after occlusion of the celiac or superior mesenteric artery) are rare causes of duodenal displacement and may simulate a mass in the head of the pancreas.
	Aortic aneurysm	Downward displacement of the third portion of the duodenum. The wall of the aneurysm is often calcified.
	Choledochal cyst	Dilatation of the common bile duct can cause a localized impression or generalized widening of the duodenal sweep. Usually in children under the age of 10.
Displacement of the duodenum	Right renal agenesis or ectopia	Abnormally posterior position of the descending duodenum and proximal jejunal loops. (DD: Right paraduodenal hernia).
	Annular pancreas, carcinoma of the head of the pancreas, postbulbar ulcer, carcinoma of the hepatic flexure of the colon.	These lesions can cause impression, mass displacement, or fixed deformity in the course of the duodenal sweep.
	Intramural duodenal hematoma	Simulates extrinsic impression of the second or third portion of the duodenum. May produce a high-grade stenosis.
	Lesser sac abscess	A retrogastric mass with an air–fluid level and *lateral* displacement of the duodenum.
	Lesser sac hernia	Retrogastric bowel loops with air–fluid levels. Anterior displacement of the stomach and *medial* displacement of the duodenum.
Abnormal position of the duodenojejunal junction (see Fig. 13, p. 64)	Malrotation	No duodenal loop (straight duodenum). Small bowel lies on the right side of the abdomen, colon on the left side. The duodenojejunal junction is paramedial.

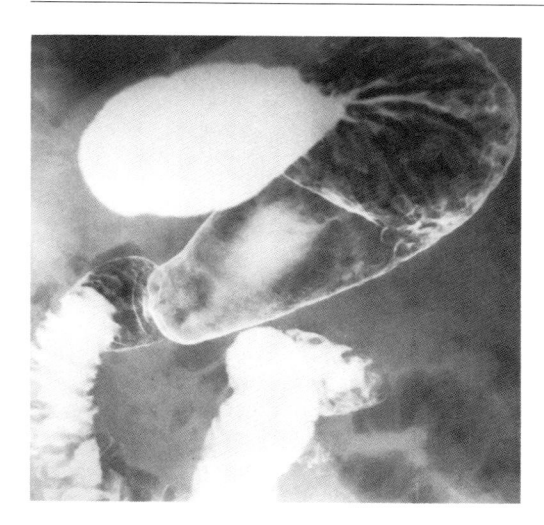

Figure 21 **Normal duodenal sweep** that appears wide when the stomach is upward displaced or horizontal, as in this overweight man.

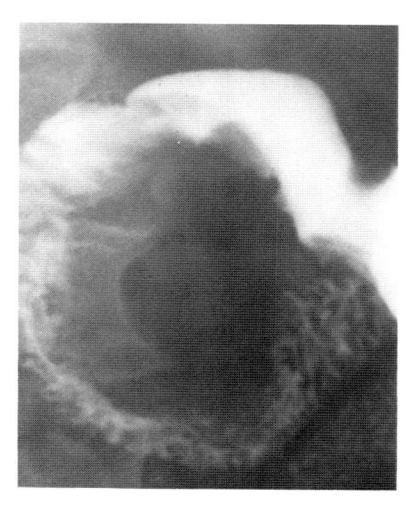

Figure 22 **Carcinoma of pancreas.** Widening and mass impression of the duodenal sweep by carcinoma of the head of pancreas.

Table 6 Separation or Displacement of Small Bowel Loops

Presentation	Associated Conditions	Radiographic Findings and Comments

Generalized separation of mobile small bowel loops (Fig. 23)	*Ascites.* Common causes include:
	  Liver cirrhosis
	  Peritonitis
	  Congestive heart failure
	  Peritoneal malignancy
		Small bowel loops floating in the ascitic fluid are separated from each other and move freely with compression or after a change in body position. Generalized abdominal haziness and other signs of abdominal fluid (e.g., lost liver edge, separation of the liver and ascending colon from adjacent flank stripe and "dog ears" over the bladder) may be present.

Separation of fixed small bowel loops (Fig. 24)	*Diseases which cause thickening of the mesentery and/or the bowel wall:*
	  Crohn's disease
	  Tuberculosis
		Thickening of the bowel wall and/or mesentery associated with narrowing of the bowel lumen create the radiologic appearance of separation of small bowel loops. Most common in the right lower quadrant.

	Intestinal hemorrhage Mesenteric vascular occlusion	Intramural or mesenteric hematoma and/or edema causes separation of bowel lumina.
	Small bowel lymphoma Amyloidosis Whipple's disease	Diffuse submucosal infiltration combined with mesenteric infiltration or enlarged mesenteric lymph nodes produce an appearance of separated bowel loops. Mucosal folds may be irregular and thickened.
	Radiation enteritis	Straightening of folds, nodular filling defects, and mucosal ulcerations with separation of adjacent bowel loops.
	Carcinoid tumor	Diffuse luminal narrowings, separation of intestinal loops, and localized abrupt angulations of the small bowel are characteristic. The primary lesion may be seen as a localized mass.
	Neurofibromatosis	Plexiform neurofibromatosis may involve the small bowel. Multiple polypoid filling defects of the mesenteric side of the bowel and thickening of the mesentery may separate bowel loops.
	Retractile mesenteritis	Fibrosis, inflammation, and fatty infiltration of the mesentery creates a diffuse mesenteric mass that separates small bowel loops.
Localized displacement of small bowel loops (Fig. 25)	*Mass in the small bowel wall* (e.g., carcinoma)	Separation of bowel loops may be visible in the region of the mass. A luminal filling defect or an intussusception are more common presentations.
	Mesenteric mass (e.g., fibroma, lipoma, fibrosarcoma, leiomyosarcoma, lymph node enlargement, mesenteric metastases)	May grow very large and still be asymptomatic. Causes displacement of adjacent small bowel loops.

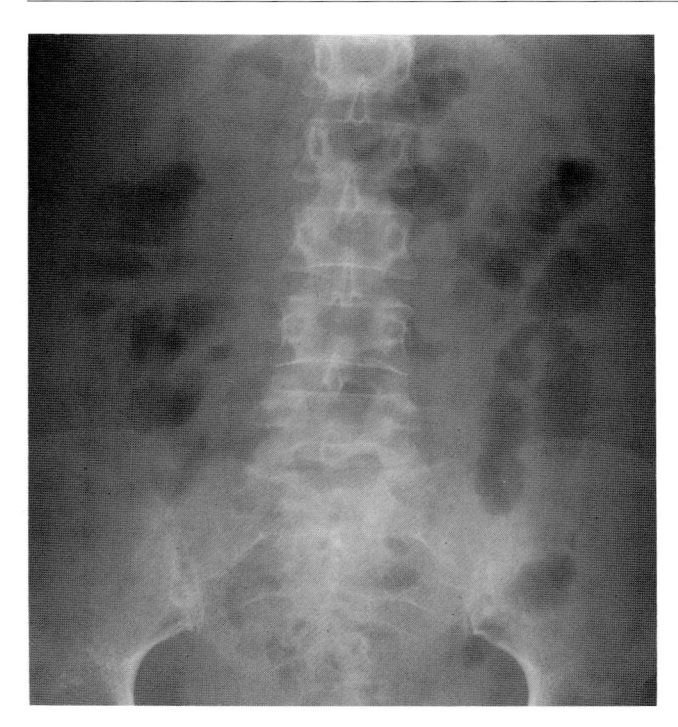

Figure 23 **Ascites.** Small bowel loops are separated from each other and have moved away from the peritoneal wall.

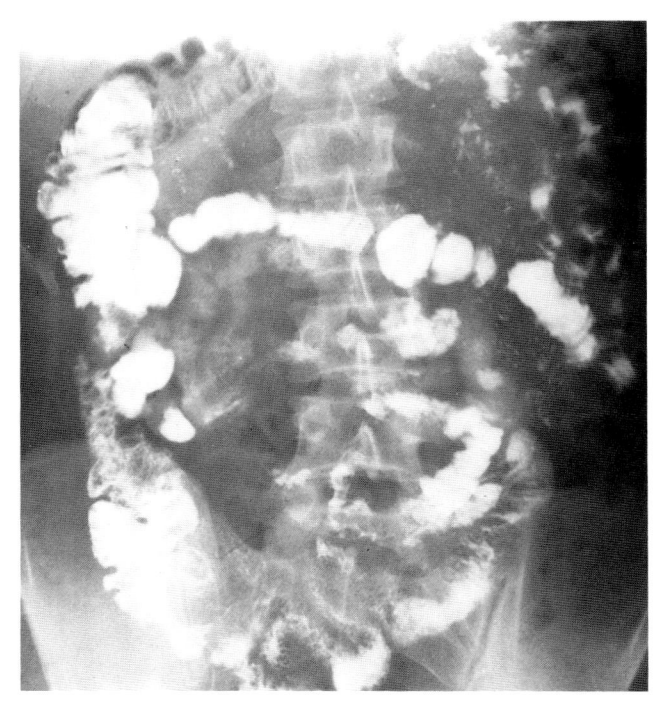

Figure 24 **Crohn's disease.** Thickened mesentery and narrow small-bowel lumen create the appearance of separation of small-bowel loops in the right lower quadrant.

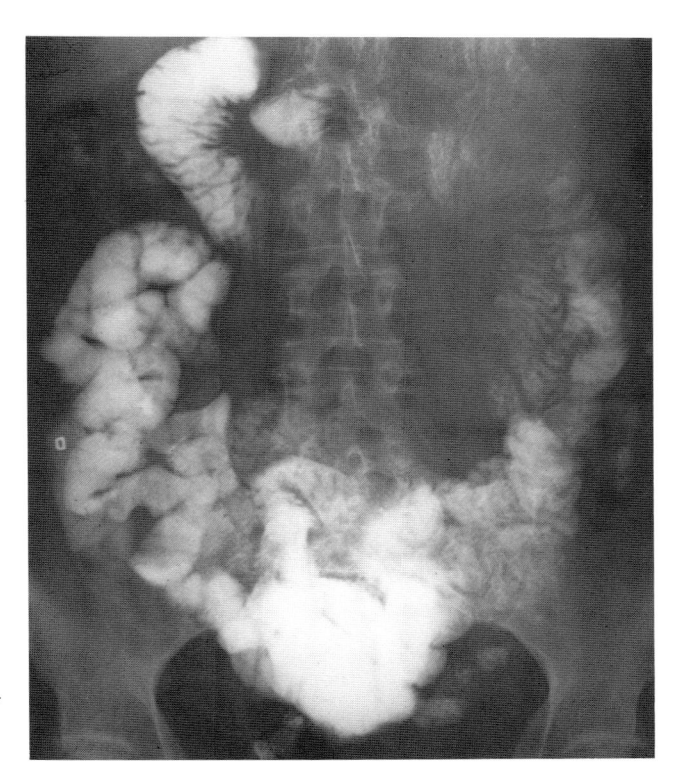

Figure 25 **Mesenteric leiomyosarcoma of the transverse mesocolon** displaces small bowel loops away from the midabdomen.

Table 6 (Cont.)   **Separation or Displacement of Small Bowel Loops**

Presentation	Associated Conditions	Radiographic Findings and Comments
(Fig. 26, 27)	*Intraperitoneal or pelvic mass* (e.g., abscess, pseudocyst of pancreatitis, ovarian tumor, enlarged urinary bladder)	A soft-tissue mass displacing and separating bowel loops. Common locations: *Appendicitis:* right pericolic gutter or pelvis *Sigmoid diverticulitis:* left pericolic gutter and pelvis *Pancreatitis, perforated gastric or duodenal ulcer:* lesser sac, central area *Ovarian tumor, enlarged bladder:* pelvis or lower central abdomen
Abnormal position of small-bowel loops	Left paraduodenal hernia	The most common among internal hernias. A bunch of small bowel loops are displaced and clustered in the left upper quadrant lateral to the distal duodenum. If partially obstructed, the loops are dilated and the transit of barium is delayed.
	Right paraduodenal hernia	Associated with incomplete intestinal rotation and low, paramedian location of the duodenojejunal junction. Jejunal loops are situated on the right side of the abdomen and extend into the right transverse mesocolon. Duodenum is dilated. May cause obstruction.
	Lesser sac hernia DD: Lesser sac abscess	Herniation of bowel and omentum through the foramen of Winslow. An acute abdominal emergency with symptoms of strangulation. Abnormal gas-filled loops of bowel can be seen along the lesser curvature medial and posterior to the stomach.
(Fig. 40, p. 79)	Inguinal or femoral hernia	Loops of bowel extend beyond the normal pelvic contour. Right-sided hernias usually contain only small bowel, left-sided hernias may include sigmoid colon. Inguinal hernias tend to be larger, but otherwise indistinguishable from femoral hernias radiographically. Air–fluid levels indicate incarceration.
	Obturator hernia	More common in females, usually right-sided. May be a cause of an acute abdomen (strangulation). Gas, or contrast material, may be seen in the bowel projecting over the obturator foramen.
(Fig. 9, p. 7)	Anterior abdominal hernia (umbilical, ventral, postoperative incisional)	Self-evident clinically, but radiography can determine the nature of contents and bowel obstruction.
	Omphalocele	Failure of complete withdrawal of the midgut from the umbilical cord during the tenth fetal week. Contains small bowel loops filled with gas.
	Spigelian hernia	A spontaneous defect just lateral to the outer border of the rectus abdominis muscle that may contain a small gas- or contrast-filled bowel loop.
	Diaphragmatic hernia	See Table **4**, p. 64.
	Malrotation	See Table **5**, p. 68.

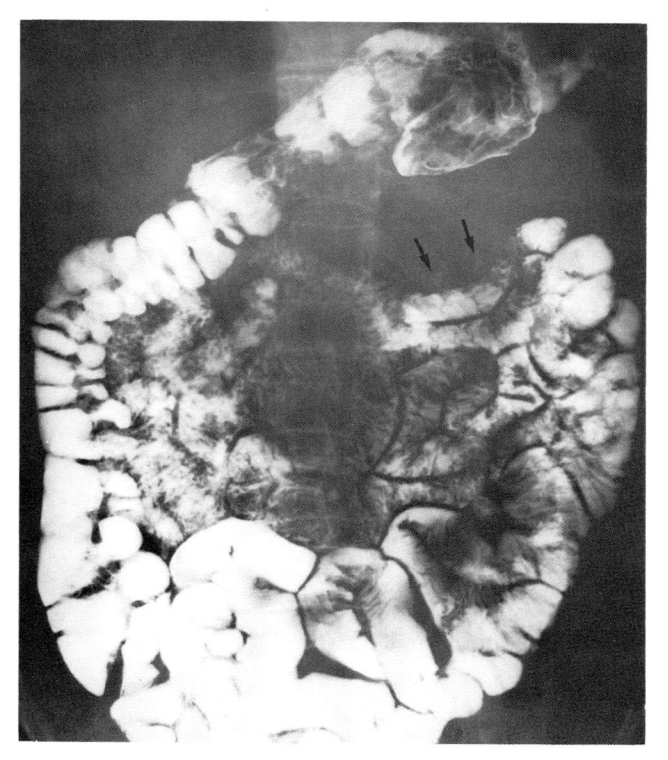

Figure 26 **Pancreatic pseudocyst** displaces the left transverse colon upward and adjacent small bowel loops downward. Pancreatic calculi (arrows) are seen in the area devoid of bowel loops.

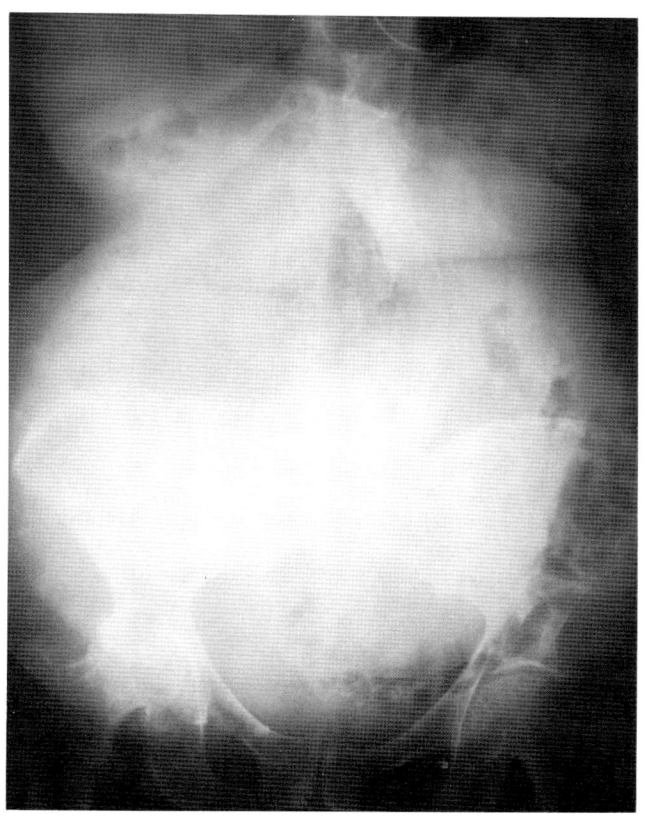

Figure 27 A large **ovarian cystadenoma** displacing all bowel loops from the central area of the abdomen.

Table 7 Displacement of the Large Bowel

Presentation	Associated Conditions	Radiographic Findings and Comments
Abnormal position of the cecum (Fig. 28)	Malrotation	The cecum is located in the right upper quadrant or on the left side.
	Mobile cecum	The position of the cecum varies from vertical to medially oriented according to body position. May be complicated by cecal volvulus.
Upward or lateral displacement of cecum (Fig. 29)	*Mass in the right iliac fossa* (e.g., appendiceal abscess, Crohn's disease, ectopic right kidney, large metastasis)	Indentation and mass displacement of the cecum. Flattening of the medial row of haustral sacculations.
	Large pelvic mass (e.g., ovarian tumor)	
Medial displacement of the cecum and/or ascending colon (Figs. 30, 31)	*Mass in the right paracolic gutter* (e.g., abscess, hematoma, retroperitoneal tumor, intraperitoneal metastasis)	Flattening of the lateral haustral row, mass displacement of the colon and possibly abscess gas.
	Pericecal hernia	Fixed loops of ileum are located posterolateral to the anteromedially displaced cecum.
(Fig. 32)	*Postsurgery* (e.g., thoracic interposition)	
Anterior displacement of cecum and/or ascending colon	*Retroperitoneal mass* (e.g., abscess, hematoma, retroperitoneal spread of pancreatitis, tumor)	Flattening of the posterior haustral row with anterior displacement of the cecum and/or ascending colon.

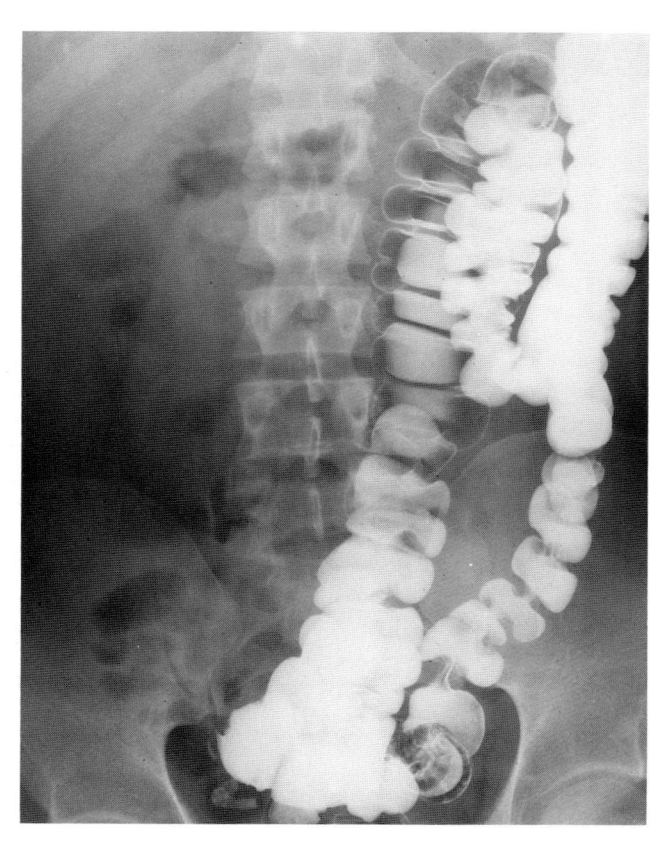

◀ Figure 28 **Malrotation.** The colon is entirely on the left side of the abdomen. Small bowel loops are located on the right side.

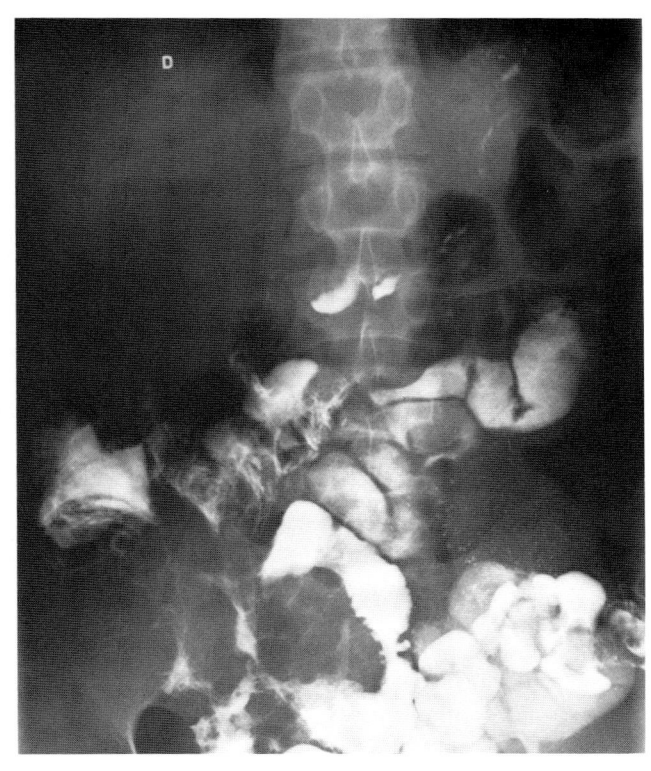

Figure **29 Crohn's disease.** A mass with multiple fistulous tracts, separation of small bowel loops, and upward and lateral displacement of the cecum is seen.

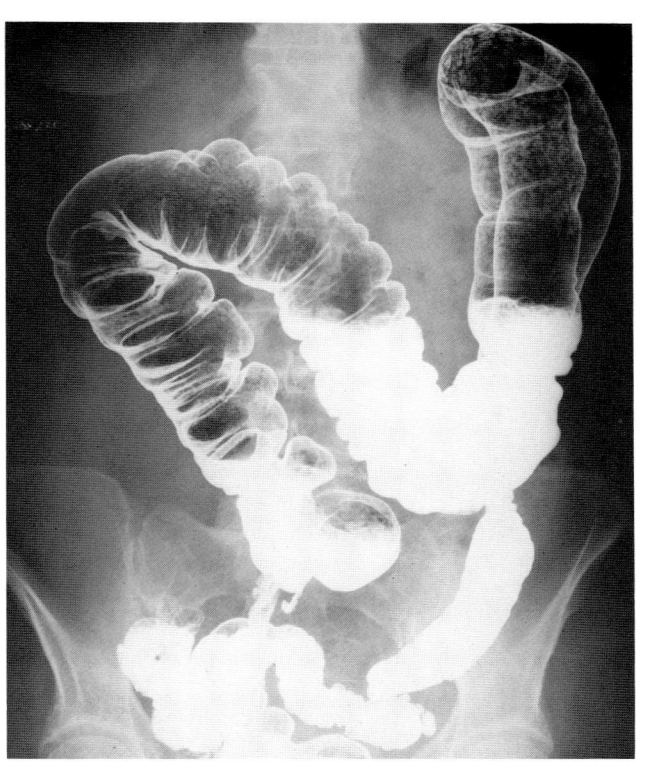

Figure **30 Retroperitoneal cyst.** A large mass causing medial displacement of the cecum and ascending colon.

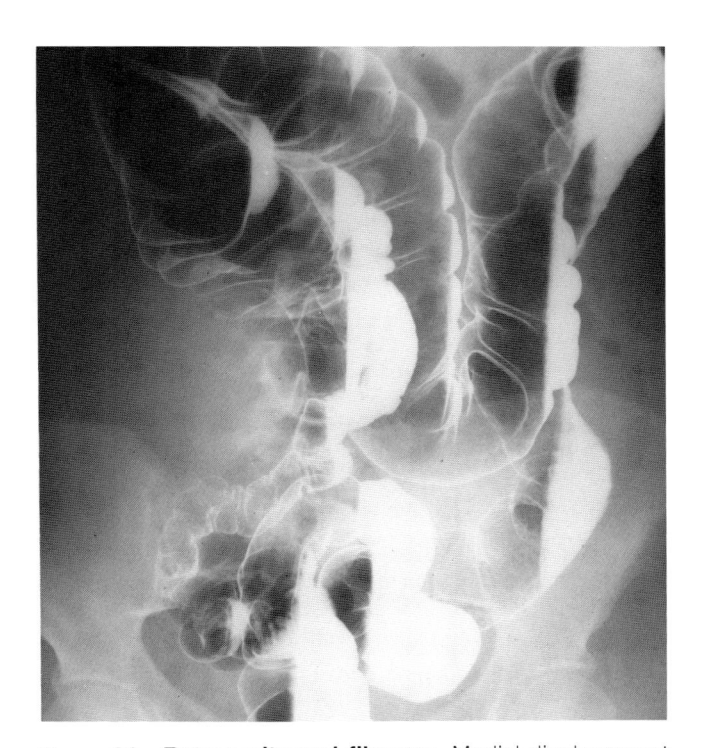

Figure **31 Retroperitoneal fibroma.** Medial displacement of the cecum and ascending colon is seen.

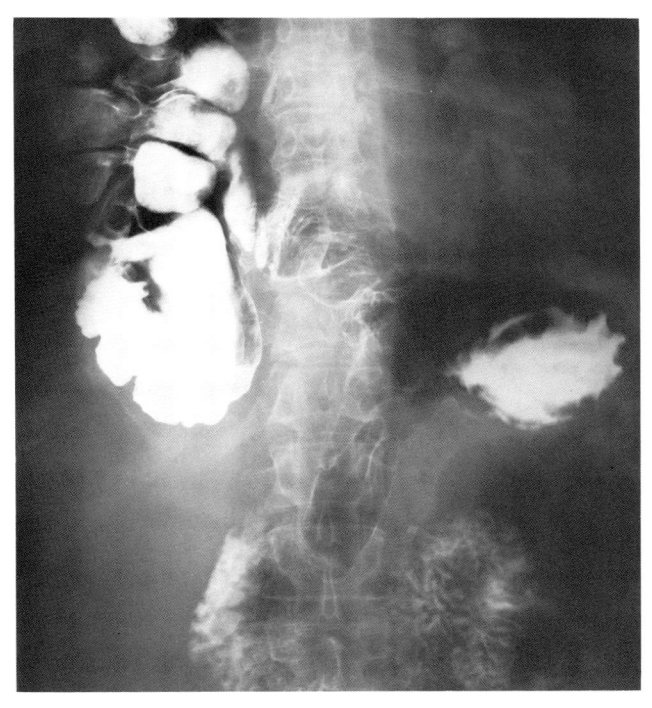

Figure **32 Thoracic interposition of the cecum and ascending colon** to replace the esophagus following lye ingestion.

Table 7 (Cont.)   Displacement of the Large Bowel

Presentation	Associated Conditions	Radiographic Findings and Comments
Displacement of the hepatic flexure: Downward (Fig. 33)	Mass in the upper pole of the right kidney or in adrenal	Inferior, medial, and anterior displacement of the segment between anterior and posterior hepatic flexures. Flattening of the superior and posterior haustral rows at this site.
	Morrison's pouch abscess	Gas and fluid containing mass with inferior displacement of the hepatic flexure and medial displacement of duodenum.
(Fig. 34) **Anterior**	Enlarged liver, liver mass	
	Mass in the lower pole of the right kidney	Elevation and anterior displacement of the colonic segment between the two hepatic flexures and compression of the inferior haustral row at this site.
	Mass of the upper descending duodenum, e. g., leiomyosarcoma	Anterior displacement of the distal hepatic flexure.
Upward (Fig. 27, p. 19)	Diaphragmatic hernia	May be associated with herniation of the liver.
	Eventration or paralysis of the right hemidiaphragm	Associated with elevation of the liver.
(Fig. 18, p. 13)	Chilaiditi syndrome	Interposition of the hepatic flexure between the right hemidiaphragm and the liver.
	Shrunken liver	Associated with cirrhosis.
Displacement of the transverse colon: Downward (Fig. 35)	Long colonic mesentery (normal)	A loop of transverse colon projects into the lower abdomen or pelvis. No mass effect, no evidence of colonic obstruction.
	Mass in the gastrocolic ligament or lesser sac (e.g., gastrocolic extension of gastric carcinoma, cyst or abscess).	Downward displacement of the involved segment of the colon with flattening of the upper row of the haustral sacculations.
Anterior	*Mass in the transverse mesocolon* (e.g., pancreatitis, pancreatic carcinoma, abscess, cyst)	Flattening of the inferior row of haustral sacculations in pancreatic carcinoma. Wrinkled sacculations of the upper haustral row may occur in pancreatitis.
	Mass in the left kidney	An upper pole mass displaces transverse colon only. A lower pole mass may displace also the descending colon. The splenic flexure is characteristically unaffected.
Upward (Fig. 45, p. 29) (Fig. 26, p. 73)	*Inframesocolic mass* (e.g., abscess, cyst, neoplasm)	Upward displacement of the transverse colon with possible displacement of the transverse or ascending duodenum.
(Fig. 14, p. 65)	Hernia of Morgagni containing colon.	See Table 4, p. 64.
Displacement of the splenic flexure Posterior	Left renal agenesis or ectopia After left nephrectomy	Displacement of the distal transverse colon and splenic flexure posteromedially into the empty renal fossa.
Anterior (Fig. 37, p. 78)	Splenomegaly	Enlarged spleen also displaces the descending colon anteromedially.
Upward (Fig. 36)	Left pleuroperitoneal foramen (Bochdalek hernia)	Bowel loops are seen in the left hemithorax. May be associated with displacement of the left kidney, spleen, and stomach into the left hemithorax.
Displacement of the descending colon Lateral	Ectopic left kidney Primary small bowel lesion Diverticulitis	Lateral displacement of the descending colon and flattening of the medial haustral row.

Displacement of Abdominal Organs 77

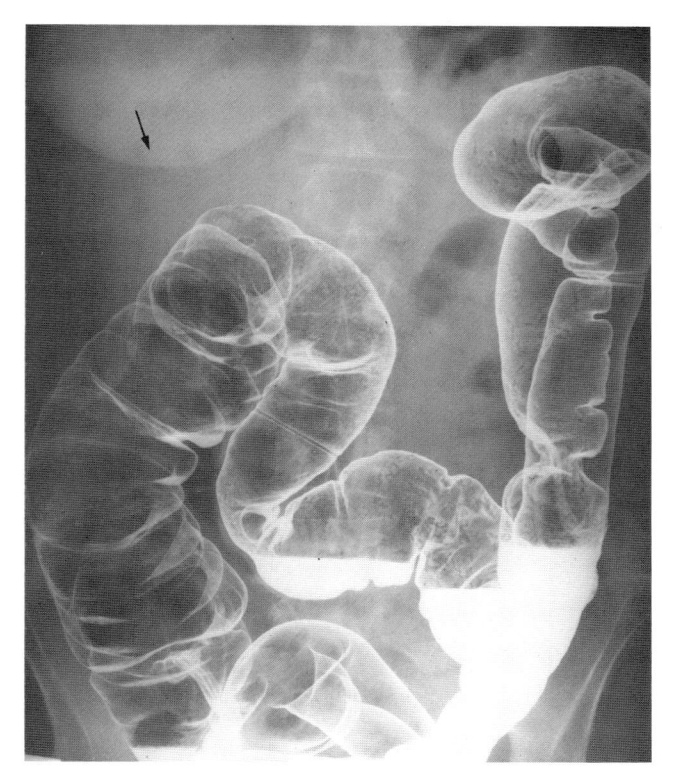

Figure 33 **Right adrenal pheochromocytoma.** Subtle downward, medial, and anterior displacement of the hepatic flexure by a mass (arrow), is seen as an increased density above the hepatic flexure.

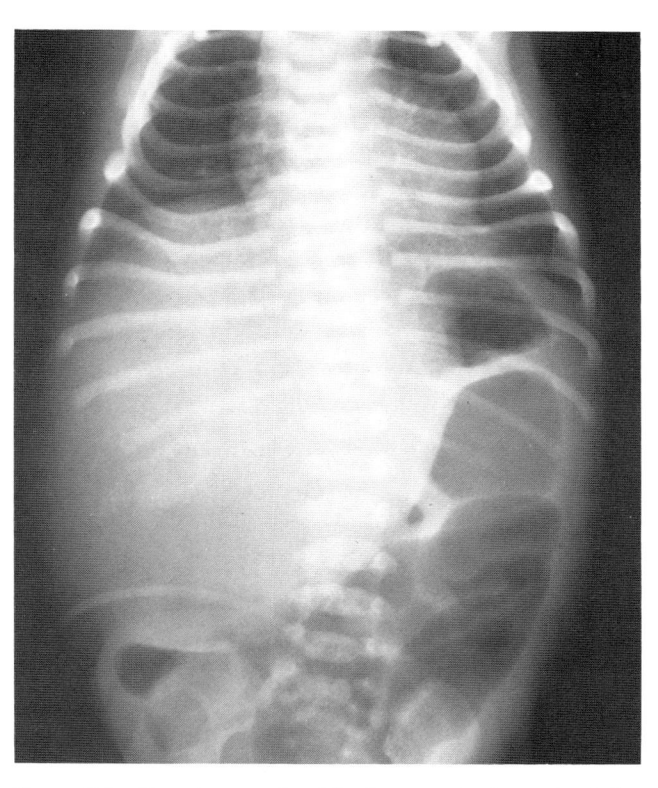

Figure 34 **Hepatomegaly.** Displacement of most of the right colon by enlarged liver in an infant is evident. The patient also had meconium peritonitis. Peritoneal calcification is seen over the liver shadow.

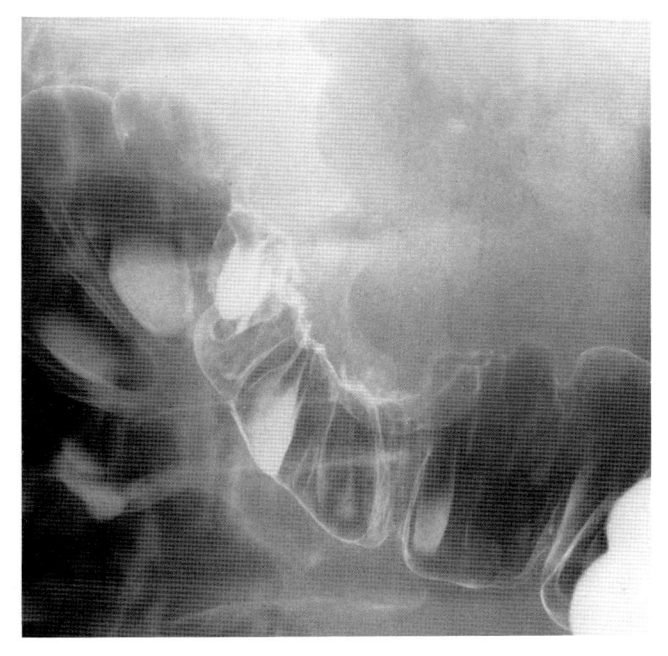

Figure 35 **Gastric carcinoma** extending along the gastrocolic ligament, displacing the transverse colon and flattening the haustral pattern.

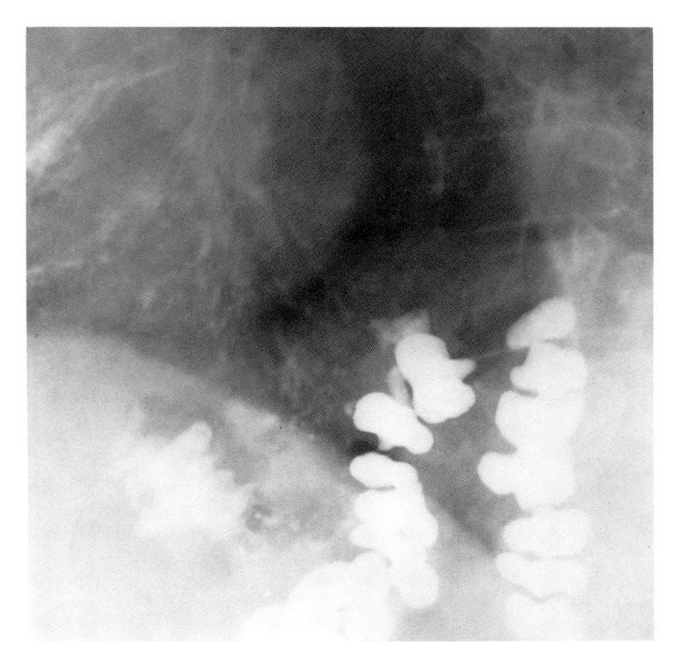

Figure 36 **Bochdalek hernia.** The splenic flexure is displaced into the left hemithorax.

Table 7 (Cont.) Displacement of the Large Bowel

Presentation	Associated Conditions	Radiographic Findings and Comments
Medial (Fig. 37)	*Left paracolic gutter mass:* (abscess, hematoma, enlarged spleen, or metastases)	Medial displacement of the descending colon and flattening of the lateral haustral row. Never caused by localized diverticulitis.
Anterior	*Primary extraperitoneal mass* Diverticulitis	Anterior displacement of the descending colon and flattening of the posterior haustral row.
Displacement of the sigmoid	Redundancy of sigmoid	A redundant sigmoid loop is usual in infants and a common variant in adults. It is associated with an increased risk of sigmoid volvulus.
Upward (Figs. 38, 39)	*Large pelvic mass* (e.g., tumor, cyst, abscess, dilated urinary bladder or pelvic lipomatosis)	Vertical elongation of the rectosigmoid and upward and usually posterior displacement of the sigmoid loop.
Downward	*Lower abdominal mass* (e.g., abscess, tumor)	Downward or lateral displacement of the sigmoid loop, depending on the localization of the mass.
(Fig. 40)	Hernia	See Table 6, p. 70.

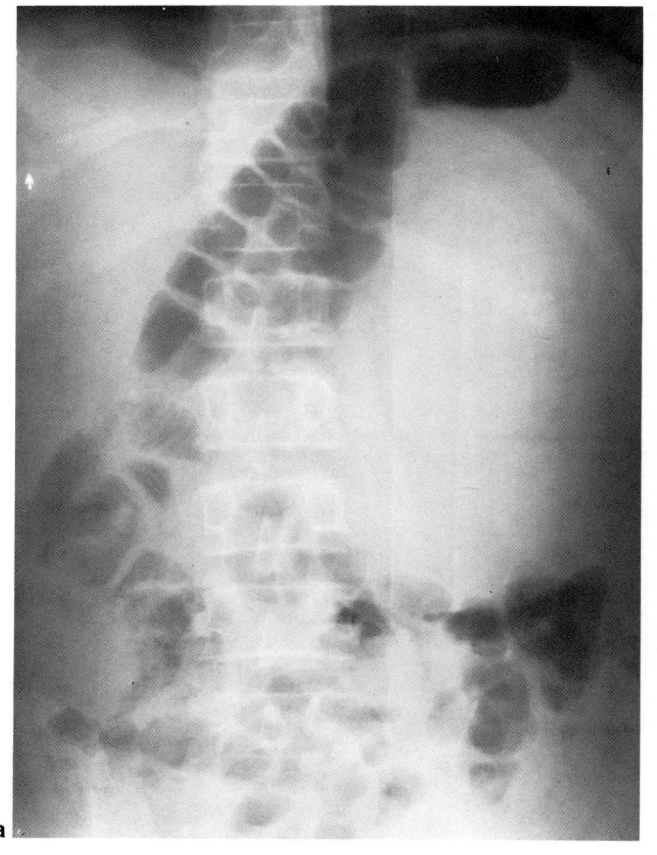

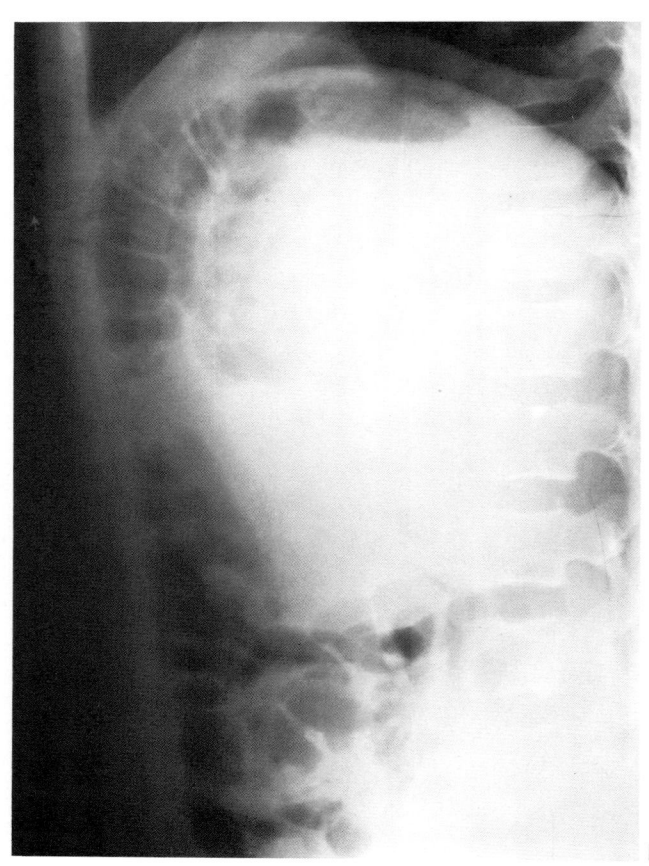

Figure **37a, b Splenomegaly (posttraumatic).** Anterior and medial displacement of the splenic flexure and the descending colon by a markedly enlarged spleen is seen.

Displacement of Abdominal Organs 79

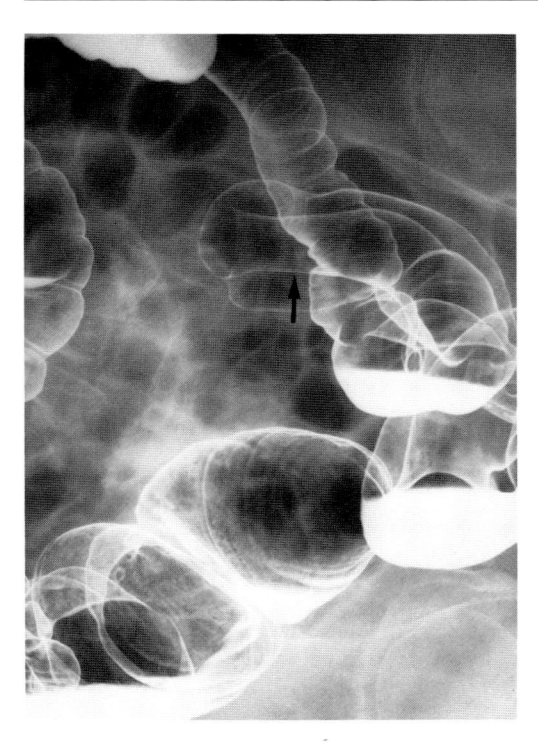

Figure **38** **Ovarian cyst** causing subtle displacement of the sigmoid loop to the left, best appreciated in a right lateral decubitus projection (arrow).

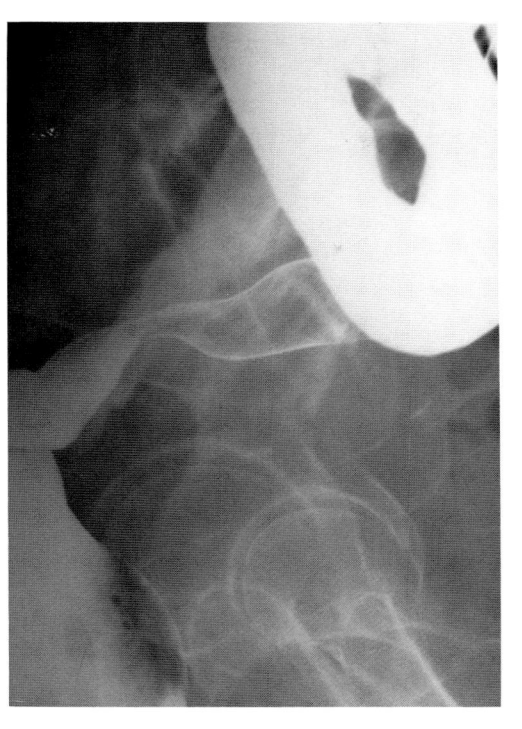

Figure **39** **Carcinoma of the uterus** causing upward and posterior displacement of the rectosigmoid. The bowel is also narrowed by compression but the mucosa appears intact.

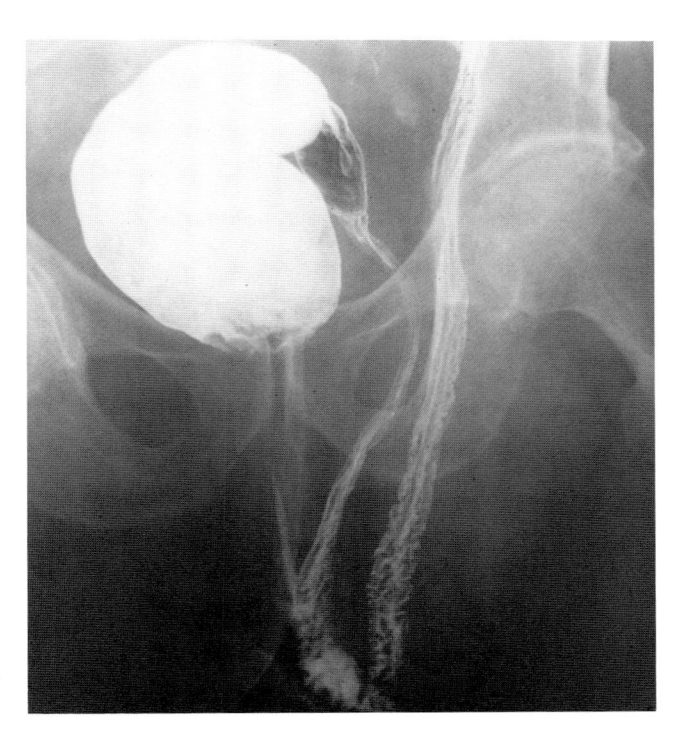

Figure **40** **Left inguinal hernia** containing a loop of redundant sigmoid colon. ▶

Table 7 (Cont.) Displacement of the Large Bowel

Presentation	Associated Conditions	Radiographic Findings and Comments
Enlargement of the retrorectal space (over 2 cm) (Fig. 41)	Normal variant	In 95% of patients the distance from the sacrum to the distended rectal wall is 0.5 cm or less, but can be up to 2 cm, especially in obese individuals.
	Ulcerative colitis	Generalized widening of the space without evidence of a focal mass, especially in severe, chronic, and extensive disease. Does not become smaller in remission.
	Crohn's disease	Diffuse widening of the retrorectal space, often associated with fistulas and sinus tracts. May decrease during remission. A perirectal abscess may occur and cause localized widening.
	Inflammatory proctitis: – Tuberculosis – Amebiasis – Lymphogranuloma venereum Radiation proctitis Ischemic proctitis	Enlarged retrorectal space and rectal narrowing in the absence of generalized bowel disease.
(Fig. 42)	Retrorectal abscess secondary to: – Infected developmental cyst – Diverticulitis – Perforated appendix – Perforation due to carcinoma – Surgery	Localized widening of the retrorectal space. If secondary to an infected developmental cyst, it is often associated with a fistulous tract.
	Benign retrorectal lesions: Developmental (dermoid) cyst Enteric (duplication) cyst Postanal (tail gut) cyst Lipoma	A soft-tissue mass behind the rectum causing indentation, but the rectal mucosa remains intact.
	Pelvic lipomatosis Cushing's disease	Massive deposition of fat in the pelvis with compression and elevation of the rectum and bladder.
(Fig. 43)	Sacrococcygeal teratoma	Retrorectal tumor with calcification, bone, or teeth in a child.
	Anterior sacral meningocele	Anomalous sacrum with an anterior soft tissue mass usually in a child.
	Neurofibroma	Enlargement of a sacral foramen associated with widening of the retrorectal space.
	Adenocarcinoma of rectum (rarely lymphoma, sarcoma, or cloacogenic carcinoma)	Enlargement of the retrorectal space associated with mucosal changes or an intraluminal mass in the rectum.
	Rectal metastases from carcinoma of prostate, bladder, ovary, or uterus	Prostatic carcinoma, in particular, may simulate rectal carcinoma by encircling the rectum Widening of the retrorectal space due to recurrent tumor or radiation effects may have identical appearances.
	Chordoma	Expansion and destruction of the sacrum, soft-tissue mass displacing the rectum, and amorphous calcification (in about 50%).
(Fig. 44)	Primary tumor of the sacrum: Osteosarcoma Chondrosarcoma Giant cell tumor Hemangiopericytoma	Bony changes in the sacrum are the dominant feature and should suggest the correct diagnosis.
	Surgery (partial sigmoid resection) Fracture of sacrum	Bleeding or scar formation into the presacral soft tissues may widen the retrorectal space.

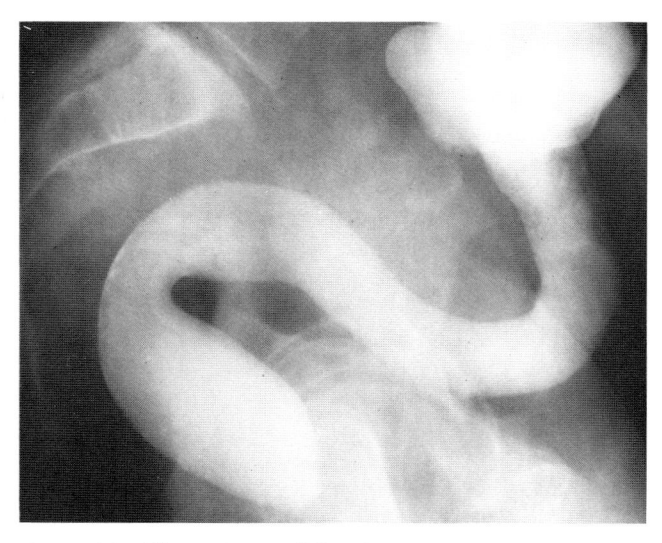

Figure **41 Ulcerative colitis.** Symmetric enlargement of the whole retrorectal space is seen.

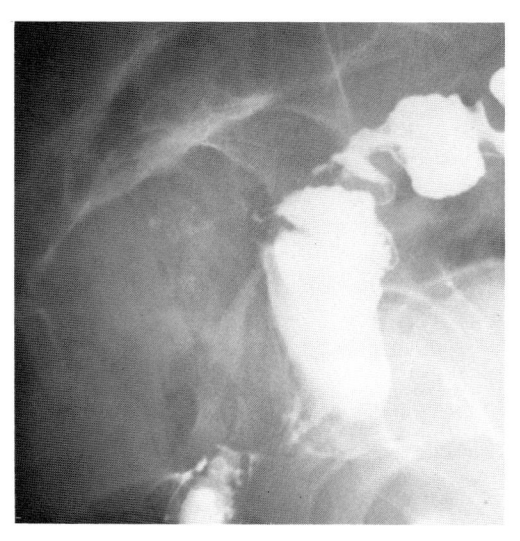

Figure **42 Retrorectal abscess.** Following surgery of the sigmoid colon a large gas-containing mass developed in the retrorectal space, displacing the rectum anteriorly.

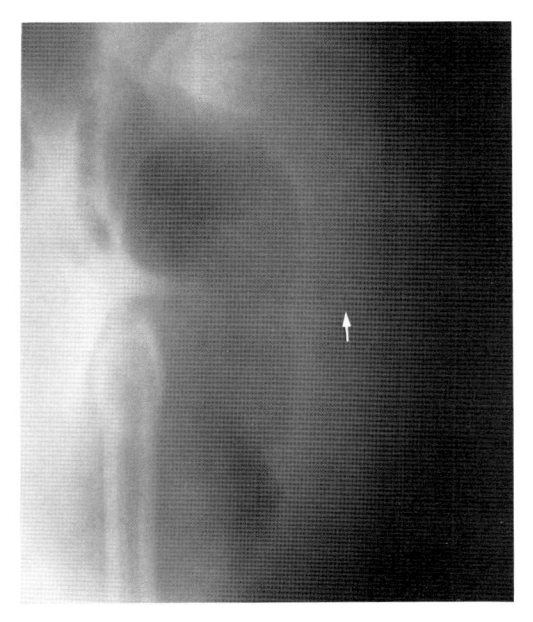

Figure **43 Sacrococcygeal teratoma** displacing the rectum anteriorly. A faint calcification is present (arrow). Age 23.

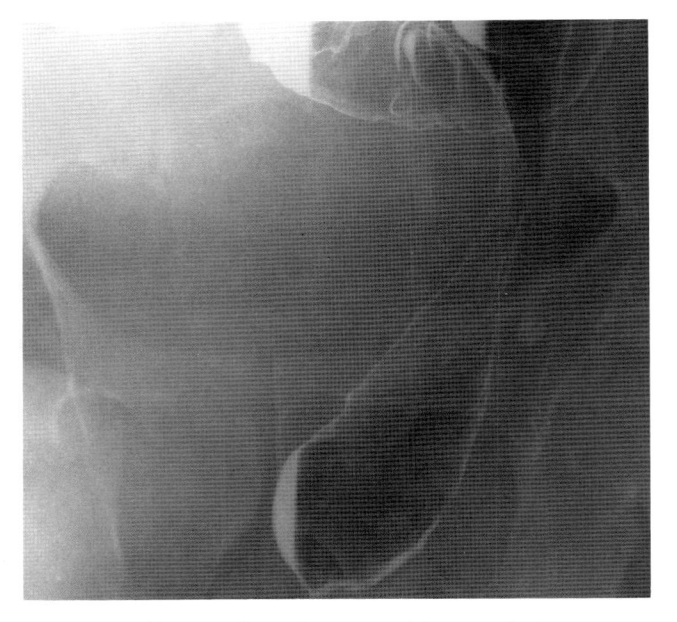

Figure **44 Hemangiopericytoma.** A large soft-tissue mass displacing the rectum forwards and to the left. Destruction of the sacrum is poorly visualized.

Chapter 4 Dilatation and Motility Disorders in the Gastrointestinal Tract

The muscular activity of the alimentary canal is responsible for the transport of food and fluid through the gut to provide mixing with the digestive juices and absorption into the blood stream. The smooth muscle of the gut is arranged in three coats: an inner muscular mucosa, a circular muscle coat, and an outer longitudinal coat. The latter two layers affect the tone and cause the peristaltic contractions in the gut.

The alimentary tract is divided into functional units by a series of sphincters and valves: the pharyngoesophageal sphincter (cricopharyngeus), the lower esophageal sphincter, the pyloric sphincter, the ileocecal valve, and the internal and external anal sphincters. Normal motility in the gastrointestinal tract is characterized by coordinated contractions and relaxations of the different muscle layers in the bowel wall and various sphincters. This is regulated by a combination of *myogenic, neural,* and *hormonal factors*. Besides a disorder affecting one of these systems, irritation of the bowel by *inflammation* or *vascular insufficiency,* or *obstruction* of the bowel lumen can result in a variety of motility disturbances affecting the alimentary canal.

Depending on the mechanism involved, a motility disorder in the gastrointestinal tract may be localized or generalized, the lumen dilated or narrowed, and the peristaltic contractions increased or decreased, and physiologically coordinated or not.

For all practical purposes an obstructive pattern has to be distinguished from adynamic ileus. Radiographic findings of purely *mechanical obstruction* reflect the increased peristalsis throughout the entire gastrointestinal tract. Distended loops of bowel containing an increased amount of gas and fluid up to the point of obstruction are evident, with a horizontal beam, as numerous relatively small air–fluid levels at different heights (stepladder formation) that change in location upon subsequent radiographic examinations. Beyond the point of obstruction, it is characteristic that little or no gas, fluid, or fecal material are present (Fig. **1**). On the other hand, *adynamic ileus* is characterized by distension of the entire gastrointestinal tract with increased gas, fluid, and solids dispersed throughout the entire bowel. Relatively long air–fluid levels at similar heights with little change between subsequent radiographic examinations are seen (Fig. **2**). Besides air–fluid levels, air and fecal material are present in the colon and particularly the rectosigmoid area.

Unfortunately these classical patterns in their pure form are rarely encountered in clinical practice, since the mechanical obstruction may be early, incomplete, intermittent, or associated with adynamic ileus, thus obscuring the radiographic findings. Correlation with clinical findings therefore appears essential to arrive at a correct diagnosis. In cases in which the diagnosis remains indefinite, barium examinations are required either to rule out a mechanical obstruction or to identify the point of obstruction.

Acute gastroenteritis with *diarrhea* can produce a picture with multiple stepladder air–fluid levels, but they are characteristically not associated with bowel dilatation, and are located in both small and large bowel, the latter being useful to differentiate this condition from small-bowel obstruction (Fig. **3**).

Colonic air–fluid levels that may or may not be associated with small bowel air–fluid levels, depending on the competency of the ileocecal valve, are also found with colonic obstruction (Fig. **4**). In this condition, the proximal colon is dilated to the point of obstruction, while the colon distal to it is collapsed. In adynamic ileus, the colon is dilated in its entire length. Long fluid levels may be found in the proximal colon, while they are rare in the distal colon. Furthermore, colonic air–fluid levels can also be the result of a cleansing enema that has immediately preceded the radiographic examination.

In the following section, functional disturbances are discussed separately for different segments of the alimentary canal.

Pharyngeal and Esophageal Dilatation and Motility Disorders

Pharyngeal dysfunction is manifested radiographically by the inability of the pharynx to clear the swallowed barium completely. The barium remains trapped in the valleculae and inferior recesses of the piriform sinus. This condition is often associated with aspiration and can be found with an obstructive lesion at the level of the cricopharyngeal muscle or the cervical esophagus and in a variety of neuromuscular diseases. Failure of the cricopharyngeus to relax properly during swallowing can produce a marked dysphagia that is termed *cricopharyngeal achalasia*. In this idiopathic disorder, the hypertrophic cricopharyngeal muscle is radiographically evident as a large hemispheric filling defect on the posterior aspect of the esophagus at the level of C5–C6. A similar radiographic picture is sometimes found in patients after *laryngectomy* in whom the hypertrophy of the cricopharyngeus is induced by developing esophageal speech. Unilateral palsy results in asymmetric deformity of the pharynx that should not be confused with neoplastic involvement.

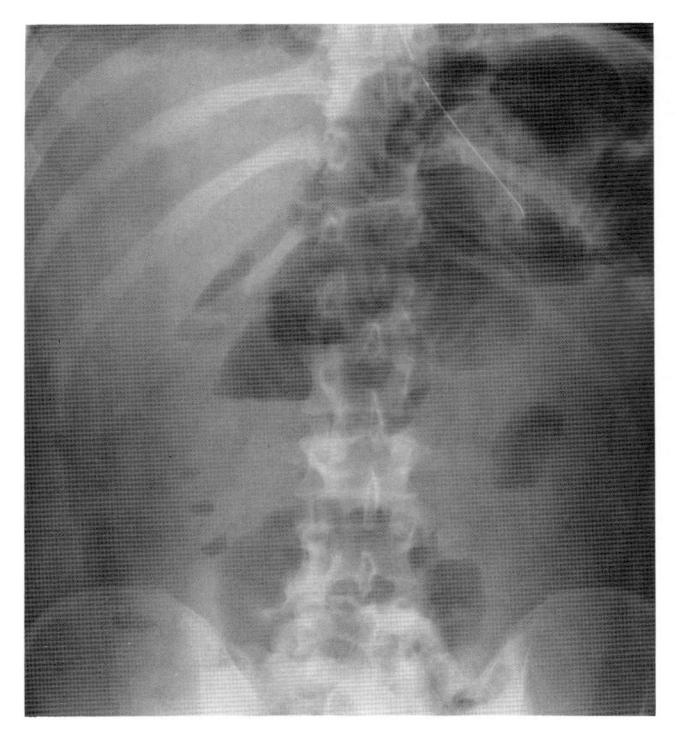

Figure 1 **Mechanical small-bowel obstruction** (upright film). Distended loops of small bowel with an inverted U-shape and multiple air–fluid levels at different levels (stepladder formation) are seen. Small gas collections retained between folds resemble a string of beads. Note also the absence of gas and fecal material in the colon.

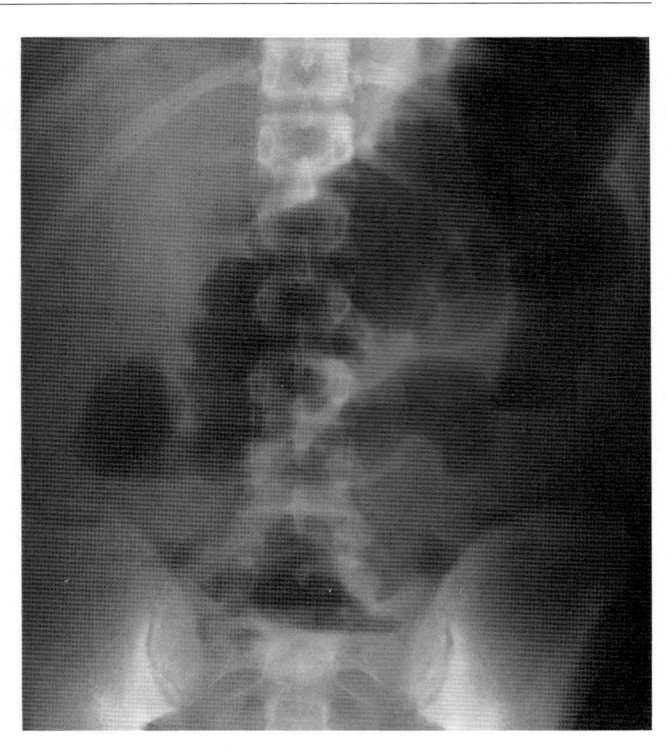

Figure 2 **Adynamic ileus** (upright film). Distended loops of both small and large bowel with multiple, relatively long air–fluid levels located at similar heights in the mid-abdomen are seen.

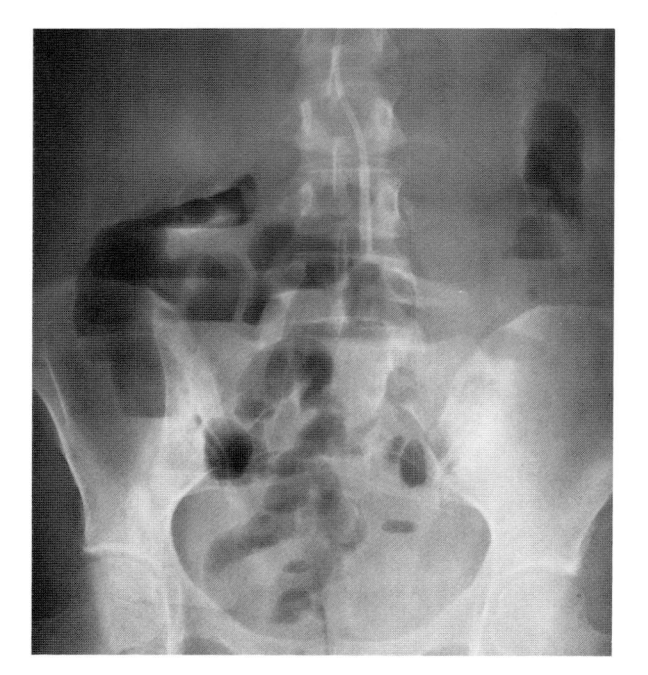

Figure 3 **Diarrhea.** Multiple small air–fluid levels at different heights are seen in nondistended small and large bowel loops. Note particularly the air–fluid levels in the descending colon.

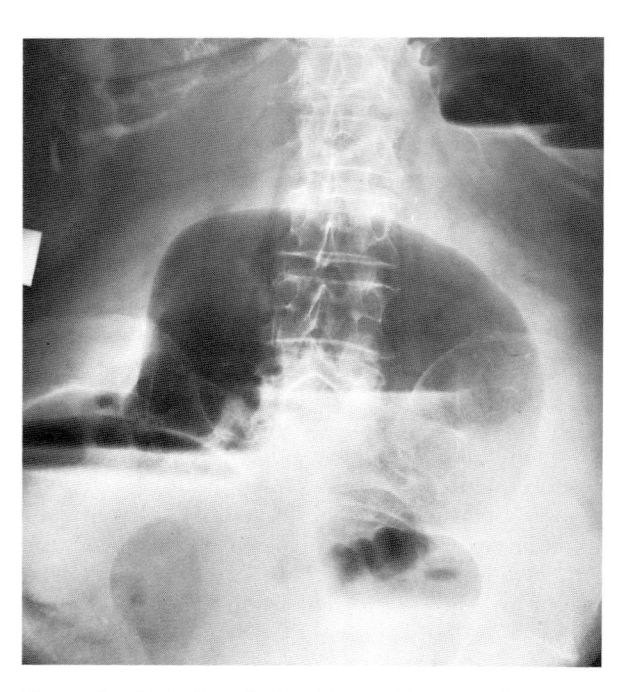

Figure 4 **Colonic obstruction** with competent ileocecal valve. A markedly distended colon with multiple air–fluid levels is seen. Note the absence of gas or fluid in the small bowel. The colonic obstruction was caused by herniation of the sigmoid into a left femoral hernia.

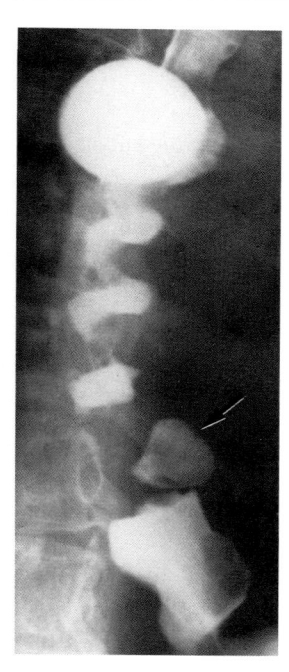

Figure 5 **Tertiary contractions.** A characteristic "cork-screw" appearance of the distal esophagus is seen. Note also the coincidental small pulsion diverticulum (arrow) and hiatal hernia.

Abnormal contractions are not uncommon in the esophagus. A contraction originating in the middle or lower third of the esophagus, spreading simultaneously upward and downward and producing radiographically an hour-glass deformity has been termed *secondary contraction*. Such contractions are rare and usually found with esophagitis.

Tertiary contractions or segmental spasms are usually limited to the lower two-thirds of the esophagus. They are irregular contractions, radiographically producing a "corkscrew" appearance, or occurring as multiple areas of severe narrowing alternating with areas of saccular distension producing a "shish kabob" appearance (Fig. 5). They are often found in asymptomatic people without any organic lesions. They may be found in the elderly without esophageal symptoms, but are often associated with other radiographic abnormalities such as dilatation *(presbyesophagus)*. However, if the contractions are associated with intermittent dysphagia, chest pain, and thickening of the esophageal wall, then the syndrome is called *idiopathic diffuse esophageal spasm*. It is most commonly found in middle-aged patients, the sex ratio being equal. In *thyrotoxicosis*, diffuse esophageal spasms can occasionally be seen combined with abnormal relaxation of upper esophageal sphincter.

Dilatation of the esophagus is found in many diseases and may or may not be associated with a motility disorder. The lumen of the normal esophagus rarely exceeds 2 cm in diameter. The differential diagnosis of a dilated and dysfunctional esophagus is discussed in Table 1.

Table 1 Dilatation and Motility Disorders of the Esophagus Including Hypopharynx

Disease	Radiographic Findings	Comments
Achalasia (Fig. 6)	Moderate to extensive dilatation of the whole thoracic esophagus tapering smoothly to a beak-like narrowing at the diaphragmatic hiatus. Peristalsis is replaced by intermittent, disorganized contractions. Small spurts of barium enter the stomach in the erect position.	Achalasia develops usually in the middle-aged, the sex ratio being equal. A positive *methylcholine test* is characteristic: 5–10 mg intramuscular or subcutaneous result in tetanic contraction of esophagus and retrosternal pain. Extensive dilatation often causes right paracardial and mediastinal mass on chest radiographs, often with air–fluid levels. The air bubble in the gastric fundus is usually small or absent.
Presbyesophagus	Mild to moderate dilatation, decreased peristaltic activity, and tertiary contractions are seen, especially in lower esophagus. Failure of lower esophageal sphincter relaxation may be associated.	In elderly patients, usually without symptoms. Rarely dysphagia while eating solids.
Obstructive lesion, extrinsic or intrinsic (Fig. 7)	Mild to moderate prestenotic dilatation of esophagus, with normal peristaltic waves. Eventually the esophagus may become aperistaltic. Radiographic appearance at the site of lesion is greatly variable, depending on location and type of obstruction.	Obstruction with prestenotic dilatation may be caused by extrinsic or intrinsic mass, stricture, web, Schatzki's ring, or foreign body.
Esophagitis	Commonly involves lower esophagus. Its caliber is only rarely increased and much more often decreased. Abnormal contractions and segmental spasm are commonly associated, whereas peristalsis is often decreased or even absent. Functional changes may precede mucosal abnormalities.	Most often caused by reflux (peptic esophagitis, usually in association with hiatal hernia), but may also be of infectious (e.g., candidiasis), caustic, or radiogenic origin.
Chagas' disease (Trypanosoma cruzi) (Fig. 8)	Moderate to extensive dilatation of entire esophagus with intermittent uncoordinated contractions. Radiographically indistinguishable from achalasia.	Virtually limited to South America. Cardiomegaly secondary to myocarditis, megacolon and megaureters are often associated. Methacholine test often positive and therefore not useful for differential diagnosis from achalasia.

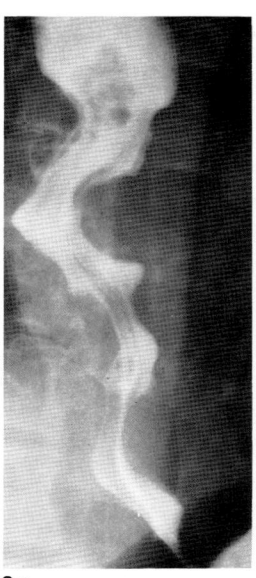

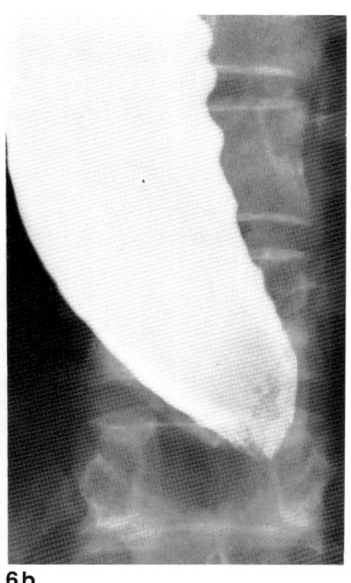

Figure 6a, b **Achalasia** (2 cases). Extensive dilatation of the esophagus, **a** with disorganized contractions and **b** with aperistalsis, is seen. Note also the smooth tapering of the distal esophagus to a beak-like narrowing at the diaphragmatic hiatus.

Figure 7 **Peptic esophagitis.** A stricture of the distal esophagus with significant prestenotic dilatation is seen.

Figure 8 **Chagas' disease.** Dilatation of the entire esophagus with smooth tapering at its distal end is seen.

Figure 9 **Scleroderma.** Moderate dilatation of a hypotonic and hypokinetic esophagus with a wide open lower esophageal sphincter is seen. Barium empties characteristically into the stomach by gravity in the upright position but pools in the esophagus in the supine position.

Table 1 (Cont.) Dilatation and Motility Disorders of the Esophagus Including Hypopharynx

Disease	Radiographic Findings	Comments
Scleroderma (Fig. 9)	Mild to moderate dilatation of the lower esophagus (below aortic arch) that is hypotonic and hypokinetic, since only the smooth muscle portion is affected. Barium empties by gravity into the stomach in upright position through the patulous lower esophageal sphincter, but pools in the esophagus in supine position. High incidence of gastroesophageal reflux leading to peptic esophagitis and stricture formation.	Abnormal esophageal motility is rarely found with other connective tissue diseases such as *Raynaud's disease, systemic lupus erythematosus, rheumatoid arthritis,* and *dermatomyositis,* that may also be associated with pharyngeal dysfunction.
Amyloidosis	Mild to moderate dilatation of the esophagus with decreased peristalsis.	Esophageal involvement is usually associated with other gastrointestinal manifestations. May be found with primary or secondary amyloidosis.
Neuromuscular diseases (e.g., cerebral disease, Parkinson's disease, multiple sclerosis, amyotrophic lateral sclerosis, familial dysautonomia, muscular dystrophy, myasthenia gravis)	Mild to moderate dilatation with decreased or absent peristalsis, primarily involving the proximal esophagus that contains predominantly striated muscle. Pharyngeal dysfunction usually much more conspicuous.	Aspiration and barium retention in hypopharynx is seen in neuromuscular disorders, but is also commonly found with a local mass lesion or a foreign body stuck in the hypopharynx. Delayed opening of the cricopharyngeal muscle is an additional feature of familial dysautonomia (Riley–Day syndrome).
Endocrine diseases (diabetes, myxedema)	Mild dilatation, decreased incidence and velocity of peristaltic waves, and nonperistaltic and nonpropulsive contractions are found.	Especially in patients with diabetic neuropathy. Clinical symptoms are, however, infrequent.
Drugs (IV anesthetics, atropine, anticholinergic drugs, curare)	Mild dilatation and depression of motor activity may involve the entire esophagus (anesthetics), the striated muscle of the proximal esophagus (curare), or the smooth muscle of the distal esophagus (atropine and anticholinergic drugs).	Changes in *chronic alcoholism* (particularly in association with peripheral neuropathy) are caused by vagal neuropathy and are similar to atropine medication. *Postvagotomy syndrome* (following vagal denervation of distal esophagus). Mild dilatation of esophagus and failure of lower esophageal sphincter to relax. Findings return spontaneously to normal within months.

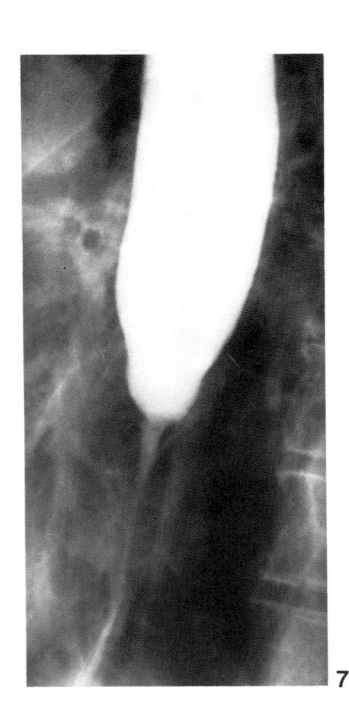

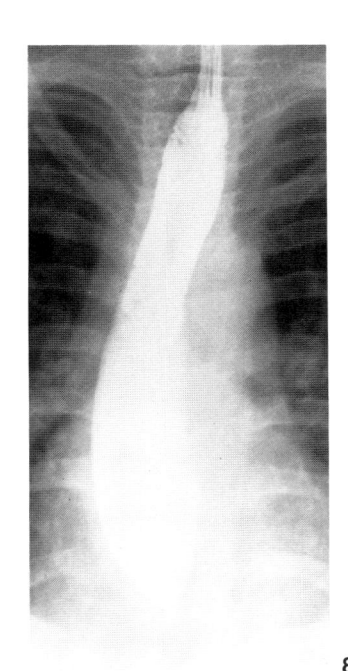

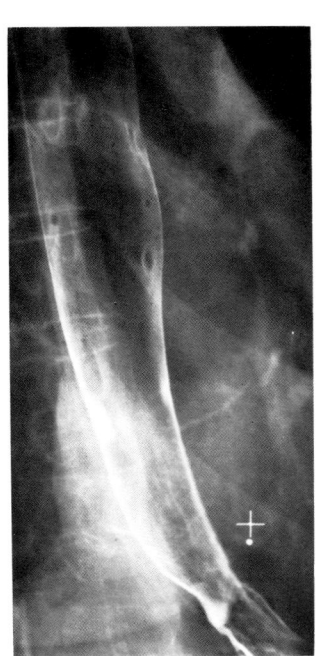

7

8

9

Gastric Dilatation

Gastric dilatation is a relatively common condition caused by *mechanical obstruction* or *functional disturbance*. In *gastric outlet obstruction*, the dilated stomach may contain up to 5 liters of fluid and a varying amount of air, resulting in a large air–fluid level when the radiograph is taken with horizontal beam. Little or no gas is characteristically found in the bowel beyond the point of obstruction. Gastric dilatation is also found with a duodenal or high small-bowel obstruction. In these cases, however, the duodenum and small bowel are also dilated up to the point of obstruction.

The leading cause of gastric outlet obstruction in adults is *peptic ulcer disease* (Fig. **10**). The narrowing of the lumen in this condition can be caused by spasm, edema, inflammation and scarring. The obstructive lesion is usually in the duodenal bulb or pyloric channel and rarely in the distal antrum.

Gastric carcinoma is the second most common cause of gastric outlet obstruction. The annular constricting lesion is usually located in the antrum. In contrast to patients with peptic ulcer disease, who have characteristically a long history of ulcer pain, primary and secondary gastric malignancies causing outlet obstruction are either not associated with pain, or the pain is of less than one year's duration.

Prolapsing antral polyps and *bezoars* are rare causes of gastric outlet obstruction, usually intermittent.

In *Crohn's disease, sarcoidosis, tuberculosis, syphilis, corrosive gastritis, pancreatitis, cholecystitis,* and other inflammatory disorders, narrowing of the gastric lumen by spasm, inflammation or stricture formation is only rarely severe enough to cause gastric outlet obstruction.

Gastric volvulus is a rare cause of mechanical obstruction that can result in dilatation of the stomach. The axis of rotation may be around a line extending from the cardia to the pylorus ("organoaxial" volvulus) or around an axis running transversely across the middle of the stomach from the lesser to the greater curvature ("mesenteroaxial" volvulus) (Figs. **11–13**). The majority of cases are associated with diaphragmatic abnormalities such as eventrations or diaphragmatic hernias. Twisting beyond 180 degrees is usually required for complete obstruction.

Hypertrophic pyloric stenosis is not a rare cause of gastric dilatation in the adult (Fig. **14**). Hypertrophy of the pyloric muscle may be idiopathic or result from previous gastritis or ulcer disease. On barium examination, elongation and concentric narrowing of the pyloric canal is found. In its mid-portion a triangular niche, the apex of which points inferiorly, is present in about 5% of cases and has to be differentiated from pyloric ulcer. On the other hand, a benign ulcer on the lesser curvature near the incisura, with concentric narrowing of the distal antrum, is found in over half of the patients with this condition.

Infantile hypertrophic pyloric stenosis is by far the most common gastric lesion during the first weeks of life. A palpable, olive-sized mass in the epigastrium combined with projectile vomiting is virtually diagnostic for this condition, which is strikingly more common among males. Radiographically, the elongated, narrowed and downward-curved pyloric channel, with symmetric and concave indentation of the duodenal bulb by the hypertrophied muscle mass, is characteristic. Other congenital lesions that rarely result in gastric obstruction

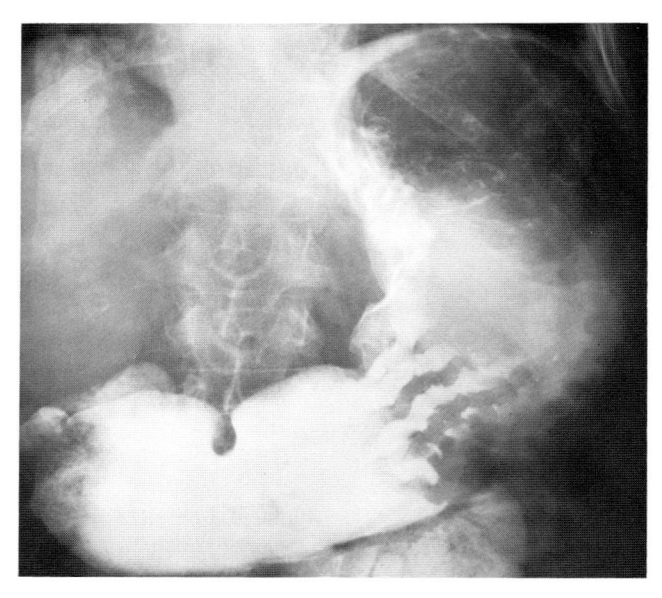

Figure **10** **Gastric outlet obstruction** caused by scarring secondary to chronic ulcer disease. A markedly dilated stomach with a large quantity of retained fluid diluting the barium is seen.

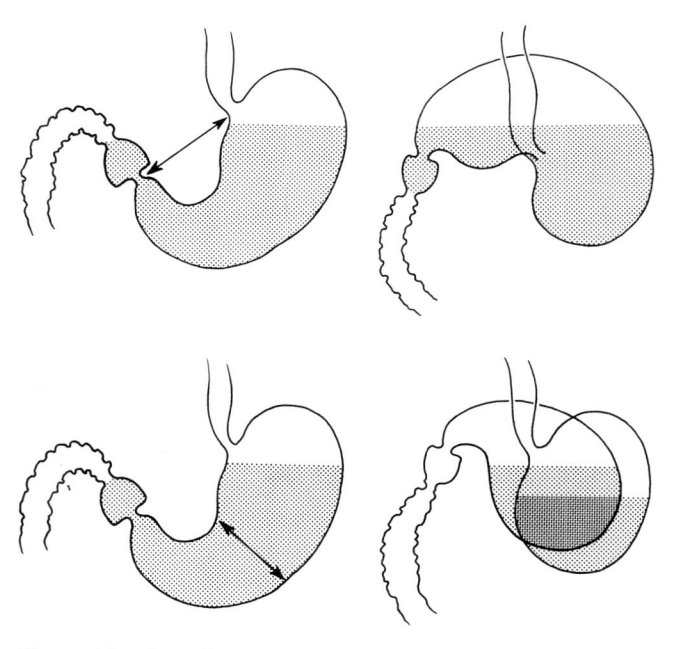

Figure **11** **Gastric volvulus.** Characteristically, the greater curvature is above the lesser curvature, cardia and pylorus are at the same level, and the pylorus and bulbus duodeni point downwards. **a** *Organoaxial volvulus.* Axis of rotation occurs along a line extending from the cardia to the pylorus. **b** *Mesenteroaxial volvulus.* Axis of rotation occurs around a line running across the middle of the stomach from the lesser to the greater curvature.

include an *antral web* (Fig. **10**), *gastric duplication*, and *annular pancreas*.

Dilatation of the stomach without mechanical obstruction is a common *postoperative complication*, but may also be found after severe *trauma*, in patients *immobolized by cast*, in *inflammatory disease* of the abdomen (e.g., acute pancreatitis, peritonitis, appendicitis, subphrenic abscess), in patients with *severe abdominal pain* (e.g. renal and biliary colics), and various *neurogenic disorders* including postvagotomy state (Fig. **15**). In *scleroderma*, gastric dilatation, decreased motor activity, and delayed emptying are seen, but the stomach is less frequently involved than other parts of the gastrointestinal tract. *Diabetes* and a variety of *drugs* (e.g., anticholinergic drugs and morphine derivatives) are common causes for gastric atony, whereas it is a relatively rare finding in *hypokalemia, uremia, porphyria,* and *lead poisoning*. Finally, a greatly distended stomach is also encountered with *aerophagia* (e.g., in psychopaths) or may be *idiopathic* in the absence of any other obvious cause. Table **2** summarizes the various causes of gastric dilatation.

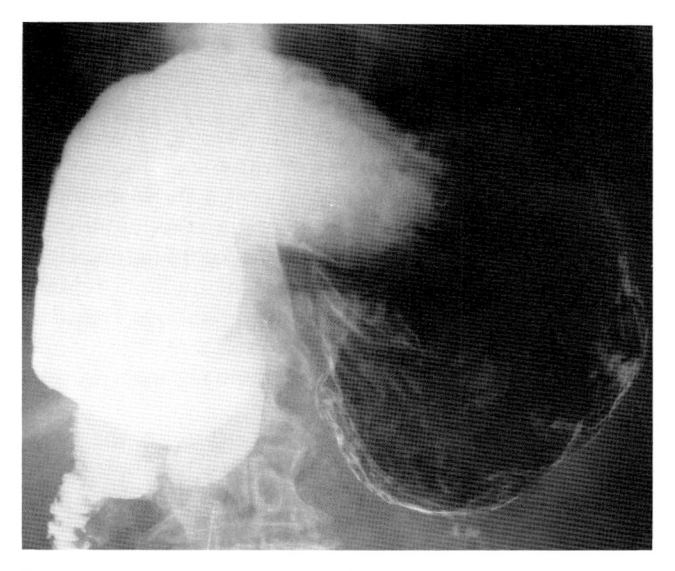

Figure **12 Organoaxial volvulus.** A markedly distended upside-down stomach with gastric outlet obstruction is seen.

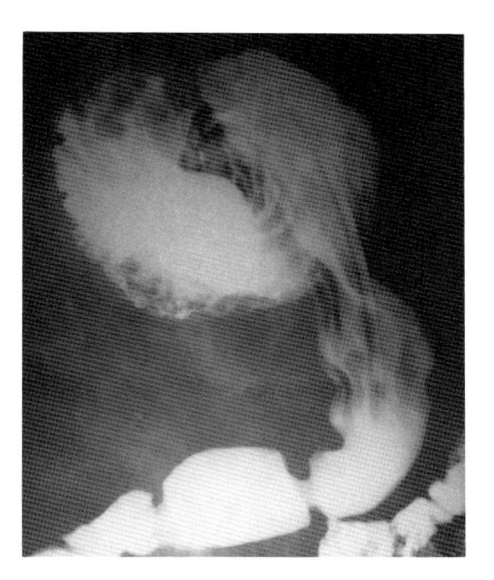

Figure **13 Organoaxial volvulus with partial diaphragmatic hernia.** The twisted proximal portion of the stomach is located in a diaphragmatic hernia, whereas the antrum and duodenal bulb are directed downwards and backwards as seen in this lateral projection.

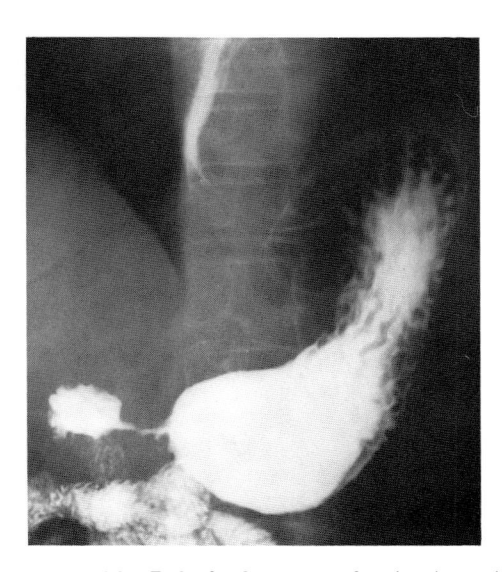

Figure **14 Pyloric hypertrophy** in the adult. Elongation and concentric narrowing of the pyloric canal is seen causing mild dilatation of the stomach.

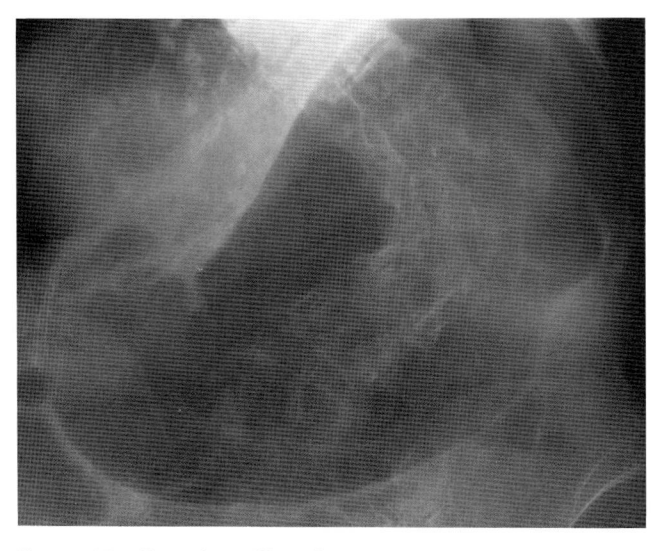

Figure **15 Gastric dilatation.** A markedly distended stomach without mechanical obstruction is seen.

Table 2 Gastric Dilatation

Cause	Disorder
Gastric outlet obstruction	Peptic ulcer disease
	Gastric carcinoma and other primary and secondary malignancies
	Prolapsing antral polyps and benign tumors
	Bezoars
	Spasm and edema secondary to an acute inflammatory condition
	Stricture formation secondary to a chronic inflammatory condition
	Gastric volvulus
	Hypertrophic pyloric stenosis (infantile and adult types)
	Congenital lesions (antral web, gastric duplication, annular pancreas)
Functional disturbance without obstruction	Postoperative (especially following abdominal surgery)
	Posttraumatic (especially with involvement of back)
	Immobilization (cast syndrome)
	Inflammatory disease (e.g., pancreatitis, peritonitis, appendicitis, subphrenic abscess)
	Pain (e.g., renal and biliary colics)
	Neuromuscular disorders
	Scleroderma
	Diabetes (especially in diabetic ketoacidosis)
	Drugs (e.g., atropine and anticholinergic drugs)
	Postvagotomy
	Electrolyte imbalance (e.g. hypokalemia, hypercalcemia, hypocalcemia)
	Coma (uremic and hepatic)
	Porphyria
	Lead poisoning
	Aerophagia
	Idiopathic

Dilatation of the Duodenum

Duodenal dilatation secondary to obstruction may be caused by *adhesions* or an *extrinsic mass* such as a neoplasm of the pancreas, aortic lymphadenopathy, and mesenteric metastases (e.g., in the ligament of Treitz) (Fig. **16**). Obstructions caused by *intrinsic mass* lesions are rare in the adult, since primary duodenal tumors, either benign or malignant, occur infrequently. Duodenal obstruction may also be secondary to *postbulbar ulcer* and *inflammatory disease* (e.g., Crohn's disease). *Congenital lesions* (e.g., annular pancreas, duodenal duplication, stenosis, and atresia) may cause obstruction in infancy but rarely in adulthood. The double-bubble sign in the newborn is virtually diagnostic of a high-grade duodenal obstruction. This appearance reflects large amounts of gas in both a markedly dilated stomach (left bubble) and in the duodenum proximal to the obstruction (right bubble).

In *midgut volvulus,* the third portion of the duodenum is obstructed, but spontaneous remissions occur. The condition is associated with malrotation and incomplete mesenteric fixation of the gut, allowing the jejunum to twist around the mesenteric root at the site of the origin of the superior mesenteric artery. The duodenojejunal junction (ligament of Treitz) is located inferiorly and to the right of its expected position, and a malpositioned cecum (e.g., in the upper left quadrant) is often present also.

In the *superior mesenteric artery syndrome,* the third portion is compressed by this artery or the mesenteric root, respectively. Both of these anatomical structures cross the duodenum anteriorly. It is characteristic for this syndrome that the duodenal dilatation diminishes considerably in prone position. This syndrome is most often found in thin patients. Duodenal compression by the superior mesenteric artery has also been observed in patients with severe burns or lying in a body cast.

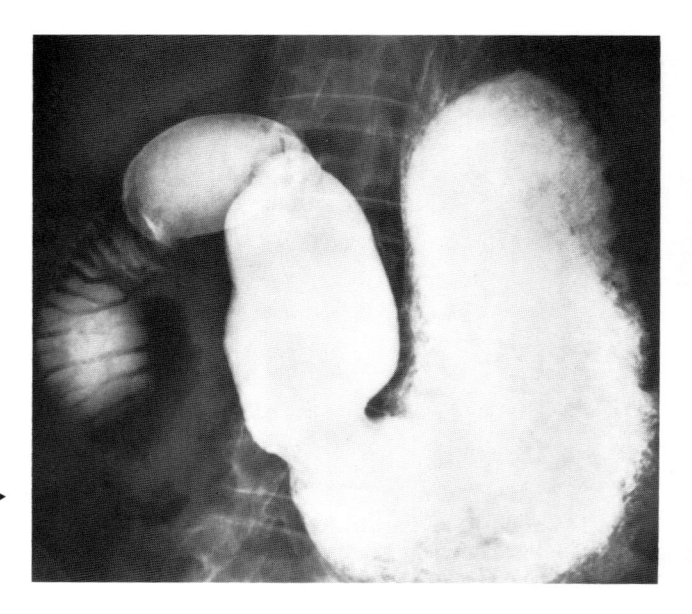

Figure **16 Pancreatic carcinoma.** Almost complete ▶ obstruction between the second and third portion of the duodenum is seen, with markedly prestenotic dilatation of the duodenum and stomach.

Duodenal dilatation is, however, much more often the result of functional disturbances than mechanical obstruction. A localized duodenal ileus is often associated with *acute pancreatitis* or *cholecystitis*. *Scleroderma* can also present with localized duodenal dilatation and delayed emptying, but more often additional radiologic and clinical findings, quite characteristic of this disorder, are associated (Fig. **17**). Similarly, a variety of *drugs* (atropine, spasmolytics, and opioids) may induce dilatation of the duodenum, but in this case it is rarely an isolated finding. An *idiopathic megaduodenum* may result from an abnormality in the myenteric plexus (Fig. **18**). Causes of duodenal dilatation are summarized in Table **3**.

Table 3 Duodenal Dilatation

Cause	Disorder
Mechanical obstruction (prestenotic duodenal dilatation)	Extrinsic mass (pancreatic carcinoma and pseudocyst, aortic or mesenteric lymphadenopathy and metastases, hematoma) Intrinsic mass (carcinoma, intramural hematoma) Postbulbar ulcer Inflammatory disease (Crohn's disease, tuberculosis, strongyloidiasis, sprue) Radiation therapy Superior mesenteric artery syndrome Midgut volvulus (infants and older) Annular pancreas (infants) Duodenal atresia, stenosis, web and duplication (infants) Congenital peritoneal or duodenal (Ladd's) bands (infants)
Functional disturbance	Pancreatitis Cholecystitis Drugs Scleroderma Idiopathic

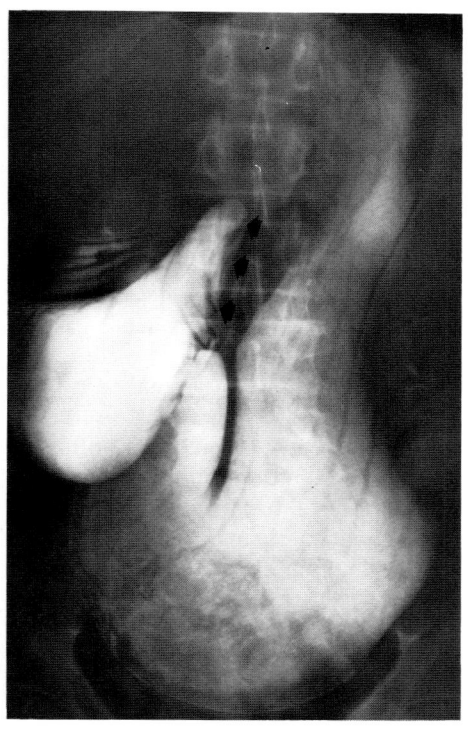

Figure **17** **Scleroderma.** A markedly dilated and atonic stomach and duodenum are seen. Barium is held up where the superior mesenteric artery crosses the third portion of the duodenum (arrows).

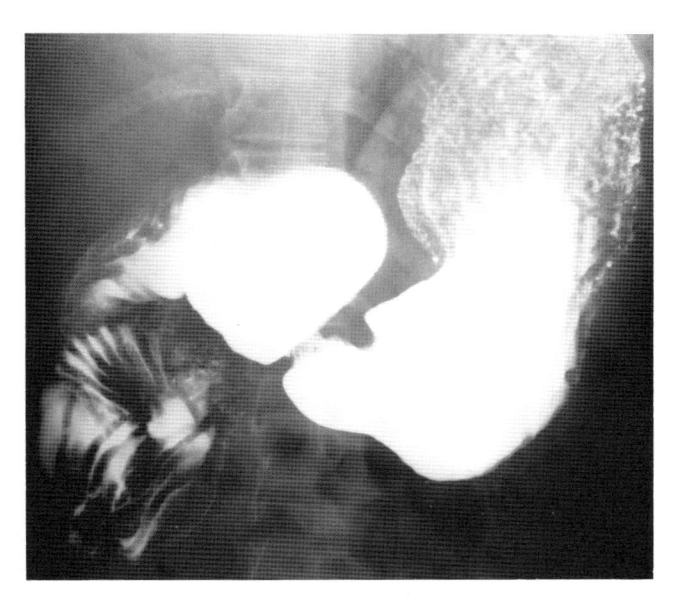

◀ Figure **18** **Idiopathic (congenital) megaduodenum.** A markedly dilated duodenal bulb and descending duodenum was complicated by intermittent retrograde small-bowel intussusceptions.

Small Bowel Dilatation

Normally only minimal amounts of gas are found in the small bowel of a healthy adult. Bedridden patients have in general an increased amount of gas in the small bowel, since the supine position facilitates the passage of gas from the stomach into the duodenum and subsequently into the small bowel.

An increase of both gas and fluid in the small bowel is found with mechanical obstruction, adynamic ileus, and gastroenteritis (diarrhea). The radiographic plain film findings of these three entities are different and produce characteristic patterns.

Small bowel obstruction is characterized by distended gas and fluid-filled loops of small bowel preferentially located in the mid-abdomen. Valvulae conniventes are often seen in the jejunum producing a characteristic spring-coil appearance. Small gas collections retained between folds may resemble a string of beads, whereas loops of small bowel containing only fluid have a sausage-like appearance. The small-bowel gas pattern changes characteristically between subsequent radiographic examinations. A minimal amount of gas and fecal material is present in the colon and if the colon is locally somewhat distended, haustral markings are recognizable. In the upright or decubitus films taken with a horizontal roentgen beam, the small-bowel loops have an inverted U-shape with multiple small air–fluid levels at different heights producing a stepladder appearance (Fig. **19**).

Mechanical *small-bowel obstruction* may be associated *with a compromised mesenteric blood supply* and in particular with compression of the venous drainage. In such cases, both the intestinal wall and mucosal folds of the involved bowel segment become rapidly edematous or hemorrhagic and appear radiographically thickened. General paresis of the gut occurs rather quickly under these circumstances, thus masking the radiographic signs of an underlying obstruction and mimicking adynamic ileus.

In *nonobstructive bowel distension* (paralytic ileus in the widest sense), the gas- and fluid-distended loops of jejunum and ileum tend to be large and contain characteristically long air–fluid levels at similar heights. The distended small bowel segments do not have a preferred location. Mucosal folds and markings are often effaced or when edematous, may appear thick. Subsequent abdominal surveys demonstrate little change in the gas pattern. The colon characteristically contains large amounts of gas and stool and may occasionally demonstrate long air–fluid levels. Gastric dilatation is often conspicuous and much more frequently seen than in mechanical obstruction (Fig. **20**).

The diarrheal bowel pattern is found in acute gastroenteritis. Increased gas and fluid is found throughout the entire bowel. Besides numerous small air–fluid levels throughout the small bowel without a preferred location, small air–fluid levels in stepladder configuration are characteristically also found in the colon (Fig. **3**, p. 84). Immediately after defecation, the colon may be completely empty and barely recognizable on the radiographs. A rapidly changing small and large bowel pattern is the hallmark of diarrhea.

The differential diagnosis of various diseases producing dilatation of the small bowel on plain film radiographs is discussed in Table **4.**

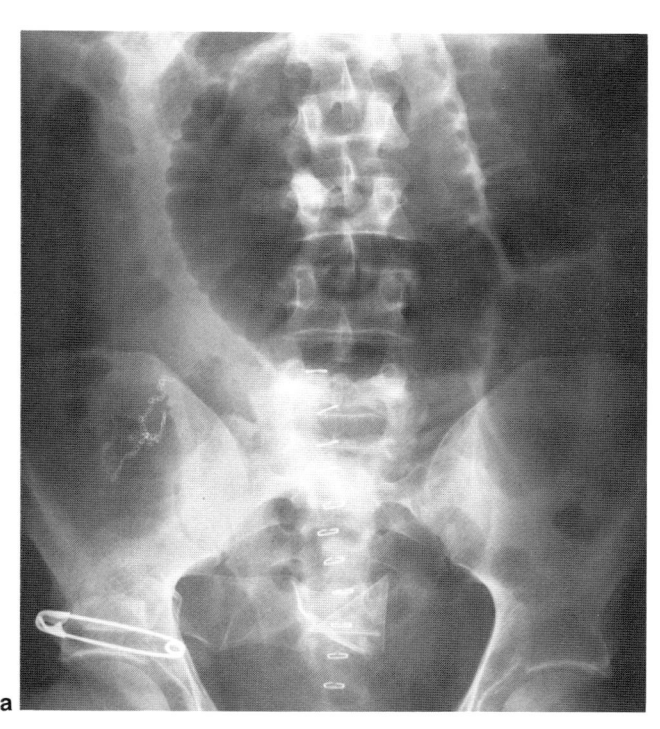

Figure 19 **Distal small bowel obstruction** in Crohn's disease **a** in supine and **b** in left lateral decubitus projections. Dilated loops of small bowel with multiple air–fluid levels at different heights and smaller air collections resembling a string of beads are seen. Note also the spring coil appearance of the valvulae conniventes in the jejunum. The colon is collapsed and contains only a minimal amount of gas.

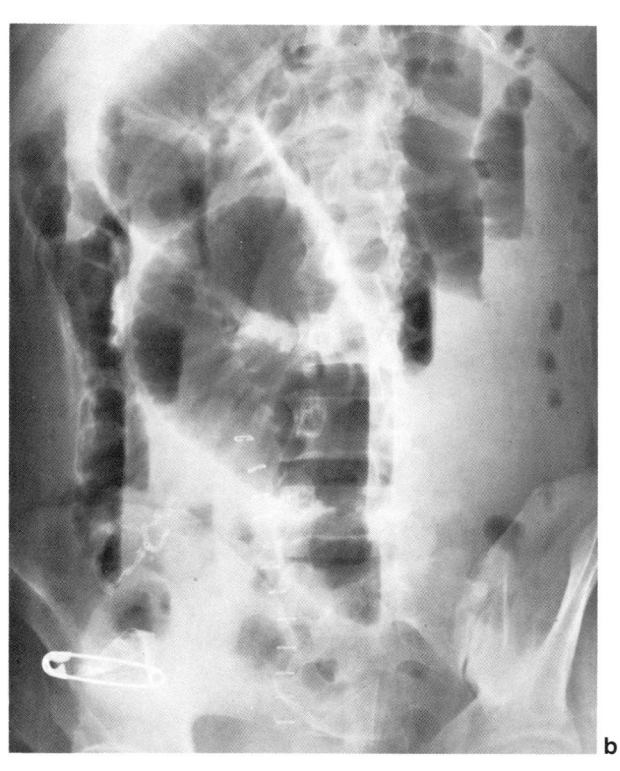

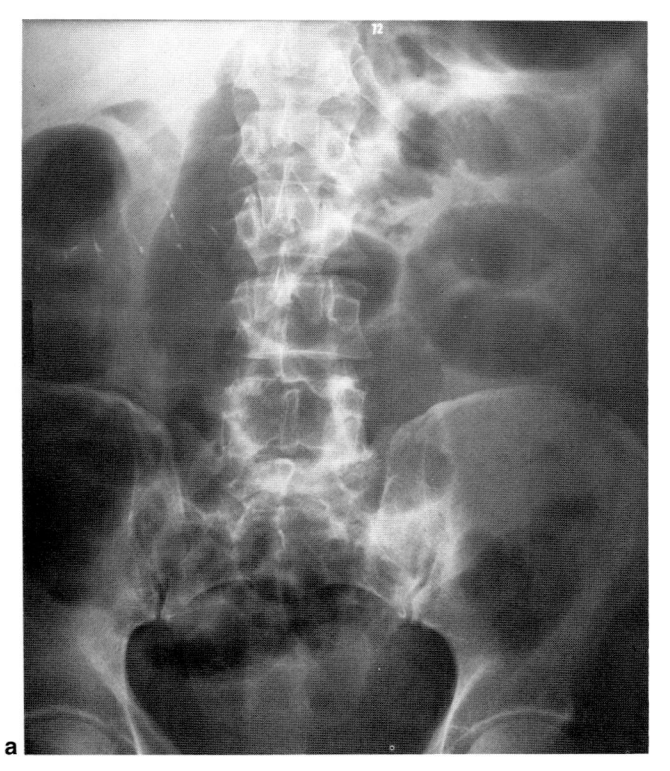

Figure 20 **Adynamic ileus (postoperative)** in **a** supine and **b** upright projections. Dilatation of the entire gastrointestinal tract is caused predominantly by air with only a few fluid levels evident on the upright film. Mucosal and haustral markings are largely effaced.

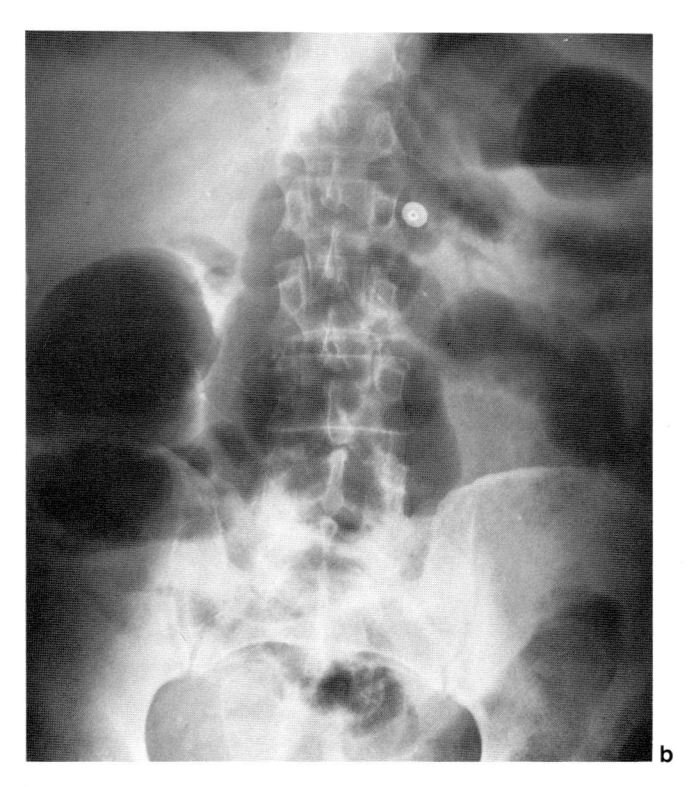

Table 4 Dilatation of Small Bowel

Disease	Radiographic Findings	Comments
Mechanical obstruction without vascular compromise		
Adhesions and bands	Obstructive pattern with site of obstruction commonly in the ileum (right iliac fossa or pelvis).	Most frequent cause of obstruction, almost always due to postoperative scarring (usually 3 weeks or later after surgery) or previous inflammatory process. Congenital bands are rare.
Neoplasm (extrinsic or intrinsic)	Obstructive pattern without predilection for location.	Most often caused by mesenteric metastases or lymphoma. Less common are benign or malignant tumors arising within the small bowel. Mesenteric cyst and endometrial implants are other rare causes of small bowel obstruction.
Strictures (Fig. 19)	Obstructive pattern without site predilection.	Neoplastic, inflammatory (e.g. Crohn's disease, tuberculosis), ischemic, posttraumatic, postoperative and post-radiation therapy.
Hematoma	Obstructive pattern without site predilection.	Intramural hematomas can occur post-traumatically or spontaneously in patients with bleeding diathesis (including anticoagulation therapy).
Parasites (e.g., ascaris)	Occasionally a cluster of linear densities representing a mass of worms outlined by gas can be seen at the site of obstruction.	Usually in children.
Foreign body	Obstruction common in terminal ileum. Foreign body may be recognizable if partially opaque.	In children and mentally disturbed or retarded patients. *Bezoars* are primarily found in mentally retarded or edentulous patients or who have undergone (partial) gastric resection.
Gallstone ileus (Fig. 21)	Obstruction most common in distal ileum. Gallstone may occasionally contain sufficient calcium to be visible radiographically. Demonstration of gas in shrunken gallbladder and/or biliary system is diagnostic.	Usually in elderly women. Caused by a large gallstone entering the small bowel via a fistula from the gallbladder or from the common bile duct to the duodenum.
Periappendiceal abscess	Extrinsic obstruction of terminal ileum. Abscess might be apparent as a right lower quadrant mass. Appendicolith is occasionally seen.	A similar right lower quadrant mass with distal small bowel obstruction can also be found with *Crohn's disease, tuberculosis, actinomycosis, lymphogranuloma venereum* and *lymphoma.*
Hernia (external and internal) (Fig. 22)	Demonstration of extraperitoneal bowel containing air and/or fluid at characteristic locations is diagnostic. If the herniated bowel contains only fluid, a mass lesion is simulated and incarceration must be strongly considered (see also under "strangulation" in this table). Whereas the diagnosis of external hernia is easily confirmed clinically, internal herniation should be suspected when bowel loops are crowded in circular arrangement in a local area.	Second most frequent cause of small bowel obstruction. External hernias are 20 times more common than internal hernias. External hernias develop in inguinal, femoral, umbilical, or obturator canals and in weakened surgical incisions. Internal hernias occur in diaphragmatic, gastroepiploic (foramen of Winslow), paraduodenal, and mesenteric defects, which may be congenital or acquired (e.g. surgical defects). The left paraduodenal hernia is the most common internal hernia, accounting for over half of all cases.

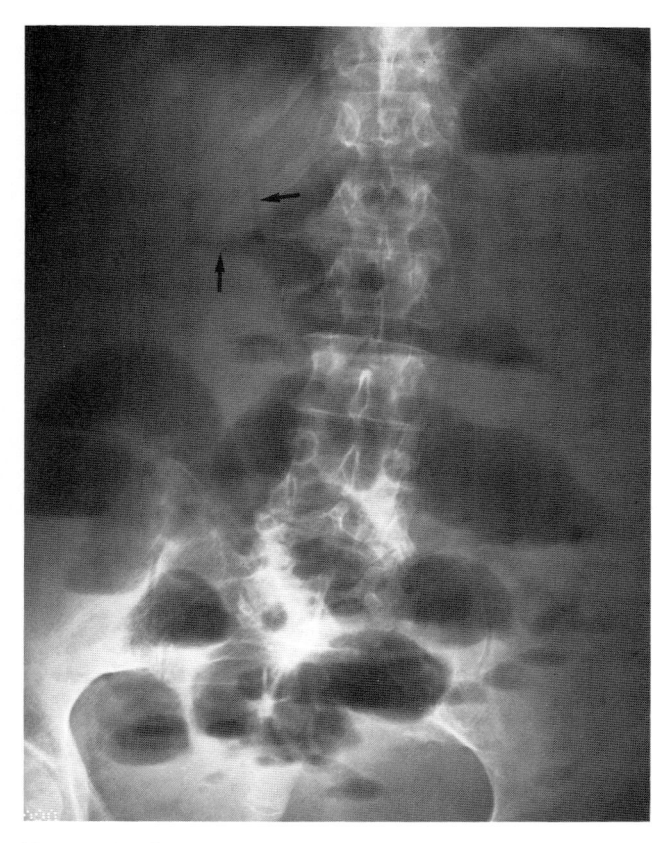

Figure **21 Gallstone ileus** in upright projection. Small bowel obstruction is caused by a nonradiopaque gallstone lodged in the distal ileum. Distended loops of bowel with inverted U-shape and multiple small air–fluid levels at different heights are seen. The colon is collapsed. The air in the larger bile ducts (arrows) is diagnostic.

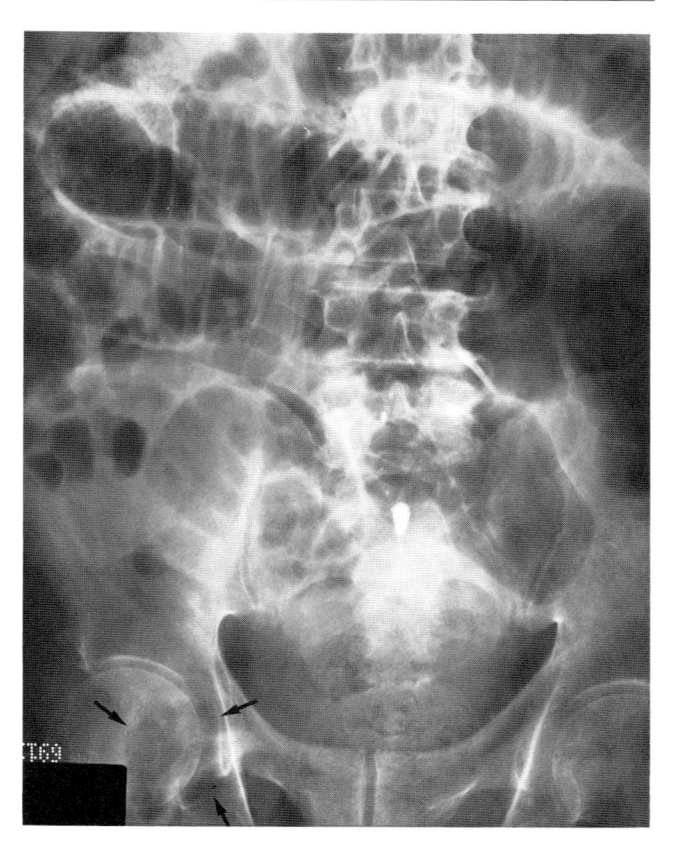

Figure **22 Right inguinal hernia** causing small-bowel obstruction in supine projection. Distended loops of small bowel with valvulae conniventes producing a spring-coil appearance are seen. Diagnostic is the herniated, air-containing, small-bowel loop projecting into the right inguinal area (arrows).

Table 4 (Cont.) Dilatation of Small Bowel

Disease	Radiographic Findings	Comments
Congenital intestinal stenosis or atresia	Triple-bubble sign is seen in infants with proximal jejunal atresia, where the gas is trapped in the stomach, duodenum and proximal jejunum.	Meconium peritonitis (often calcified) is a common complication of small bowel atresia.
Meconium ileus	Obstruction of the distal ileum in infants by meconium evident as bubbly mass in the right quadrant. Microcolon is also present.	Ileal inspissation with abnormal sticky meconium is commonly associated with cystic fibrosis. May be complicated by stenosis, atresia or volvulus of the small bowel.
Meckel's diverticulum	Obstruction in distal ileum.	Obstruction may be caused by 1 intussusception, 2 internal herniation through congenital band extending from Meckel's diverticulum, and 3 sequelae of chronic inflammation.
Colonic obstruction	Small bowel dilatation occurs with incompetent ileocecal valve. The cecum and to a lesser degree the remaining colon proximal to the obstruction are characteristically distended also.	For differential diagnosis of colonic obstruction, see Table 5, pages 99–103.
Mechanical obstruction with vascular compromise		
Strangulation	External obstruction of both the afferent and efferent limb of a bowel loop with compromise of mesenteric vessels at the site of obstruction. *Incomplete* strangulation is indistinguishable on plain radiography from simple mechanical obstruction. *Complete* strangulation: little or no gas but extensive fluid accumulates in the strangulated bowel loop presenting often as mass lesion with characteristically polycyclic outline. Air–fluid levels in prestenotic bowel are initially short and located at different levels, but with rapidly occurring paresis become longer and located at similar levels.	The most common cause of a strangulating obstruction is an *incarcerated hernia*.
Intussusception	Dilated ileum often has beak-like termination at the intussusception site. Intussusception may produce a mass lesion with convex defect in the air column of ascending or transverse colon. On barium examination the classic coiled-spring appearance (barium trapped between the intussusception and the surrounding bowel wall) may be evident.	Common in children between 6 months and 2 years of age ("idiopathic" form). In older children and adults, intussusceptions are much less common and result usually from an associated mass lesion. Ileocolic intussusceptions account for 90% of cases, whereas ileoileal (6%) and colocolic (4%) intussusceptions are rare.
Volvulus	Thickened folds may appear as radiating stripes converging towards center of the torsion. On upright films, torqued loops may demonstrate long air–fluid levels indicating paresis. The distended small bowel loops often appear disarranged and have a tendency to be located in the right upper quadrant as opposed to a simple mechanical obstruction, where the distended loops are somewhat more often seen in the left upper quadrant.	More common in infants and children than adults. Small bowel volvulus is often associated with anomalies of the mesentery and malrotation. In the latter case, cecum and terminal ileum are usually placed upwards and to the left.

Table 4 (Cont.) Dilatation of Small Bowel

Disease	Radiographic Findings	Comments
Nonobstructive dilatation		
Adynamic ileus, localized ("sentinel loop")	Localized dilatation of small and/or large bowel loops adjacent to an acutely inflamed organ, or associated with point tenderness.	Found with acute processes involving the appendix, gallbladder, pancreas, or part of urogenital system.
Adynamic ileus, generalized 1. Postoperative, posttraumatic 2. Shock, sepsis 3. Acute disease in abdomen, pelvis, chest (pneumonia, myocardial infarction) 4. Electrolyte imbalance (uremia, hypokalemia) 5. Drugs (atropine and substitutes, morphines and derivatives, barbiturates, phenothiazines, and hexamethonium) 6. Pain (especially colics caused by ureteral or common bile duct stones, torsion of uterine fibroid, or ovarian tumor) 7. Neurogenic or neuromuscular disorders (myotonic dystrophy, parkinsonism, spinal cord lesions, tabes dorsalis) 8. Endocrine disorders (diabetes, hypothyroidism, hypoparathyroidism, adrenal insufficiency)	Dilatation of entire gastrointestinal tract without mucosal or intestinal wall abnormalities is characteristic. Small bowel distension is caused predominantly by air and less by fluid.	Causes of adynamic ileus that clinically mimic small-bowel obstruction by frequently being associated with colicky abdominal pain include: 1 *Pelvic surgery* 2 *Urinary retention* 3 *Biliary and ureteral colics* 4 *Lead poisoning* 5 *Acute porphyria* 6 *Idiopathic intestinal pseudo-obstruction* 7 *Neonatal adynamic ileus* Conditions simulating adynamic ileus, with gastric dilatation being usually the most prominent finding, are: 1 *Aerophagia* 2 *Assisted ventilation*
Peritonitis	Findings similar to adynamic ileus, although colonic distension is often very prominent. Restricted diaphragmatic movements, pleural effusions and particularly ascites are associated. *Ascites* may be evident as increased density in pelvis with "dog ears" on urinary bladder, obliteration of hepatic and splenic angles, medial displacement of the liver, spleen, ascending and descending colon from radiolucent (fat) flank stripes which may become thinned, and separation and central location of small bowel loops.	Primary peritonitis (without underlying cause such as perforation or surgery and without evidence of infection elsewhere) is essentially limited to young children and adults with liver cirrhosis. With conventional technique, usually 200 ml or more intraperitoneal fluid is required for a diagnosis. Smaller amounts can however, easily be demonstrated with ultrasonography and computed tomography.
Scleroderma	Dilatation most prominent in duodenum and jejunum. Air in the esophagus and/or colonic outpouchings (pseudodiverticula) is virtually diagnostic when present.	Disease of middle age with female sex predominance of 3 : 1. Honeycombing in the lung bases may be observed.

Table 4 (Cont.) Dilatation of Small Bowel

Disease	Radiographic Findings	Comments
Sprue, tropical and nontropical	Predominantly small bowel dilatation. Pneumatosis and intussusception occur with increased frequency.	Tropical sprue is limited to the Far East, India, and Puerto Rico. Nontropical sprue (adult celiac disease) is an important dietary-related cause of chronic malabsorption in response to the ingestion of gluten found in temperate climates.
Ischemic bowel disease (Fig. 23)	Localized or generalized "adynamic ileus" pattern. Submucosal edema or hemorrhage may be evident as "thumb prints." Gas may be seen in bowel wall (streaky appearance as opposed to the bubbly appearance of pneumatosis), portal vein system including intrahepatic branches, and/or peritoneum (poor prognostic sign).	Mesenteric infarction can result from an embolus or thrombus in the superior or inferior mesenteric artery and less commonly from venous thrombosis. Nonocclusive mesenteric ischemia is 5 times more common in the bowel supplied by the inferior mesenteric artery (descending colon and sigmoid) than superior mesenteric artery. *Neonatal necrotizing enterocolitis* in premature or dehydrated infants is the counterpart of the mesenteric infarction in the elderly.
Acute gastroenteritis and food poisoning	Increased motor activity characteristically causes numerous small air–fluid levels at different heights throughout small and large bowel.	Caused by bacterial, viral, and toxic agents.

Dilatation of the Colon (Megacolon)

A dilated colon (megacolon) can be diagnosed when the colonic diameter exceeds 8 cm. This may be the result of obstruction with prestenotic dilatation, paralysis, or disintegration of the bowel wall. The most important complication of a megacolon is perforation regardless of the etiology of colonic distension (obstruction versus nonobstruction). Colonic rupture can occur when the diameter of the colon exceeds 10 cm. Since the cecum is generally the widest segment of the colon, perforation takes place most often at this site.

Differential diagnosis of a local or generalized dilatation of the colon is discussed in Table **5**.

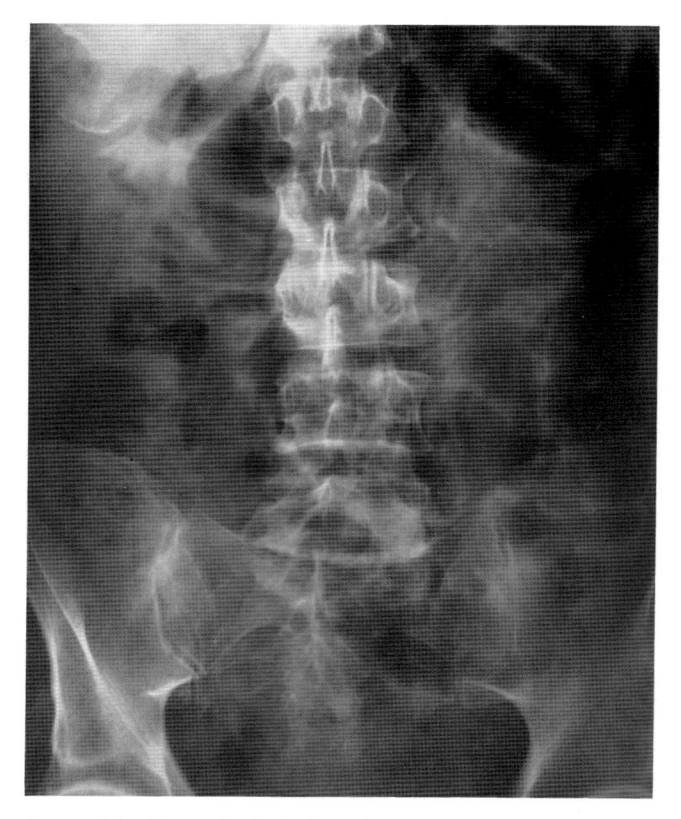

Figure **23 Mesenteric infarction** (supine projection). A generalized adynamic ileus pattern with dilatation of both small and large bowel is seen. In addition, streaky and to a lesser degree mottled radiolucencies are seen scattered throughout small bowel loops indicating intramural gas. Gas is also seen in the portal system of the liver as irregular peripheral radiolucencies. A close-up view of the liver in this patient is shown in Fig. **2**, p. 84.

Table 5   Dilatation of the Colon

Disease	Radiographic Findings	Comments
Obstruction		
Fecal impaction (Fig. 24)	Large masses of mottled-appearing stool in rectosigmoid area and other colon segments with distension of proximal large and small bowel.	Usually in elderly or bedridden patients. Other rare causes of colonic obturation include foreign bodies, gallstones, and parasites.
Tumor (intrinsic or extrinsic) (Fig. 25)	Chronic rather than acute colonic obstruction. Large quantities of fecal material, fluid, and gas distend the colon proximal to the obstruction.	Carcinoma of the colon is by far the most common intrinsic tumor. Extrinsic colonic obstruction may be caused by the invasion of malignant pelvic tumors or metastases (e.g., from carcinomas of stomach or pancreas).
Diverticulitis	Virtually limited to lower descending and sigmoid colon. Obstruction may result from an intramural or intraperitoneal abscess and is usually incomplete and chronic in nature. Abscess may present radiographically as mass that sometimes contains gas within the lesion. Fistulas between sigmoid and bladder (pneumaturia), vagina, flank, or thigh occur. Gas-filled diverticula are occasionally seen but not diagnostic.	*Granulomatous colitis* (Crohn's disease) rarely results in colonic obstruction.
Periappendiceal abscess	Mass in ileocecal area producing small bowel obstruction is characteristic. Rarely, obstruction of the sigmoid colon might occur. Appendicolith may be seen.	
Pelvic abscess	Most often originating from the female genital system. Developing within tubes or pelvic recesses. May obstruct rectum by extrinsic compression.	Commonly gonococcal infection, less often streptococcus, staphylococcus, and tuberculosis.

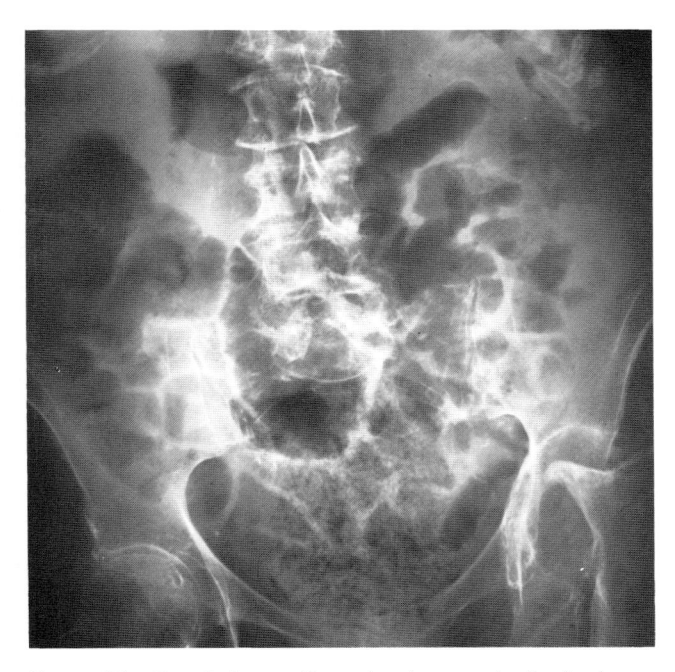

Figure **24 Fecal impaction** (supine projection). Large amounts of fecal material is seen in the rectosigmoid area. Distension of the colon and to a lesser degree the small bowel is evident in this immobilized patient with advanced rheumatoid arthritis causing destruction of the left hip.

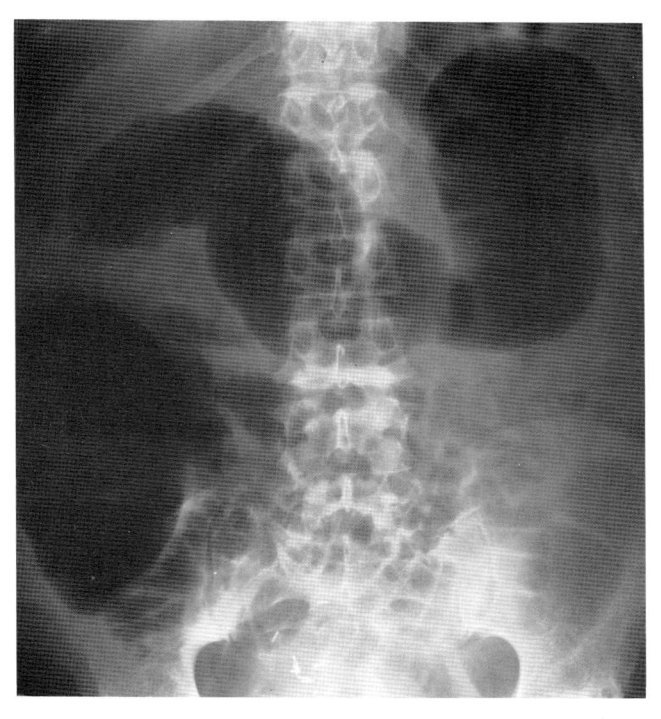

Figure **25 Colonic obstruction** (supine projection). Marked distension of the entire colon, with the exception of the rectosigmoid area, was caused by a metastatic ovarian carcinoma invading the sigmoid.

Table 5 (Cont.) Dilatation of the Colon

Disease	Radiographic Findings	Comments
Pancreatitis	Strictures occur rarely in the transverse or proximal descending colon, which may simulate primary or metastatic carcinoma, but are usually reversible.	Such a stricture has to be differentiated from an adynamic ileus of the transverse colon in pancreatitis producing the "colon cut-off sign." See under localized adynamic ileus of the colon in this table.
Lymphogranuloma venereum	Rectal strictures are late sequelae of the disease causing chronic obstruction.	In women and homosexual men following an evanescent primary genital lesion with subsequent enlargement of inguinal lymph nodes and fistula formation.
Volvulus (Figs. 26, 27)	Marked dilatation of twisted colonic segment with only mild to moderate dilatation of prestenotic bowel. Barium column from enema terminates characteristically as beak at point of obstruction. *Sigmoid:* Walls of dilated segment converge in 3 separate lines toward twisted mesenteric root, evident as soft-tissue density. Adjacent medial walls form a thicker central line, while each lateral wall forms a thinner peripheral line ("coffee bean" sign). Massively dilated, closed loop tends to project into the right upper abdomen. *Cecum:* Depending on torsion axis, markedly dilated cecum presents as single sac preferentially located in the midabdomen ("bag" type), or may have the shape of a kidney located in the left mid to upper quadrant, with the twisted mesentery simulating a dense renal hilum. *Transverse colon:* Twisted loop characteristically to the left of midline. A distended redundant and ptotic transverse colon (*"pseudovolvulus"*) must be differentiated by the fact that the walls do not converge towards a twisted mesentery.	Involves colon with mobile mesentery, most commonly the sigmoid, less frequently the cecum, and rarely the transverse colon. Usually in elderly patients, often from nursing homes or mental institutions. Characteristic is acute onset, but may be intermittent or occasionally even chronic. Compromised blood supply leads to bowel necrosis and subsequent perforation when not promptly treated.
Hernias (external and internal)	Similar to small bowel hernias (see Table 4, page 94) but less common, since only sigmoid and transverse colon have sufficient mobility to herniate.	Interposition of colon (or occasionally small bowel) between liver and diaphragm occurs in asymptomatic patients, but may rarely cause abdominal pain *(Chilaiditi syndrome)*.

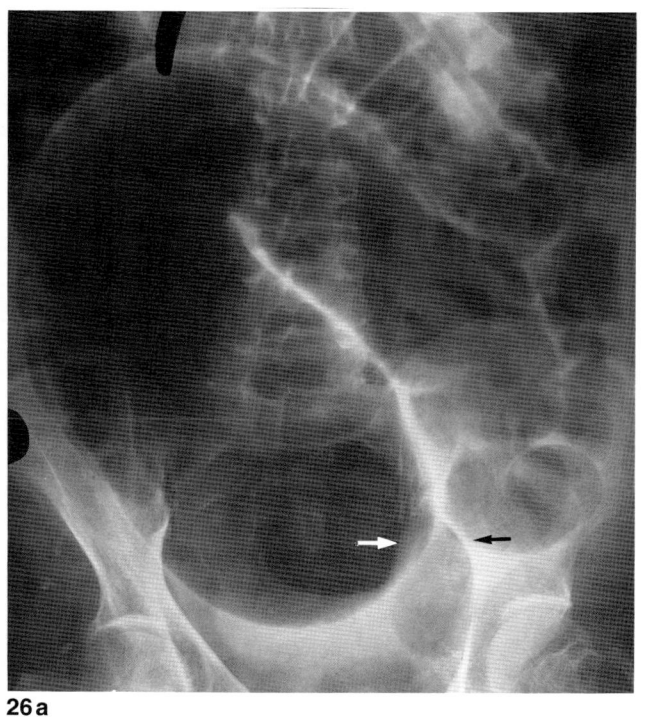

Dilatation and Motility Disorders in the Gastrointestinal Tract 101

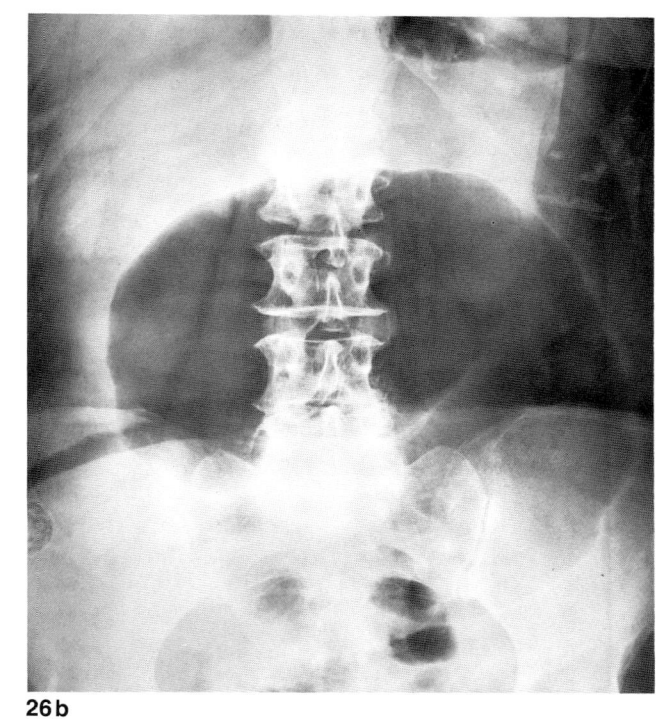

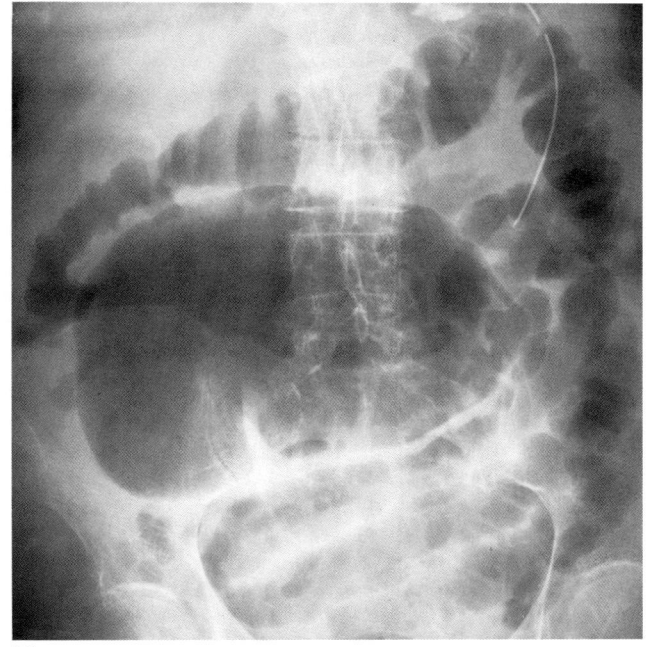

Figure **26a–c** **Volvulus of the colon** (supine projections). **a** Sigmoid volvulus resembling a "coffee bean". **b** Cecal volvulus assuming the shape of a kidney. **c** Cecal volvulus ("bag" type).

Figure **27a–c** **Volvulus of the colon. a** Sigmoid volvulus. Walls of dilated segment converge in 3 separate lines towards twisted mesenteric root (arrows). The adjacent medial walls form a thicker central line while each lateral wall forms a thinner peripheral line. The overall appearance resembles a coffee bean. Note also the moderate prestenotic colon dilatation and the absence of gas and fecal material in the distal sigmoid and rectum. **b** Cecal volvulus. The appearance resembles a kidney with the twisted mesentery simulating a dense renal hilum. Note also the collapsed poststenotic colon. **c** Cecal volvulus ("bag" type). The dilated cecum presents as sac-like lesion in the midabdomen. Note also the collapsed poststenotic colon.

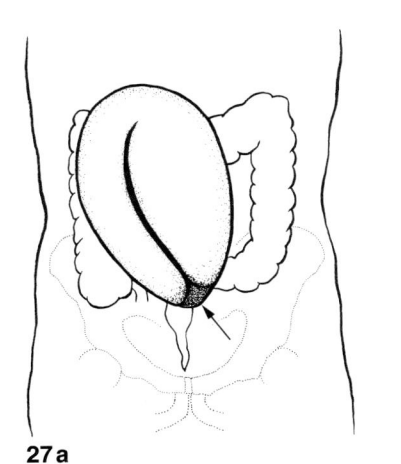

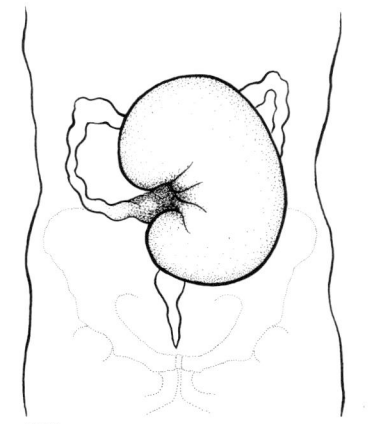

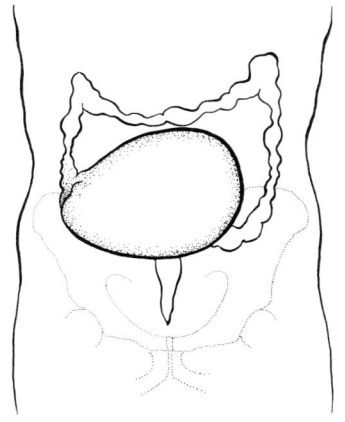

Table 5 (Cont.) Dilatation of the Colon

Disease	Radiographic Findings	Comments
Strictures (postoperative, postirradiation, posttraumatic, postinflammatory, postischemic) (Fig. 28)	Obstruction of involved segments, of varying length, is caused by circumferential narrowing (edema, hematoma, or fibrosis).	Postoperative obstruction at a stoma site (colostomy, iliostomy) can be difficult to differentiate on plain films from postoperative adynamic ileus, since dilatation of the bowel down to the stoma is present in both conditions.
Adhesions	Extrinsic or circumferential narrowing of a short segment.	Usually postoperative or postinflammatory, rarely developmental.
Nonobstructive		
Adynamic ileus, localized ("sentinel loop")	Localized colonic distension adjacent to acutely inflamed organ.	For example, terminal ileum and cecum in appendicitis, hepatic flexure in cholecystitis, transverse colon in pancreatitis, and descending colon in diverticulitis. The term "colon cut-off sign" was originally associated with the absence of gas in the transverse colon in pancreatitis, but was later used to describe the adynamic gaseous distension of part or the entire transverse colon with abrupt collapse ("cut-off") of its distal part or the splenic flexure.
Adynamic ileus, generalized	Colonic dilatation is part of generalized gastrointestinal tract dilatation.	See Table 4 (page 97) for various causes.
Peritonitis	Findings similar to adynamic ileus, but colonic dilatation usually prominent. Signs of ascites.	See Table 4, page 97.
Toxic megacolon (Fig. 29)	Dilatation of entire colon occurs, but transverse colon is usually the most affected segment, demonstrating marked distension, thinning of the wall, and loss of haustral markings. In less involved segments, haustra may even appear thickened. A few long air–fluid levels in the colon are usually found on upright or decubitus films. Pseudopolyps recognizable in the air-distended segments are virtually diagnostic for ulcerative colitis.	Characterized clinically by abdominal pain, fever, leukocytosis, and shock. Relatively common (5%) and life-threatening complication of *ulcerative colitis* and rare in other forms of enterocolitis (e.g., *amebiasis, cholera, typhoid fever, bacillary dysentery* and *Crohn's colitis*). *Ischemic colitis* can also present with identical clinical and radiographic findings.
Ischemic colitis	Most common presentation is a localized or generalized adynamic ileus. Haustra may be edematous and appear thickened. Intraluminal gas may outline multiple rounded soft tissue densities representing submucosal edema and hemorrhage ("thumb prints"). Presence of streaky gas in bowel wall and portal system is a very ominous sign (Fig. 23, page 98). Rapidly progressive ischemia may progress to "toxic megacolon" syndrome and perforation. Healing may occur with formation of a stricture and sacculations (pseudodiverticula).	Splenic flexure (at junction of superior and inferior mesenteric artery) is the most common location, followed by descending and sigmoid colon (supplied by inferior mesenteric artery), but every segment can be involved. Similar radiographic findings (adynamic ileus and "thumb printing") may occasionally be seen in a variety of bleeding disorders (e.g., *purpura Henoch–Schönlein, idiopathic thrombocytopenic purpura, anticoagulation therapy*) and *hereditary angioneurotic edema*.
Jejunoileal bypass	Chronic dilatation of entire colon. Cause unknown.	For examples, for morbid obesity. Abdominal distension and pain developing 1–3 years following bypass surgery.
Colonic pseudoobstruction (Ogilvie's syndrome or colonic ileus) (Fig. 31)	Disproportionate gaseous distension of the colon without organic obstruction. Massive cecal dilatation is often the dominating feature.	Usually associated with major systemic diseases or following abdominal or pelvic surgery. Cecostomy may be necessary to prevent perforation.

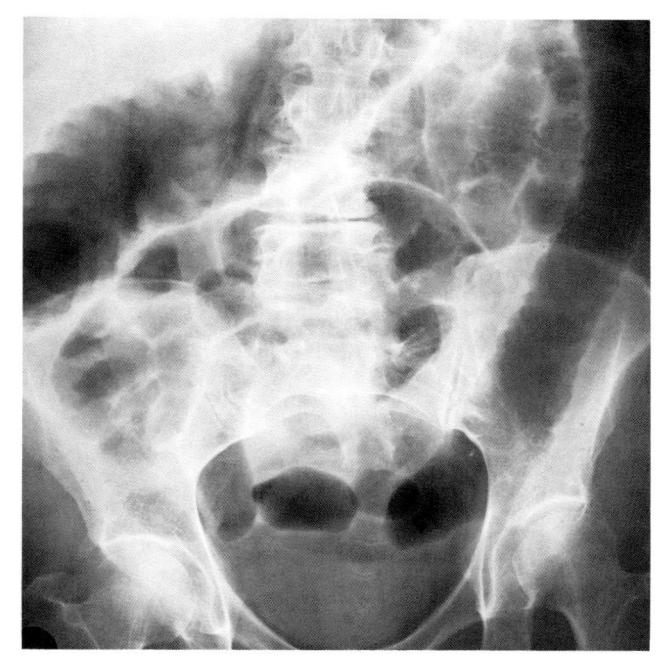

Dilatation and Motility Disorders in the Gastrointestinal Tract 103

Figure 28 **Inflammatory stricture of the sigmoid colon** (supine projection). A markedly dilated colon down to the sigmoid area is seen, whereas the rectum appears empty (virtually complete absence of gas and fecal material in this area).

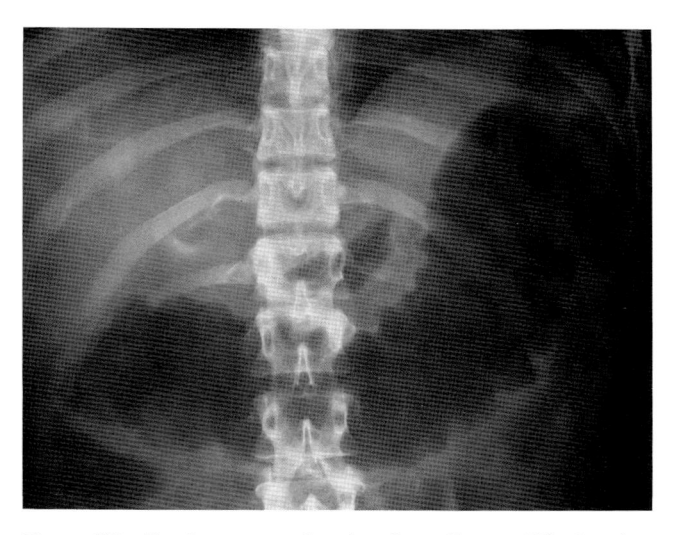

Figure 29 **Toxic megacolon in ulcerative colitis** (supine projection). Marked dilatation of the transverse colon, loss of haustral markings and pseudopolyps outlined by air are seen.

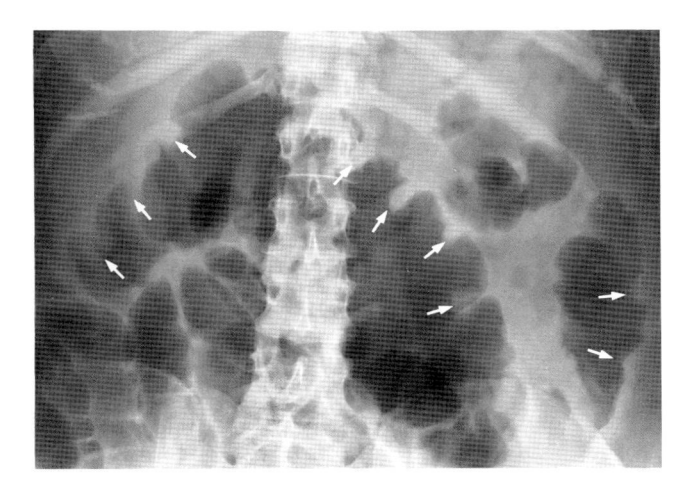

Figure 30 **Ischemic colitis.** A distended transverse colon with thickened haustra and "thumbprinting" (arrows) caused by submucosal edema and hemorrhage is seen.

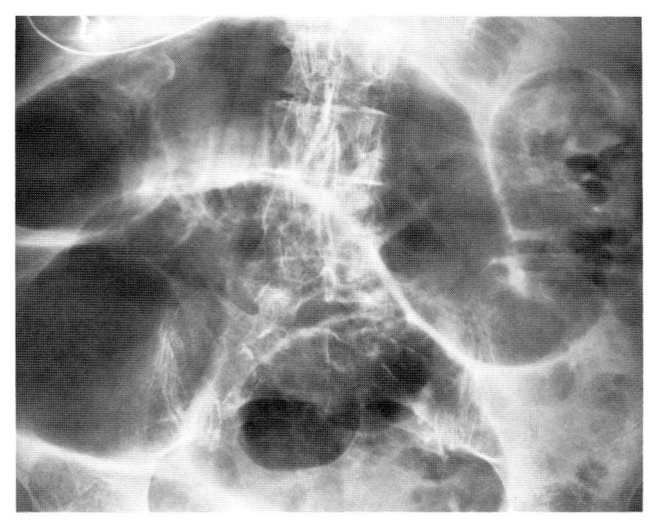

Figure 31 **Colonic pseudo-obstruction** (supine projection). Dilatation of the entire colon is seen, but is most pronounced in the cecum followed by the transverse colon.

Table 5 (Cont.) **Dilatation of the Colon**

Disease	Radiographic Findings	Comments
Hirschsprung's disease (aganglionosis) (Fig. 32)	Chronic dilatation of proximal colon with normal- or narrowed-appearing rectum and/or sigmoid representing the aganglionic segment.	Although characteristically a disease of childhood, it can be seen in adults, presenting with chronic constipation and progressive abdominal distension.
Chagas' disease	Besides megaesophagus, megacolon is most common manifestation.	Caused by *Trypanosoma cruzi,* which damages the ganglion cells in the myenteric plexus. Limited to South America.
Scleroderma	Findings usually more pronounced in esophagus and small-bowel. Colonic dilatation and loss of haustra occur. Sacculations (pseudodiverticula) on antimesenteric border (as in ischemic colitis) are quite characteristic.	Middle-aged women most commonly affected (male–female ratio, 1:3).
Amyloidosis	Colonic dilatation occurs only in rare cases.	Radiographic findings simulate more often ulcerative colitis (narrowing and thickening of bowel wall, absent haustral markings and multiple polypoid mass lesions).
Muscular dystrophies	Colonic dilatation may be segmental or complete.	Extracolonic findings are much more conspicuous.
Hypothyroidism	Although entire gastrointestinal tract may be affected, atony and dilatation (acute or chronic) is most striking in the colon.	Nonspecific symptoms of bloating, flatulence, and constipation are frequently present.
Idiopathic ("psychogenic" constipation, or "functional constipation")	Chronic dilatation of entire colon and rectum not associated with any disease.	May result from faulty bowel habits or may be the "functional" sequela of a completely healed disease.

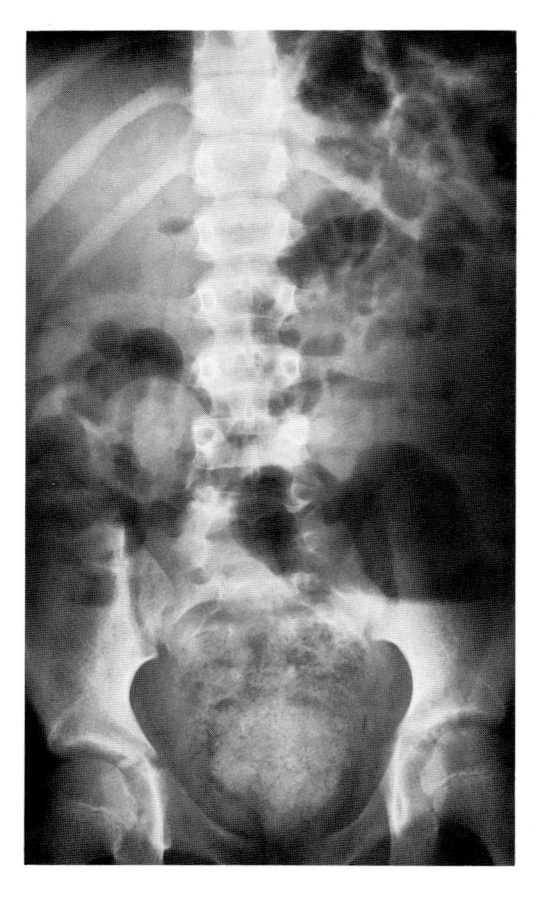

Figure **32 Hirschsprung's disease** (upright projection). Chronic dilatation of the colon with a few air–fluid levels and a large amount of fecal material in the rectosigmoid area is seen. The aganglionic segment was limited in this case to the distal rectum.

Chapter 5 Abnormal Mucosal Pattern in the Gastrointestinal Tract

The mucosal pattern of the gastrointestinal tract is best evaluated with a double-contrast examination, i.e., gaseous distension and mucosal coating with a thin layer of high density barium.

The fully distended normal *esophagus* has a smooth mucosal surface (Fig. **1**). As the esophagus collapses, the mucosal folds become visible as longitudinal, straight, and narrow folds (Fig. **2**). Rarely, delicate transverse folds appear in the mid-esophagus. They may represent contraction of the muscularis mucosae. Abnormal mucosal patterns include nodularity, superficial ulcerations, and abnormal mucosal folds. They usually represent esophagitis or varices, rarely a superficially spreading carcinoma.

In a fully distended *stomach* with good mucosal coating, the areae gastricae (the surface pattern) are visualized (Fig. **3**). The areae gastricae are most frequently seen in the antrum, in some patients also in the proximal body and fundus. The normal diameter of areae gastricae is about 2 to 3 mm in the antrum, somewhat larger in the body and fundus. The lack of visualization of areae gastricae may be due to technical factors and is not necessarily indicative of disease (Fig. **4**). An unusually coarse surface pattern may represent nonspecific inflammation (gastritis), intestinal metaplasia, or rarely, lymphoid hyperplasia of the gastric antrum. The coarse surface pattern is therefore indicative of a benign form of mucosal inflammation with questionable histological specificity (Fig. **5**).

In an incompletely distended stomach (Fig. **6**) and in conventional barium examination, the rugal folds of the stomach are well demonstrated, but they will flatten after proper gaseous distension. Persistence of the antral folds despite adequate distension is almost always due to antral gastritis. Large normal rugal folds in the body and fundus may be difficult to distinguish from those infiltrated by tumor or those caused by dilated veins of the gastric wall. Abnormal folds tend to be stiffer than normal and therefore resist effacement or gaseous distension. Localized abnormalities of the mucosal pattern are usually due to erosions, ulcers, polyps, carcinoma, or lymphoma.

The surface of the *duodenal bulb* is smoother than that of areae gastricae, representing the fine villous pattern of the duodenal mucosa. Nodularity in the mucosa of the duodenal bulb represents hyperplasia of Brunner's glands, duodenitis, or lymphoid nodular hyperplasia. Radial folds usually represent duodenal ulcer scars.

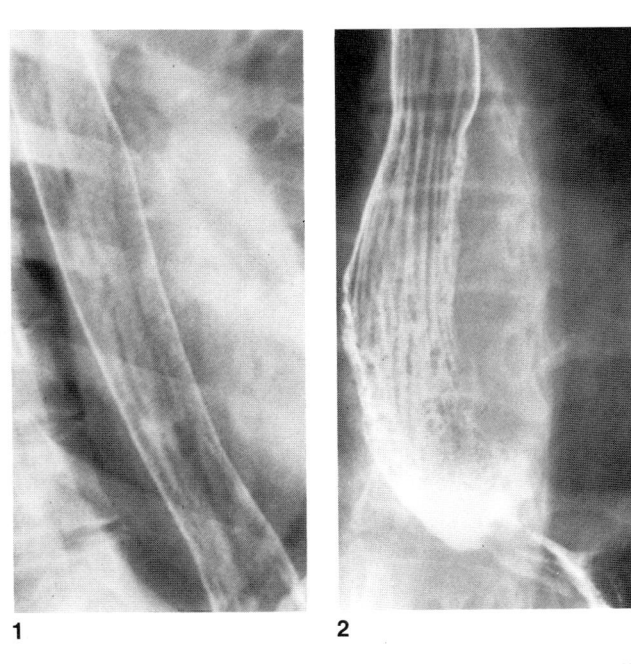

Figure **1 Normal smooth mucosal surface of the well-distended esophagus.**

Figure **2 Longitudinal mucosal folds in the normal esophagus** appear when gaseous distension decreases.

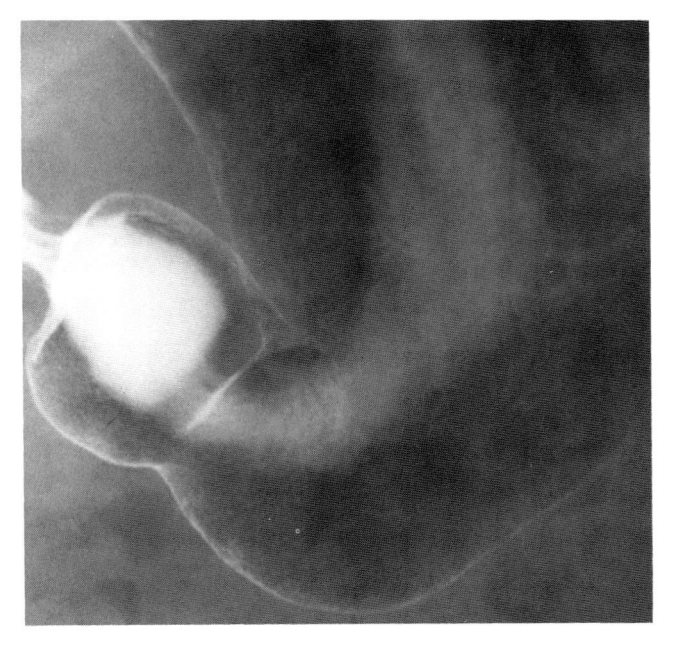

Figure **3 Normal surface pattern of a well-distended stomach** in double-contrast examination. The areae gastricae have a diameter of 2 to 3 mm in the antrum. They are slightly larger in the body.

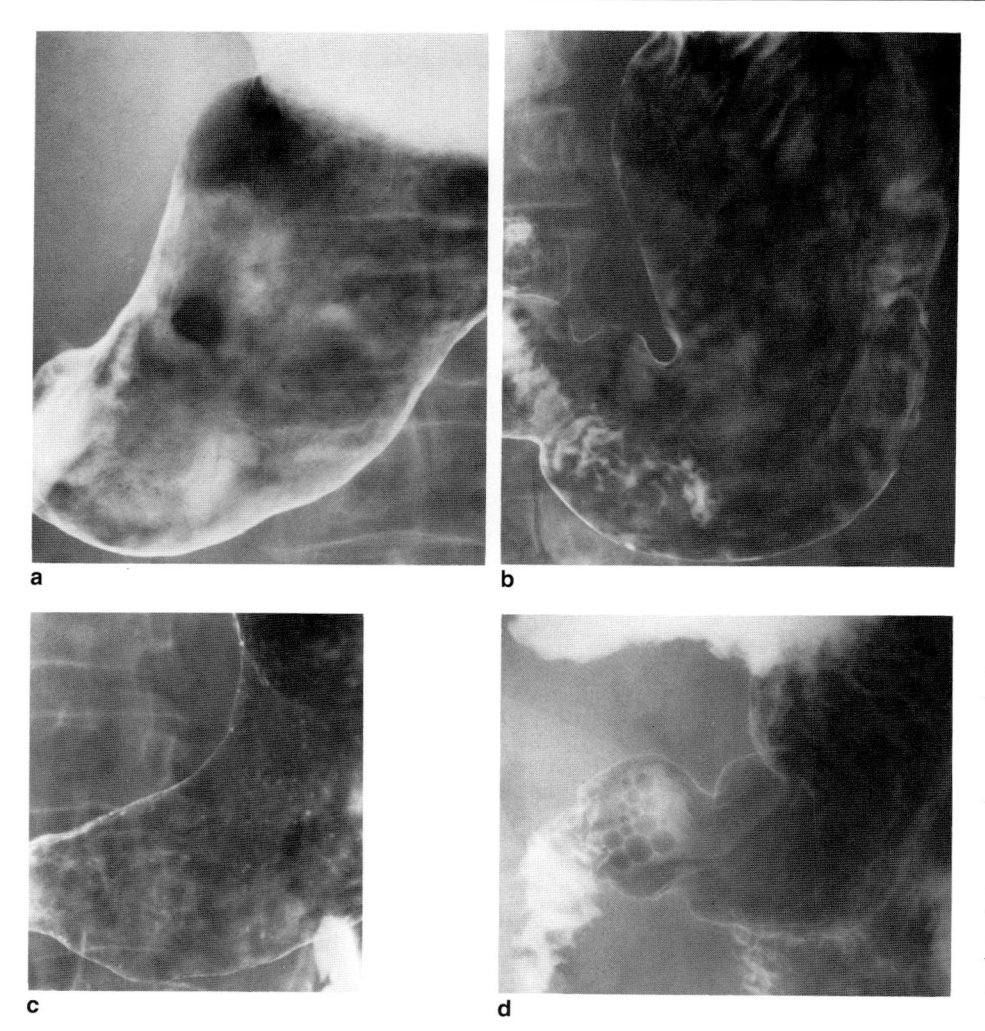

Figure 4a–d **Some artifactual surface patterns of the stomach** which should be distinguished from disease: **a** lack of visualization of the surface pattern due to too viscous barium suspension, **b** uneven coating of the mucosal surface may create ulcer like appearances, **c** small stippled densities over the mucosa from improper mixing of the contrast suspension. The densities represent unsuspended barium sulfate aggregates, **d** gas bubbles may resemble polyps but they, unlike polyps tend to aggregate together and finally coalesce.

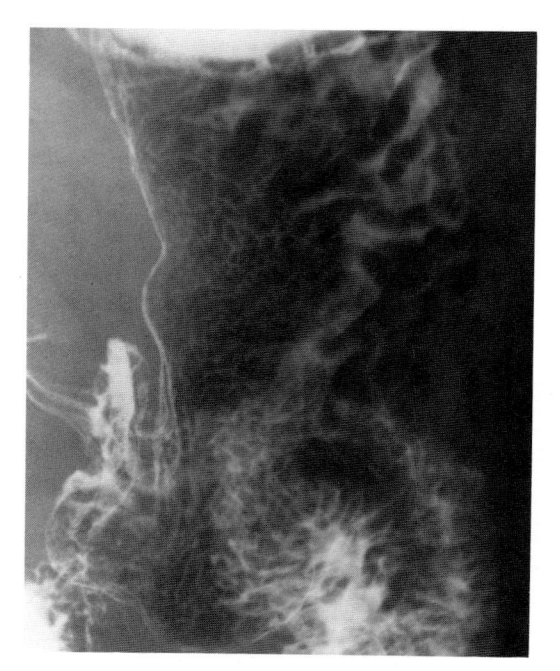

Figure 5 **Enlarged areae gastricae** (coarse surface pattern), a sign of benign mucosal inflammation without histologic specifity.

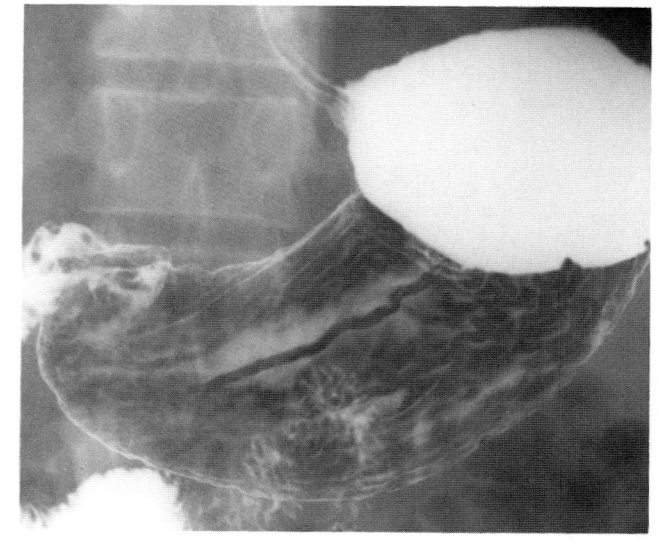

Figure 6 **Rugal folds** in a normal incompletely distended stomach.

The major landmarks of the *duodenal loop* are the circular valvulae conniventes and the papilla (ampulla of Vater) with its associated longitudinal folds (Fig. 7). Deformation of valvulae conniventes should raise a suspicion of a postbulbar duodenal ulcer, Crohn's disease, or pancreatic disease, especially carcinoma. Thickened or nodular folds point toward duodenitis.

Flocculation of contrast agent may create problems in the interpretation of the *small-bowel* mucosal pattern, especially in a single-contrast examination. A double-contrast examination with duodenal intubation enables the examiner to distend the whole small bowel. Combined with compression, this method makes it possible to study fold shapes more closely (Fig. 8). Valvulae conniventes are fewer and less pronounced in the ileum than in the jejunum. With the bowel distended, they run relatively straight across the long axis. Sometimes they may crowd together to create a triangular pattern, which has no diagnostic significance. Normal jejunal folds are about 2 mm thick, ileal folds about 1.5 mm thick. Fold thickness exceeding 2.5 mm in the jejunum and 2 mm in the ileum is considered to be pathological. Usually two to three folds are seen per centimeter in the jejunum and one to three folds in the ileum, depending on the degree of distension. The height of folds has little diagnostic significance. Numerous 2–3 mm rounded elevations, representing lymph follicles, may normally be present in the terminal ileum of children and adolescents (Fig. 9).

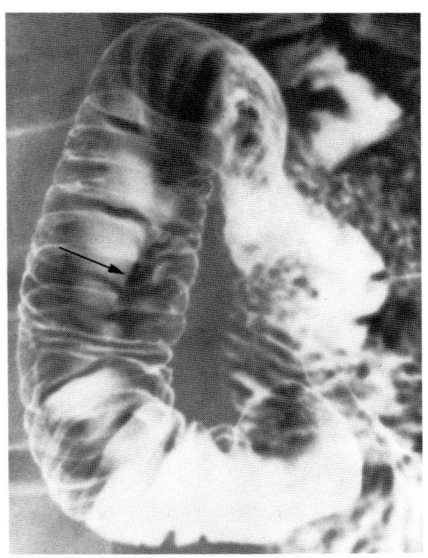

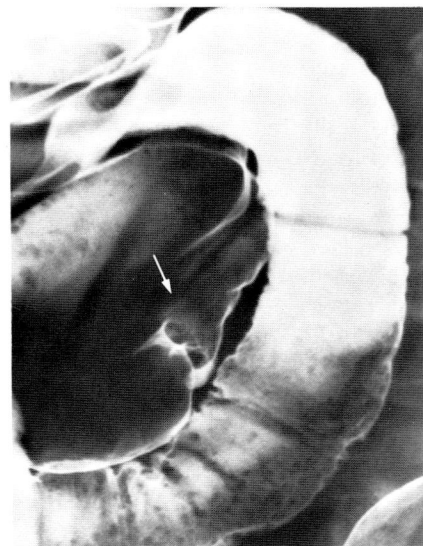

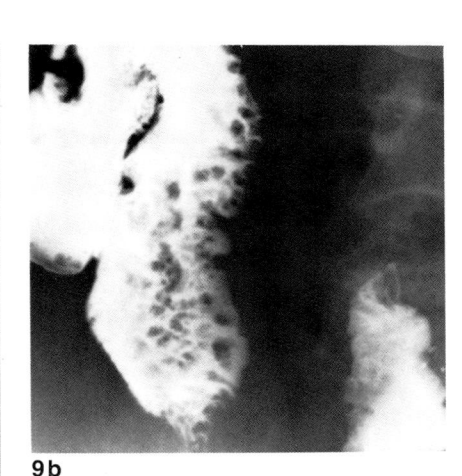

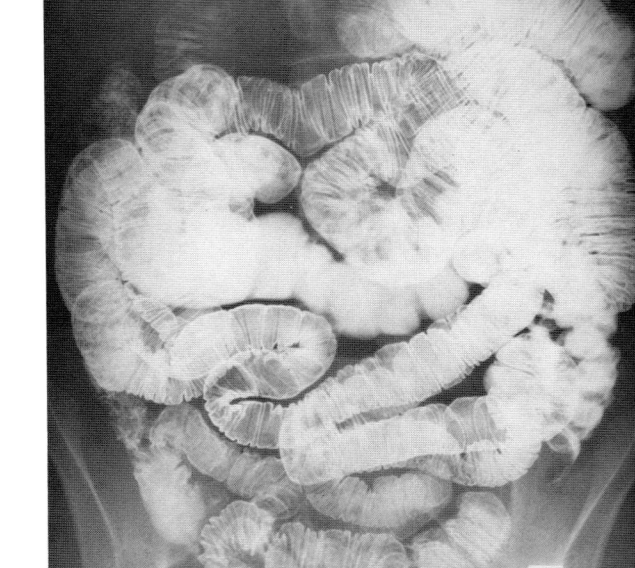

Figure 7 **Normal mucosal fold pattern of the duodenum.** The longitudinal fold in the posteromedial wall (arrow) is associated with the duodenal papilla.

Figure 8 **Normal mucosal fold pattern of the small bowel** in a double-contrast study. The diameter of small bowel, fold thickness, and the number of folds all decrease from proximal jejunum to distal ileum.

Figure 9a, b **Nodular lymphoid hyperplasia. a** Lymph follicles. 2–3-mm-wide rounded elevations are seen in the distal ileum. The film also demonstrates a typical postappendicectomy deformity in the distal end of the cecum (white arrow). **b** Enlarged lymph follicles. Age 17.

Abnormalities of the mucosal pattern of the small intestine include thickening of folds, with or without nodular appearances. These patterns can be combined with variable degrees of dilatation of the bowel and increase of intestinal fluid. The latter is often considered an unreliable sign, since technical factors may cause poor coating and flocculation of barium, mimicking increased fluid content. The diameter of an undistended, barium-filled small bowel is not more than 2.5 to 3 cm. In a duodenal intubation study, the diameter of the small bowel exceeding 4.5 cm in the upper jejunum, 4 cm in the mid-small bowel, and 3 cm in the distal ileum is considered abnormal.

Inflammatory bowel disease (e.g., Crohn's disease) and malignant tumors (with the exception of small bowel lymphoma) generally produce localized lesions (stenosis, dilatation, or ulceration) rather than diffuse mucosal abnormality.

In the *colon,* the mucosal pattern is best evaluated with the double contrast examination. The normal colonic mucosa is thin, smooth, and straight, essentially featureless except for the haustral markings (Fig. **10**). A series of tightly spaced circular folds may be seen as a transient phenomenon in some patients, most frequently in children. The colonic mucosa may be studded with tiny nodules, 1 to 2 mm in diameter. They represent lymph follicles, and are usually unrelated to disease. Large, umbilicated lymph follicles may represent a response to infection, allergy, or an immunologic deficiency state. Such changes are rare in adults. Abnormal mucosal patterns are encountered in colonic polyposis, diverticulosis, ulcerative colitis, Crohn's disease, and other less common forms of colitis. Granular mucosa, ulceration and inflammatory polyps alone or in combination, and possibly associated with strictures and fistulas may be seen. Flocculation and cracking of the barium sulfate layer on the colonic mucosa represents drying of the suspension on the mucosa and the effect of peristalsis and should be distinguished from a true mucosal abnormality (Fig. **11**).

In the *rectum* there are usually three prominent folds, called the valves of Houston. In a partially collapsed rectum, the columns of Morgagni may be seen in the distal portion. The surface pattern of the rectal mucosa is smooth, similar to that of the colon. Mucosal abnormalities of the rectum are seen in the same diseases which affect the colon. In addition, hemorrhoids may appear as tortuous or polypoid filling defects similar to esophageal varices.

Conditions associated with abnormal mucosal pattern in the gastrointestinal tract are presented in Tables **1** through **5.**

Table 1 Abnormal Mucosal Pattern in the Esophagus

Disease	Radiographic Findings	Comments
Reflux esophagitis (Figs. 12 and 13)	Mild forms are radiographically negative. Earliest findings in double-contrast studies consist of streaks or dots of barium in superficial mucosal erosions, or of a diffuse granular or cobblestone pattern. In a single-contrast study, the mucosa is hazy or serrated, possibly with erosions or widened, edematous longitudinal folds.	Reflux may not be demonstrated during the examination. Predisposing conditions include hiatal hernia, prolonged or repeated vomiting, chalasia of infancy, pregnancy, scleroderma, drugs (such as anticholinergics, nitrites, beta-adrenergic agents, and tranquilizers), and esophageal or gastric surgery. Ulcer or stricture may be seen in more severe disease.
Infectious esophagitis (Figs. 14–16)	Small marginal filling defects with fine serrations may progress to an irregular cobblestone pattern, deep ulcerations, and sloughing of mucosa. Usually the whole esophagus is involved.	The most common cause is *candidiasis* affecting patients with malignancy (especially leukemia, lymphoma, or AIDS) or as a complication of radiation therapy, chemotherapy, corticosteroids, or other immunosuppressive agents. Diabetes mellitus, systemic lupus erythematosus, primary hyperparathyroidism, and renal failure are other predisposing conditions. *Herpetic* esophagitis usually produces an identical radiographic pattern. Rarely, *tuberculous esophagitis* or esophageal *Crohn's disease* may be the cause of a cobblestone pattern.

Abnormal Mucosal Pattern in the Gastrointestinal Tract 109

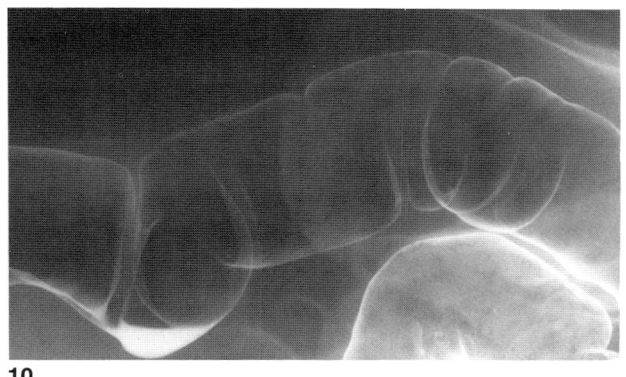

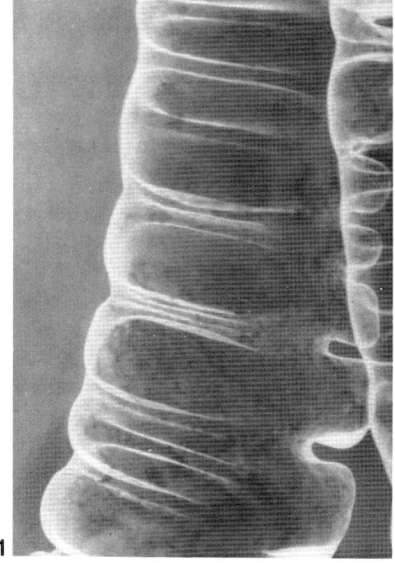

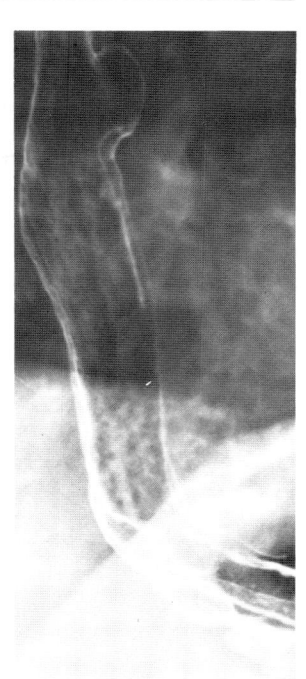

Figure 10 **Normal mucosa of the colon.** Only haustral markings are recognizable.

Figure 11 **Flocculation and cracking of the barium sulfate** layer covering the large bowel mucosa. It should not be confused with a mucosal abnormality. This phenomenon increases with time as water is resorbed from the barium suspension.

Figure 12 **Reflux esophagitis.** Thickened folds with irregular barium coating of the mucosa represents surface erosions. A traction diverticulum is demonstrated in the midesophagus.

Figure 13 **Reflux esophagitis** with a flat cobblestone pattern.

Figure 14 **Esophageal moniliasis** in a patient receiving cancer chemotherapy. Multiple marginal filling defects and fine serrations are seen.

Figure 15 **Esophageal moniliasis.** Large filling defects and ulcerations as well as sloughing of the mucosa are seen.

Figure 16 **Esophageal moniliasis** in an AIDS patient. Severe mucosal edema with deep longitudinal ulcerations.

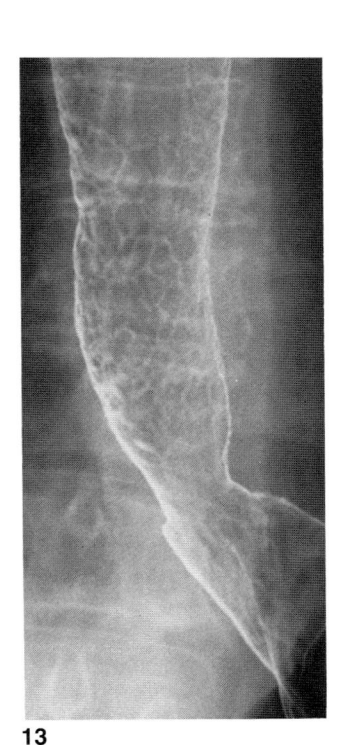

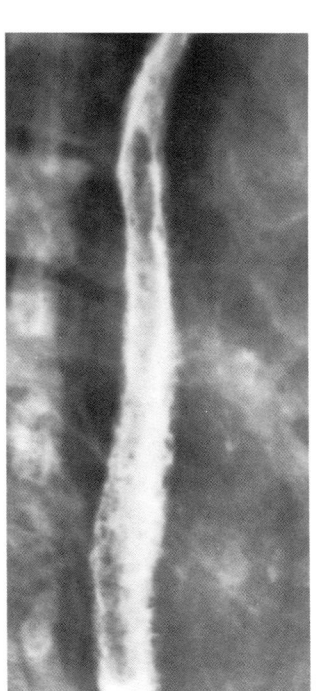

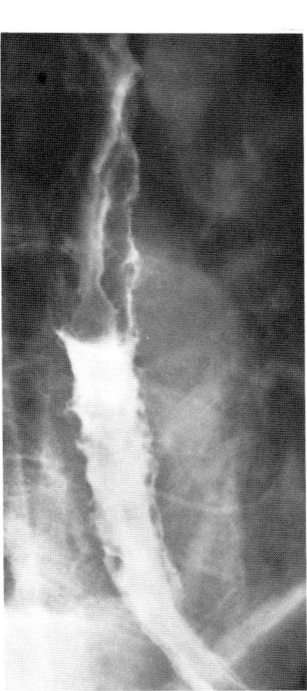

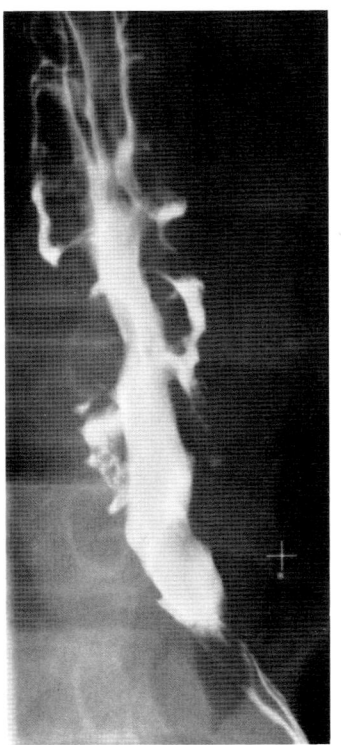

Table 1 (Cont.) Abnormal Mucosal Pattern in the Esophagus

Disease	Radiographic Findings	Comments
Esophageal carcinoma (with superficial spread) (Fig. 17)	Multiple nodular filling defects associated with impaired distensibility of the wall of the esophagus.	Nodular, submucosal spread is a rare manifestation of esophageal carcinoma. A filling defect, ulcer, or local narrowing are more common manifestations.
Corrosive esophagitis	Mucosal edema and/or a diffusely granular pattern may be present in early phase.	Alkali tends to produce more severe esophageal injuries than acid. Mucosal ulceration is followed by gradual narrowing of the esophagus within a few weeks.
Radiation esophagitis	Serrations, small marginal filling defects, or a cobblestone pattern; identical to esophageal candidiasis.	Doses greater than 45 Gy frequently lead to severe esophagitis and stricturation. Even doses less than 20 Gy can cause esophagitis if combined with chemotherapy (especially adriamycin or actinomycin D therapy).
Leukoplakia	Small, superficial filling defects with somewhat poorly defined borders, usually in the middle esophagus. Peristalsis is not impaired.	Small round foci of epithelial hyperplasia. Usually found only in esophagoscopy, radiographic presentation is rare.
Acanthosis nigrigans	Multiple verrucous proliferations throughout the mucosa, similar to skin changes. May produce a radiographic appearance of finely nodular filling defects.	A premalignant skin disorder characterized by papillomatosis, pigmentation, and hyperkeratosis, which may involve the esophagus.
Intramural esophageal pseudodiverticulosis	Numerous 1–3 mm outpouchings, mimicking multiple ulcers, but appear as a chain of beads. May be associated with a smooth stricture in the upper esophagus and/or candidiasis.	An extremely rare disorder of unknown origin with dilated ducts of the submucosal esophageal glands.
Esophageal varices (Fig. 18)	Initially mild thickening of folds and irregularity of esophageal outline, easily hidden behind complete filling with barium. Later tortuous, ribbon-like defects involve the distal esophagus. Early varices are generally situated in the right anterolateral wall of the distal esophagus.	Associated with portal hypertension, superior vena cava obstruction and rarely with noncirrhotic diffuse liver disease or congestive heart failure. Small varices may mimic mild chronic esophagitis (thick folds). Pliability of the wall and the varices can be used to differentiate the condition from varicoid esophageal carcinoma.

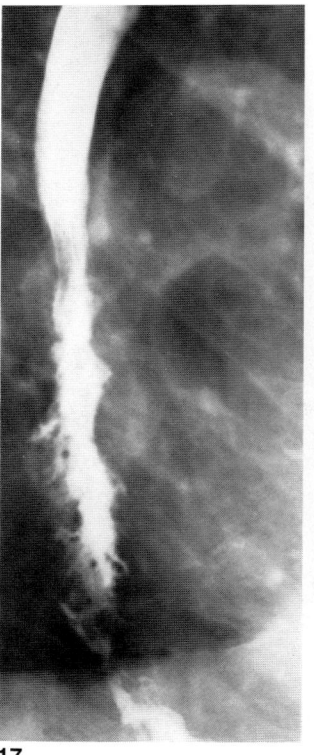

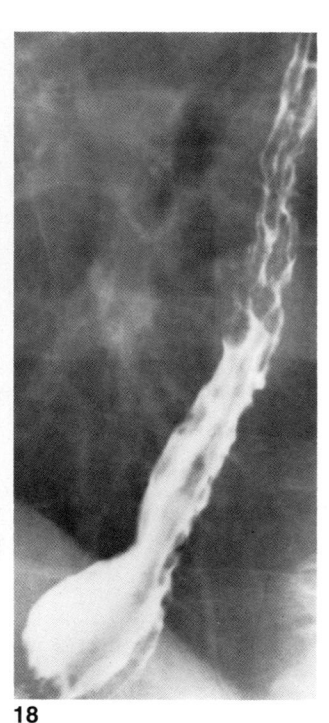

Figure 17 **Esophageal carcinoma.** Filling defects and ulcerations in the narrow esophagus resemble severe esophagitis. The lesion is localized whereas esophagitis usually involves the whole esophagus.

Figure 18 **Esophageal varices.** Tortuous, smooth filling defects are pliable and involve the distal esophagus only.

Table 2 Abnormal Mucosal Pattern in the Stomach

Disease	Radiographic Findings	Comments
Normal variant Hypertrophic gastritis Alcoholic gastritis	Apparent thickening of the mucosal folds, which may be over 5 mm wide in the fundus and proximal body. The folds stretch evenly and appear thinned when the stomach is distended.	Thickening of folds is more common in association with gastritis than in normal population but transient gastritis (e. g., alcoholic) or so-called hypertrophic gastritis cannot be differentiated from normal variant radiographically. Histological evidence of gastritis if often present without radiographic abnormality.
Viral gastritis (Fig. 19)	Occurs in association with viral gastroenteritis, and is seen as a nonspecific thickening of mucosal folds.	Cytomegalovirus gastroenteritis may complicate AIDS and immunosuppressive therapy.
Antral gastritis	Thickening of mucosal folds is localized to the antrum. Often associated with lack of normal antral distension, asymmetric peristaltic waves, or mucosal wrinkling.	A controversial entity most likely representing one end of the spectrum of peptic ulcer disease.
Corrosive gastritis	Thickened gastric folds, mucosal ulcerations, atony and rigidity of the antrum and lower body.	Usually results from ingestion of acids or highly concentrated alkali.
Infectious gastritis	Thickened gastric folds possibly gas in the wall of the stomach (if gas-forming organism).	May be associated with botulism, diphtheria, dysentery, typhoid fever, or anisakiasis
Radiation gastritis	Thickened gastric folds followed by rigidity or luminal narrowing.	A diagnostic possibility if the patient has received more than 45 Gy to the upper abdomen.
Peptic ulcer disease	Thickening of gastric folds, increased gastric fluids despite fasting, and a peptic ulcer may be present.	The degree of enlargement of gastric folds in the body and fundus have a positive correlation to the level of acid secretion. Very prominent folds are characteristic of *Zollinger–Ellison syndrome,* in which ulcers of the distal duodenum are common.

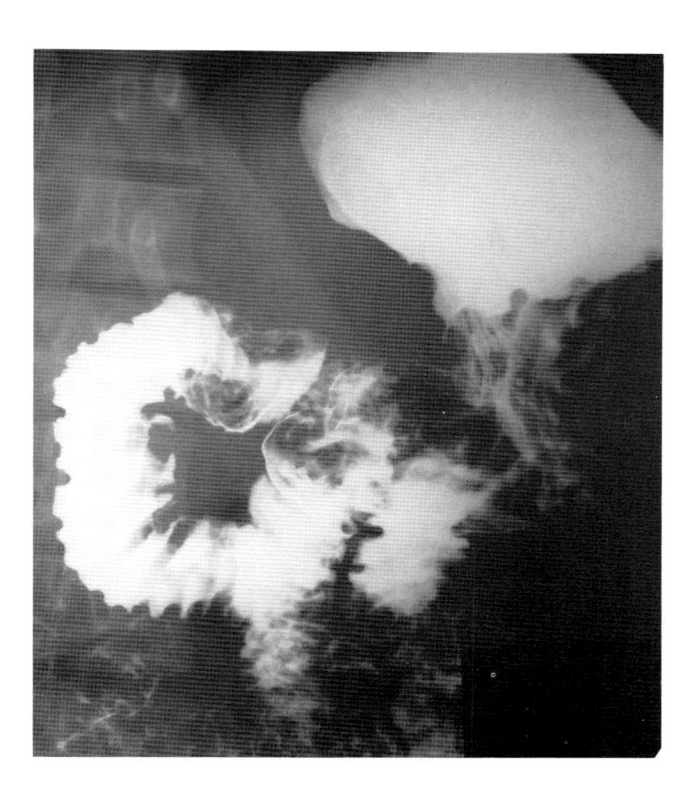

Figure **19** **Cytomegalovirus gastroenteritis** in an AIDS patient. Gastric and small-bowel folds are thick and irregular.

Table 2 (Cont.) Abnormal Mucosal Pattern in the Stomach

Disease	Radiographic Findings	Comments
Gastric scarring (Fig. 20)	Abnormal course of gastric folds, with or without fold enlargement. DD: Gastric carcinoma.	May be secondary to peptic ulcer disease, corrosive gastritis or trauma (surgery).
Ménétrier's disease	Massive enlargement of irregular rugal folds, particularly in the greater curvature. Folds may mimic polyps. Excessive mucus may produce mottled mucosal surface.	Hyperplasia and hypertrophy of the gastric glands. May be the cause of a protein-losing enteropathy. Increased incidence of adenocarcinoma of the stomach.
Uremia (Fig. 21)	Enlarged rugal folds.	Uremia is often associated with enlargement of gastric and duodenal folds, although not as extensive as in Ménétrier's disease.
Gastric lymphoma (Fig. 22)	Thickening, distortion, or nodularity of gastric rugal folds. Often associated with a polypoid and ulcerated lesions, a retrogastric mass, or an enlarged spleen.	May mimic Ménétrier's disease, but often involves also the distal portion of the stomach, the lesser curvature, and even duodenum.
Pseudolymphoma	Enlarged gastric rugal folds, often associated with a large gastric ulcer.	A benign proliferation of lymphoid tissue that can be mistaken histologically for malignant lymphoma.
Gastric carcinoma	Enlarged, tortuous, and coarse gastric folds simulating lymphoma are an unusual presentation of gastric carcinoma. Colloid carcinoma and mucinous adenocarcinoma may contain punctate calcifications (psammoma bodies). A polypoid gastric cancer may have a surface pattern comparable to surrounding areae gastricae, if only the submucosa is involved.	Due to variable radiographic patterns of gastric carcinoma, all mucosal abnormalities require endoscopic verification.
Gastric varices (Fig. 23)	Multiple, pliable, smooth, lobulated filling defects in the fundus projecting between curvilinear, crescenting collections of barium. Concomitant esophageal varices are common. May involve the lesser curvature, unlike Ménétrier's disease. Varices do not cause wall rigidity as does malignancy.	Associated with *portal hypertension*. Gastric varices without esophageal varices indicate isolated splenic vein occlusion (e.g., *pancreatitis* or *pancreatic carcinoma*).
Eosinophilic gastritis	Thickening of folds usually in the distal half of the stomach.	A rare diffuse infiltration of the rugal folds by eosinophilic leukocytes associated with blood eosinophilia.
Granulomatous disease, amyloidosis	Rugal enlargement may precede antral narrowing and rigidity.	A rare presentation of *Crohn's disease, sarcoidosis, tuberculosis, syphilis,* or amyloidosis.
Pancreatitis	Selective prominence of the mucosal folds of the posterior wall and the lesser curvature.	Becomes evident a few days after clinical onset of pancreatitis and returns to normal when clinical symptoms improve. Not present in mild pancreatitis.
Pancreatic carcinoma	Enlarged folds predominantly in the greater curvature may be seen.	Caused by direct metastatic invasion.

Abnormal Mucosal Pattern in the Gastrointestinal Tract 113

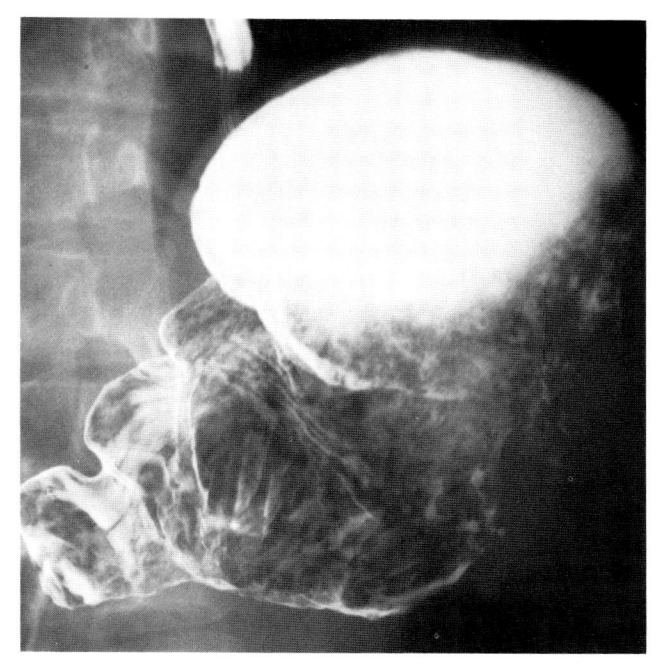

Figure 20 **Gastric scarring secondary to peptic ulcer.** The gastric folds take an abnormal course and the involved area appears rigid, mimicking carcinoma.

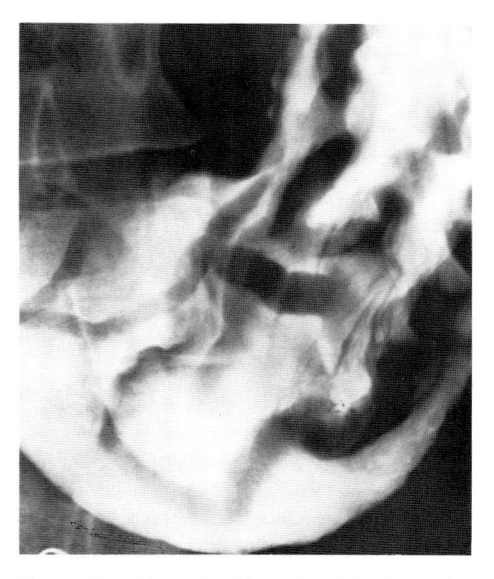

Figure 21 **Uremia.** Hypertrophic, irregular gastric folds are seen.

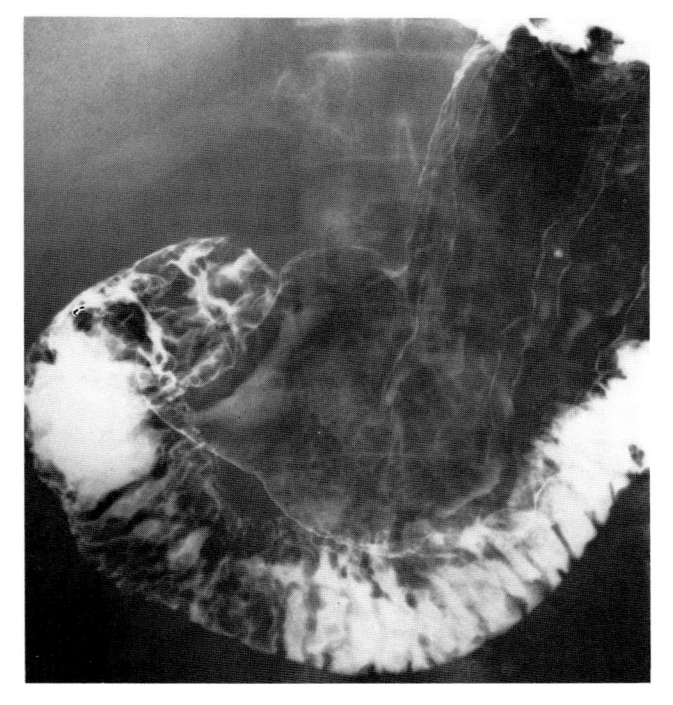

Figure 22 **Gastric and duodenal lymphoma.** Thick gastric folds, do not efface even with good gaseous distension. The surface pattern is coarse and irregular.

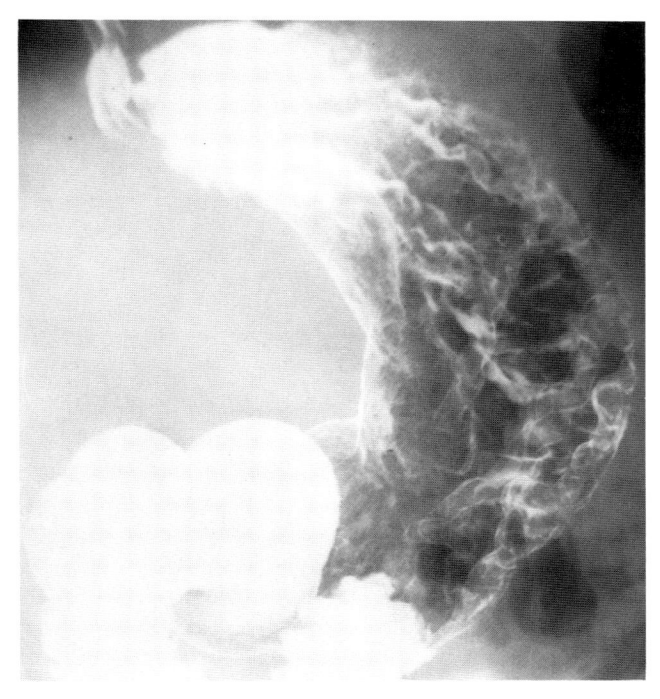

Figure 23 **Gastric varices** (carcinoma of pancreas with splenic vein thrombosis). Smooth, enlarged gastric folds in the body and fundus of the stomach are seen. The gastric wall is not rigid. There is no evidence of esophageal varices.

Table 2 (Cont.) Abnormal Mucosal Pattern in the Stomach

Disease	Radiographic Findings	Comments
Gastric polyposis (hyperplastic polyposis, familial adenomatous polyposis, Gardner's syndrome, Peutz–Jeghers syndrome, Canada–Cronkhite syndrome, Cowden's disease) Fig. 24)	Multiple polypoid filling defects in the gastric mucosa, often associated with polyposis in the colon. Hyperplastic polyps are small (less than 1 cm) and uniform in size. Adenomatous polyps tend to be larger (over 2 cm).	Multiple hyperplastic polyps may result from excessive regeneration of the epithelium in chronic gastritis. Numerous small polyps of the stomach are found in patients with familial adenomatous polyposis of the colon and in Gardner's syndrome (polyposis, osteomas in facial bones), Peutz–Jeghers syndrome (hamartomatous polyposis of small bowel and mucocutaneous pigmentation), Canada–Cronkhite syndrome (diarrhea, alopecia, atrophy of the nails, skin pigmentation, and diffuse gastrointestinal polyposis). Cowden's disease is characterized by multiple hamartomatous polyps, circumoral papillomatosis, and nodular gingival hyperplasia. Filiform gastric polyposis is a rare presentation of *Crohn's disease*.
Enlarged areae gastricae (Fig. 25; Fig. 5, p. 106)	A coarse surface pattern caused by prominent areae gastricae.	Associated with nonspecific inflammation, intestinal metaplasia, or benign lymphoid hyperplasia.
Erosive gastritis (Fig. 25)	Tiny flecks of barium representing erosion, surrounded by a radiolucent halo representing a mound of edematous mucosa. May not be seen in single-contrast examination. Incomplete erosions may not have surrounding reaction and tend to remain undetected.	May be "idiopathic" or associated with predisposing conditions (e.g., alcohol, anti-inflammatory drugs, analgesics, emotional stress). Aphthoid ulcers of Crohn's disease or candidiasis may have an identical appearance.

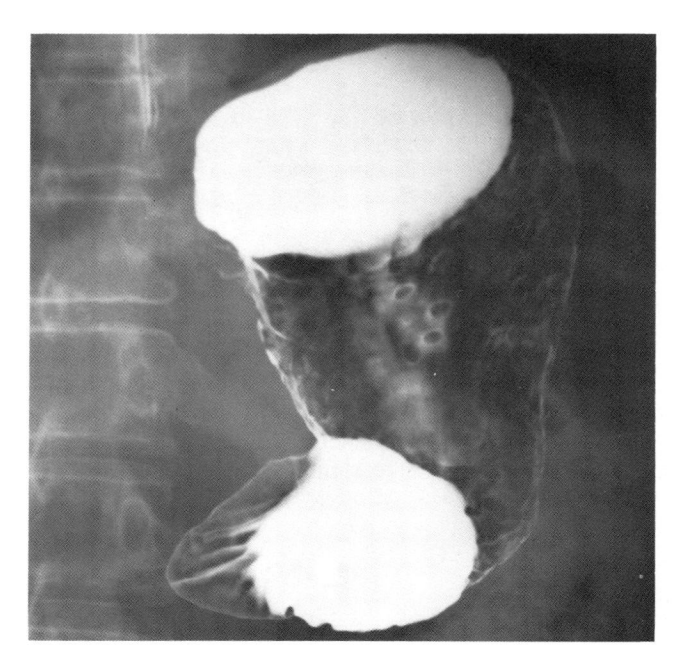

Figure 24 **Gastric polyposis.** Multiple polypoid filling defects in the gastric mucosa.

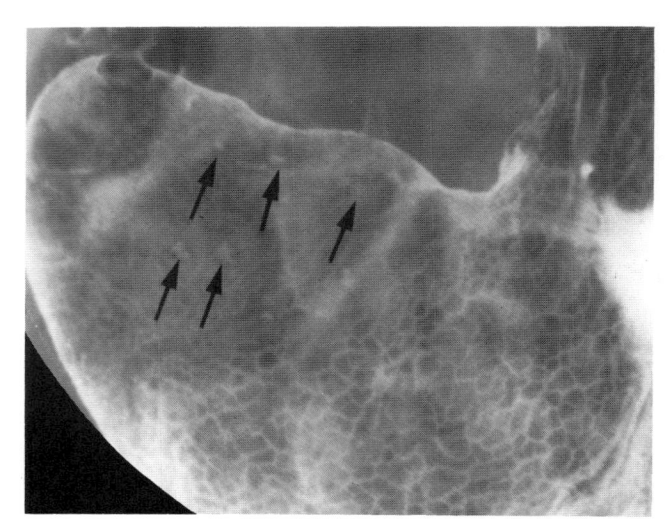

Figure 25 **Erosive gastritis.** The erosions are seen as tiny flecks of barium surrounded by a radiolucent halo. The surface pattern is coarse (enlarged areae gastricae).

Table 3 Abnormal Mucosal Pattern in the Duodenum

Disease	Radiographic Findings	Comments
Brunner's gland hyperplasia	Multiple nodular filling defects or nodular thickening of folds in the duodenal bulb and in the proximal half of the second segment of the duodenum.	Probably represents a response of the duodenal mucosa to peptic ulcer disease.
Benign lymphoid hyperplasia (Fig. 9, p. 107)	Innumerable tiny nodular defects evenly scattered throughout the duodenum without wall rigidity.	Proliferation of lymphoid aggregates without known cause or associated with hypogammaglobulinemia.
Peptic ulcer disease	Duodenal fold thickening may represent mucosal edema or diffuse hyperplasia of Brunner's glands (nodular thickening).	If associated with enlarged gastric rugal folds and distal ulcerations of the duodenum, one should consider the *Zollinger–Ellison syndrome* (non-beta islet cell tumor of pancreas with elevated gastric secretion).
Pancreatitis	Edematous thickened folds in the periampullary region and proximal descending duodenum.	Similar changes can be associated with other types of adjacent periduodenal inflammation, e.g., *cholecystitis*.
Uremia	Irregular, swollen, and stiffened folds in the duodenal bulb and second portion of the duodenum. High incidence of hyperplastic polyps in the same area.	Fold thickening may simulate changes caused by pancreatitis, a frequent complication of uremia.
Crohn's disease	The early lesions consist of superficial erosions, aphthoid ulcers and fold thickening, usually in the bulb and proximal second segment. Later findings consist of narrowing and scarring.	Duodenal involvement has been reported in 1% to over 20% of patients with Crohn's disease. Similar changes occur rarely in duodenal *tuberculosis* or *strongyloidiasis*.
Giardiasis (Fig. 26)	Nodular thickening and edema of duodenal and jejunal folds. Increased secretions.	A bizarre pattern of nodular fold thickening in the duodenum may represent an early stage of *nontropical sprue*.
Lymphoma (Fig. 27)	Coarse, nodular, irregular folds, with or without mass lesions.	A mass lesion is a more common presentation.
Pancreatic carcinoma	May cause localized nodular impressions and thick folds due to impaired lymph drainage.	*Metastases to peripancreatic lymph nodes* can have a similar appearance.

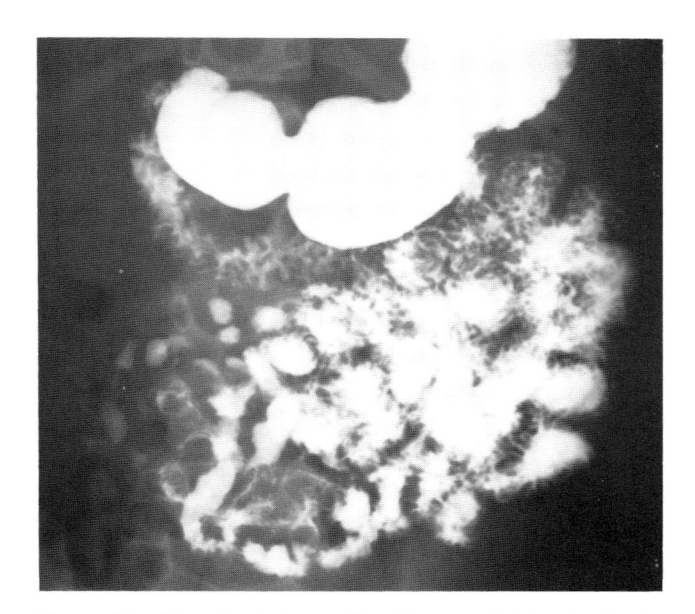

Figure 26 **Giardiasis** in a child. Mucosal thickening in the duodenum and proximal jejunum with increased secretions seen as poor coating of the mucosa.

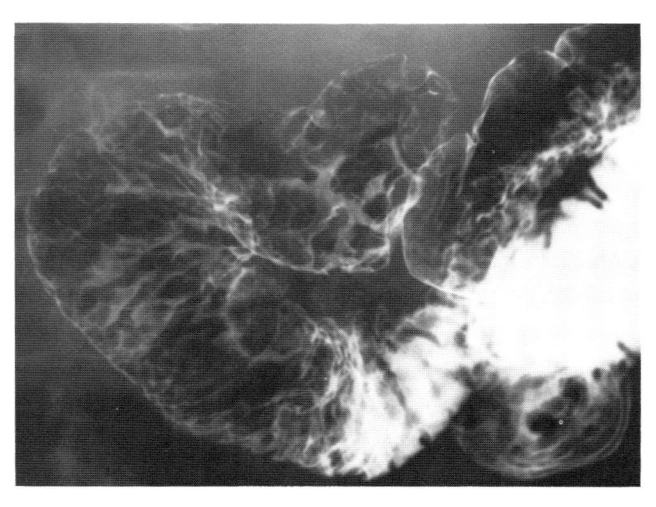

Figure 27 **Lymphoma.** Coarse, nodular, irregular folds of the duodenal sweep and large, smooth nodular filling defects in the duodenal bulb.

Table 3 (Cont.) Abnormal Mucosal Pattern in the Duodenum

Disease	Radiographic Findings	Comments
Whipple's disease **Amyloidosis** **Mastocytosis** **Eosinophilic enteritis** **Intestinal lymphangiectasia**	Thickening of duodenal folds in association with diffuse small bowel disease.	See Table 4, p. 117.
Vascular impressions (duodenal varices, mesenteric arterial collaterals)	Small varices or enlarged arteries may cause a diffuse polypoid or serpiginous mucosal pattern, mimicking fold thickening or Brunner's gland hyperplasia.	Varices are secondary to portal hypertension. Esophageal varices are usually present. True mucosal fold thickening may be present due to venous congestion. Collateral circulation through the gastroduodenal and pancreaticoduodenal arteries is caused by mesenteric arteriosclerotic occlusive disease.
Duodenal hemorrhage	"Stacked coins" appearance of mucosal fold thickening, associated with an intramural mass.	May be a complication of trauma to the upper abdomen or caused by anticoagulant therapy.
Cystic fibrosis (Mucoviscidosis)	Thickened, coarse, proximal duodenal folds, often associated with nodular indentations and distorted, contour of the duodenal sweep.	The cause of these changes is not known.
Erosive duodenitis	Central collections of barium surrounded by a radiolucent halo, most frequently seen in the duodenal bulb.	Erosive changes are only demonstrated by double contrast technique. Erosive, hemorrhagic duodenitis may be associated with a *duodenal ulcer* or be a complication of *myocardial infarction* or *congestive heart failure*.
Duodenal polyposis	Multiple polypoid filling defects in the duodenal mucosa associated with polyps elsewhere in the intestine.	Duodenal polyposis may occur in association with gastrointestinal polyposis syndromes (see Table 5, pages 132–133). Polypoid mucosal hyperplasia in the proximal duodenum occurs frequently in association with uremia.

Table 4 Abnormal Mucosal Pattern in the Small Bowel

Disease	Radiographic Findings	Comments
A. Thickened Folds and Small Bowel Dilatation		
Ischemic bowel disease	Dilated bowel with thickening of the mucosal folds due to edema and/or hemorrhage. A plain film may show an ileus pattern.	May be caused by venous insufficiency, thromboembolic disease, or hypoperfusion due to atherosclerosis or low cardiac output. Bowel dilatation without thickening of mucosal folds is a less common presentation.
Metastases Crohn's disease Tuberculosis Radiation enteritis	Dilatation of small bowel that shows thickened folds and edema (secondary lymphangiectasis). May lead to bowel obstruction.	Involvement of the mesentery results in this pattern.
Zollinger–Ellison syndrome	Proximal jejunal dilatation, fold thickening, and increased fluid content with large gastric folds and ulcers in atypical locations. Distal jejunum and ileum are normal.	Acid secretions produce chemical enteritis. 50% of gastrin-secreting tumors are malignant. May be associated with *multiple endocrine adenomatosis*.
B. Thickened Folds and Gastric Involvement		
Lymphoma	Thick, irregular, or distorted folds in the small bowel with or without separation of small bowel loops. Large gastric folds with intraluminal masses, ulceration, or nodular lesions.	Small bowel dilatation may occur in advanced disease.
Ménétrier's disease with hypoproteinemia	Thickened, regular small bowel folds associated with massively enlarged gastric folds. Increased intestinal fluid content.	Extensive protein loss from the stomach may create hypoproteinemia and small bowel changes similar to that seen in cirrhosis and ascites.
Eosinophilic gastroenteritis	Thick, regular, distorted, or nodular folds in the proximal small bowel associated with thickened antral folds, antral narrowing, and occasionally ulcers. Rigidity of the wall may mimick carcinoma or Crohn's disease.	Diffuse small bowel involvement alone occurs as well. Eosinophilia is common. Symptoms and signs follow the ingestion of specific foods.
Zollinger–Ellison syndrome	Enlarged gastric folds and ulcers. Thickened small bowel folds. Increased fluid content.	Proximal small bowel dilatation is often present.
Crohn's disease	A broad spectrum of small bowel abnormalities (ulceration, fold thickening, cobblestoning, strictures, fistulas) may be associated with antral rigidity and deformity mimicking gastric carcinoma	Crohn's disease in the distal ileum is almost always present.
Cirrhosis	Prominent gastric rugae or nodular fundal masses in association with regular thickening of small bowel folds.	Seen in patients with severe liver disease and hypoproteinemia. Esophageal varices are usually present.
Intestinal amyloidosis Whipple's disease	Thickened folds both in the stomach and small bowel, possibly with antral narrowing.	Intestinal amyloidosis may be associated with nonspecific immunoglobulin abnormalities. Both are rare causes of combined gastric and small bowel involvement.
C. Thickened Irregular Folds		
Hemorrhagic bowel disease	Usually localized, regular thickening of small bowel folds with sharply delineated margins ("stack of coins" appearance). Scalloping and thumbprinting may be present. The radiographic pattern varies according to the clinical course.	Associated with several conditions including: *Ischemic bowel disease* (atherosclerosis, infarction, trauma, radiation endarteritis) *Vasculitis* (connective tissue diseases, thromboangitis obliterans, Henoch–Schönlein purpura) *Hemophilia* *Idiopathic thrombocytopenic purpura* (acute in children) *Trauma* *Secondary coagulation defects* (liver disease, leukemia, lymphoma, multiple myeloma, metastatic carcinoma, anticoagulant therapy)

Table 4 (Cont.) Abnormal Mucosal Pattern in the Small Bowel

Disease	Radiographic Findings	Comments
Intestinal edema (Fig. 28)	Regular thickening of several or all small bowel folds with increased intestinal fluid (flocculation, dilution, poor coating).	The most common cause is *hypoproteinemia* with albumin level below 2 g/100 ml. Causes of hypoproteinemia include liver cirrhosis, nephrotic syndrome, protein-losing enteropathies (such as Ménétrier's disease, Crohn's disease, Whipple's disease, lymphoma, carcinoma, ulcerative colitis or intestinal lymphangiectasia, constrictive pericarditis, burns, and allergic reactions). *Lymphatic blockage* by tumor or radiation and *angioneurotic edema* are other causes of intestinal edema. Angioneurotic edema tends to cause more localized changes, which rapidly revert to normal.
Intestinal lymphangiectasia (Fig. 28)	Regular thickening of mucosal folds due to intestinal edema (see above) and lymphatic dilatation.	*Primary:* Congenital lymphatic blockage; usually a young patient with no evidence of liver, kidney, or heart disease. *Secondary:* A complication of inflammatory or neoplastic lymphadenopathy.
Abetalipoproteinemia	Mucosal fold thickening is most marked in the duodenum and jejunum. Small bowel dilatation, irregularity of folds or even nodular folds may occur.	A rare recessively inherited disease manifested by malabsorption of fat, progressive neurologic deterioration and retinitis pigmentosa. Jejunal biopsy is diagnostic.
Eosinophilic enteritis **Amyloidosis** **Pneumatosis intestinalis**	True or apparent regular thickening of mucosal folds may be a feature in these conditions.	Irregular, distorted folds are a more common presentation of eosinophilic enteritis. Radiolucent gas cysts are diagnostic of pneumatosis intestinalis.

D. Irregular Folds without Small Bowel Dilatation

Disease	Radiographic Findings	Comments
Whipple's disease (Fig. 29)	Extensive thickening and distortion of folds is seen predominantly in the duodenum and jejunum.	Infiltration of the lamina propria by large periodic acid–Schiff stain positive macrophages and Gram-positive bacilli. Diarrhea, arthritis, fever, and lymphadenopathy are common. Jejunal biopsy is diagnostic.
Giardiasis (Fig. 26, p. 115)	Irregular, distorted, thickened mucosal folds in the duodenum and jejunum. Hypersecretion and hypermotility of the bowel is common. Associated nodular lymphoid hyperplasia points towards an underlying immunodeficiency state.	Symptomatic (gastroenteritis, cramping, malabsorption) usually among children, post-gastrectomy patients, travelers to endemic areas, and patients with gastrointestinal immunodeficiency. Cysts in the stool or a jejunal smear demonstrating *Giardia lamblia* are diagnostic.
Lymphoma	Thickening or obliteration of mucosal folds. Segmental constrictions, ulcers, or polypoid masses may occur. May be localized to one or several segments or diffusely involve most of the small bowel. Most frequent in the ileum.	May represent *primary* intestinal lymphoma or be a manifestation of a disseminated lymphomatous process that affects many organs (*secondary*). Primary intestinal lymphoma may be a complication of sprue.
Amyloidosis (Fig. 30)	Sharply demarcated thickening of folds throughout the small bowel have either regular or irregular appearance. Jejunization of the ileum is characteristic. Nodularity and tumor-like defects may occur. Ulceration, intestinal infarction, or impaired peristalsis may occur.	Small-bowel involvement occurs in at least 70% of cases of generalized amyloidosis, which can be either primary or secondary to a chronic disease (tuberculosis, osteomyelitis, ulcerative colitis, rheumatoid arthritis, multiple myeloma and other malignant diseases, familial Mediterranean fever). Rectal or jejunal biopsy are diagnostic.
Eosinophilic enteritis	Thickened, initially regular, folds, which are most prominent in the jejunum, become irregular with more extensive disease. Bowel wall may have a saw-toothed contour and become rigid.	May simulate Crohn's disease radiographically, but peripheral eosinophilia and gastrointestinal symptoms related to ingestion of specific foods are characteristic.

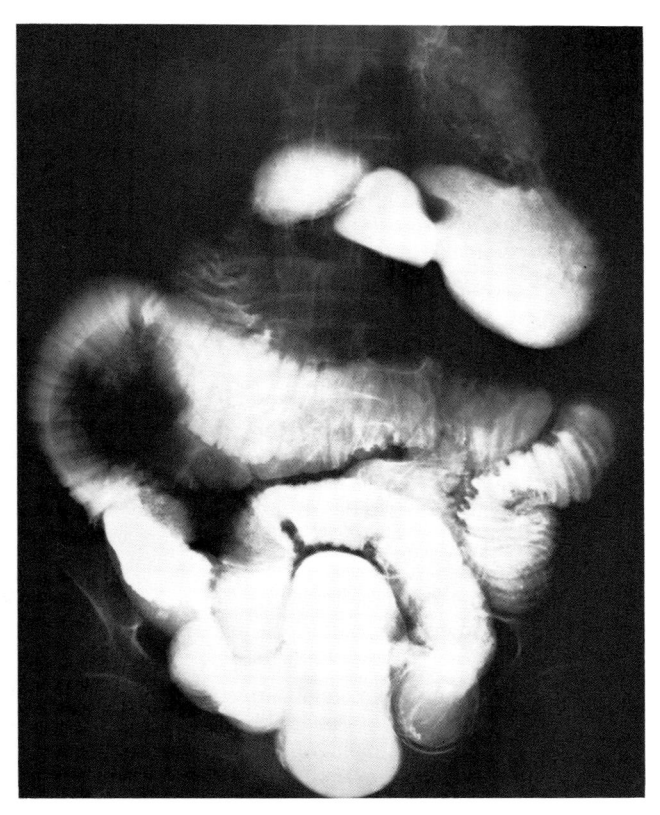

Figure 28 **Intestinal edema** (secondary intestinal lymphangiectasia). Regular thickening of mucosal folds, dilatation of small-bowel loops, and increased fluid content of the small bowel are seen.

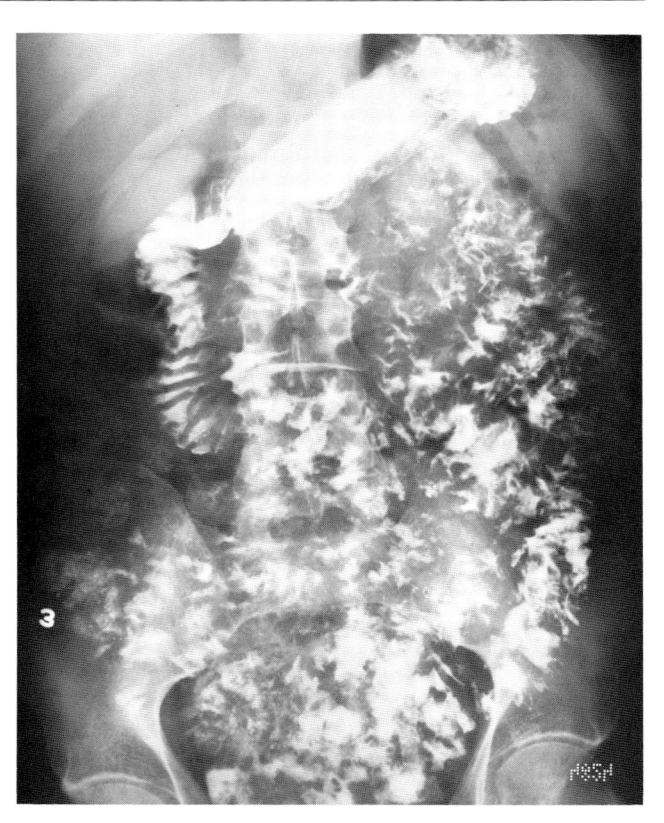

Figure 29 **Whipple's disease.** Extensive thickening and distortion of the mucosal folds in the whole small bowel are evident.

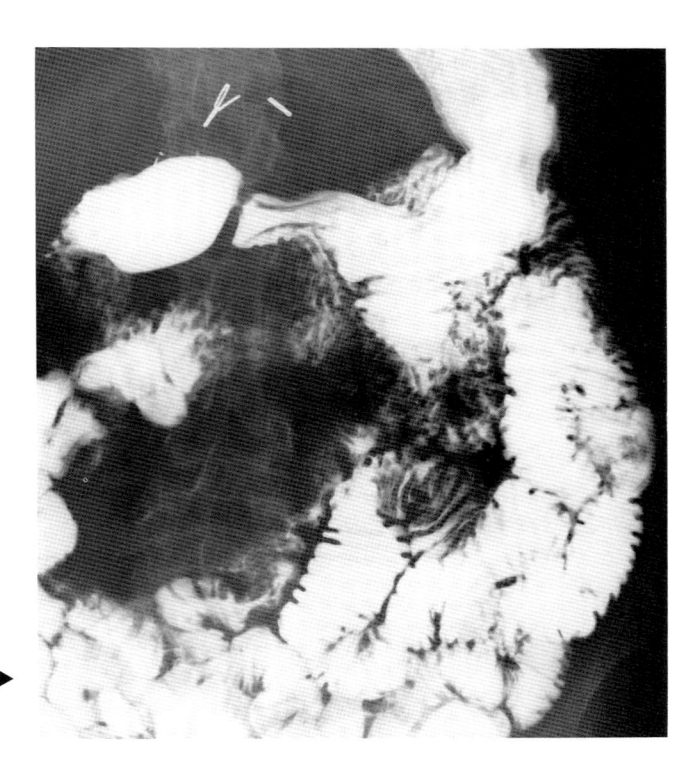

Figure 30 **Amyloidosis.** Sharply dermarcated, thick small-bowel folds and a few small nodules are seen, but the diameter of the small bowel is normal.

Table 4 (Cont.) Abnormal Mucosal Pattern in the Small Bowel

Disease	Radiographic Findings	Comments
Crohn's disease (Fig. 31)	The radiographic mucosal changes in their usual sequence of appearance are: Irregular thickening and distortion of the valvulae conniventes. Rough cobblestone appearance of the ulcerated, thick mucosa. Rigid thickening of the bowel wall with narrowing of lumen and loss of mucosal pattern (string sign). The terminal ileum is most commonly involved, but diseased segments occur commonly elsewhere.	Other common radiographic findings include intramural tracking, separation of bowel loops, and fistulas. *Tuberculosis* may produce an indistinguishable pattern, but is usually localized in the ileocecal region only.
Mastocytosis (urticaria pigmentosa) (Fig. 32)	Generalized irregular, distorted and thickened folds. Sometimes a diffuse pattern of sand-like nodules is present.	Mast cell proliferation in the reticuloendothelial system and skin. Lymphadenopathy, hepatosplenomegaly, peptic ulcer, and sclerotic bone lesions may be associated.
Strongyloidiasis (Fig. 33)	Irritability of bowel and irregular thickening of the duodenal and proximal jejunal folds, eventually the whole intestinal tract.	May be asymptomatic or mimic acute tropical sprue. Worms or larvae are detected in duodenal secretions.
Yersinia enterocolitica	Coarse, irregular thickening of small bowel mucosal folds is the most common finding, but nodular filling defects and ulceration producing a cobblestone appearance as in Crohn's disease may occur. The changes are usually localized in a short segment of the terminal ileum.	In children, Yersinia infection usually causes acute enteritis, in adolescents and adults an acute terminal ileitis or mesenteric adenitis is the usual presentation.
Typhoid fever	Irregular thickening and nodularity of the terminal ileum. The lesion is symmetric. Skip areas and fistulas do not occur.	An acute illness caused by *Salmonella typhosa* can be distinguished radiographically from Crohn's disease of the terminal ileum. Splenomegaly is common.
Alpha chain disease	Coarsely thickened irregular mucosal folds, possibly with nodules throughout the small bowel.	A disorder of immunoglobulin peptide synthesis causes in defective secretory IgA production, and results in diarrhea and malabsorption.

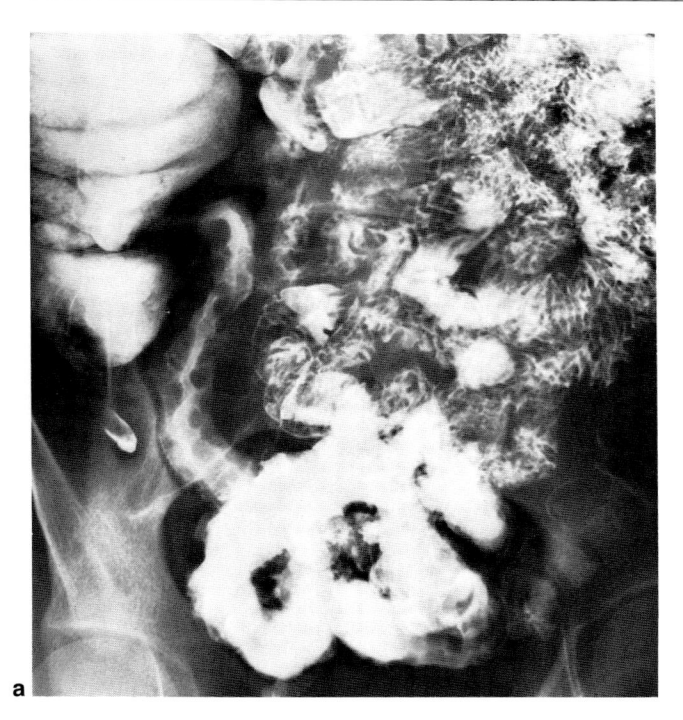

Figure **31 a, b Crohn's disease. a** Irregular thickening, distortion and disappearance of valvulae conniventes. The distal small bowel wall appears rigid and thickened. Cobblestone pattern is seen in the distal ileum. **b** Loss of mucosal folds and increased secretions in the distal ileum of another patient.

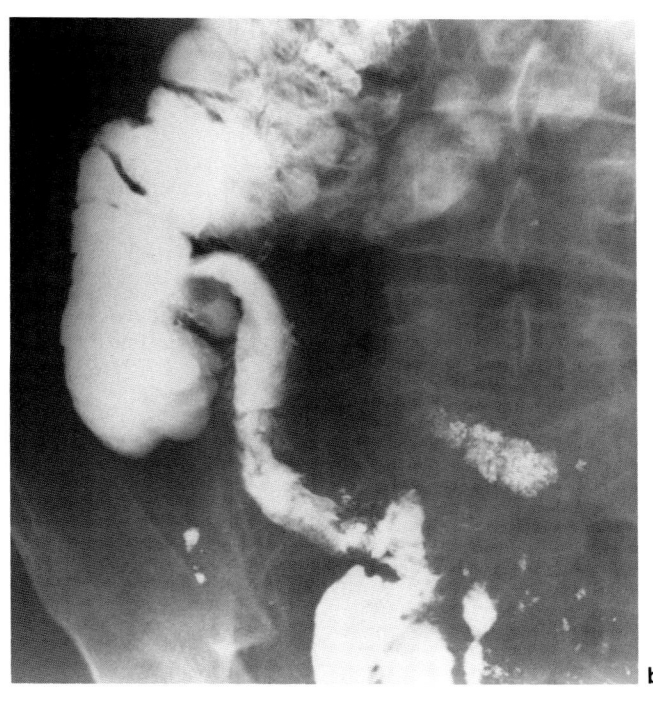

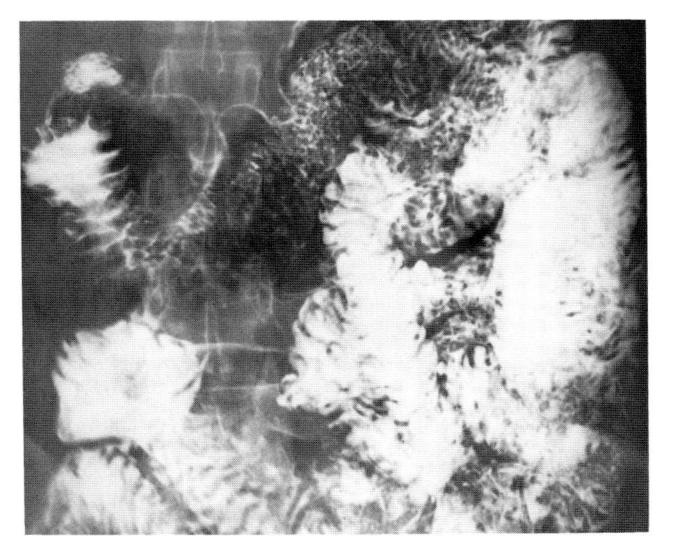

Figure **32 Mastocytosis.** Small nodules are seen in the small-bowel mucosa. Mucosal folds are slightly irregular, and the duodenal folds are thick.

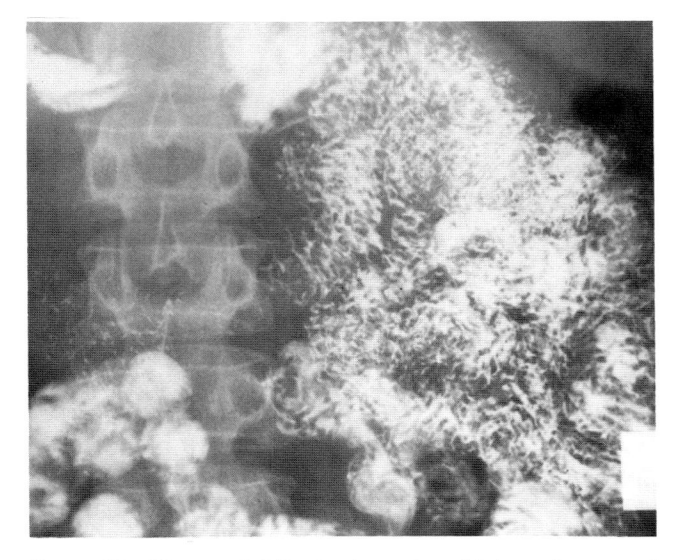

Figure **33 Strongyloidiasis.** Irregular, thickened mucosal folds are present in the jejunum.

Table 4 (Cont.) Abnormal Mucosal Pattern in the Small Bowel

Disease	Radiographic Findings	Comments
Radiation enteritis (Fig. 34)	Thickened and/or irregular folds, loss of mucosal pattern, separation of bowel loops, spasticity. Ulcerations and fistulas may occur.	Changes occur at the site of radiation therapy. They may mimic Crohn's disease.

E. Small Bowel Polyposis

Disease	Radiographic Findings	Comments
Peutz–Jeghers syndrome	Multiple polyps (hamartomas) are seen throughout the small bowel and may occur elsewhere in the gastrointestinal tract.	This is the most common small bowel polyposis syndrome. Multiple gastrointestinal polyps are associated with mucocutaneous pigmentation. Hyperpigmentation of the buccal mucosa is characteristic. Increased incidence of adenocarcinoma of duodenum or jejunum and of ovarian cysts and tumors.
Gardner's syndrome	Multiple adenomatous polyps are occasionally seen in the small bowel, predominantly in the distal portion.	Diffuse colonic polyposis associated with osteomas, soft-tissue tumors and eventual colorectal carcinoma.
Familial polyposis	Multiple adenomatous polyps may be seen throughout the gastrointestinal tract.	Extraintestinal lesions of the Peutz–Jeghers or Gardner's syndrome are absent. A very rare condition with a high risk of gastrointestinal carcinoma.
Juvenile gastrointestinal polyposis	Polyps (hamartomas) are present throughout the gastrointestinal tract.	If associated with alopecia, nail dystrophy, hyperpigmentation, and malabsorption, it is called the *Canada–Cronkhite syndrome*. The latter disorder presents in later life, unlike other juvenile polyposis syndromes.
Multiple hemangiomas	The combination of phleboliths and multiple filling defects in the small bowel is pathognomonic.	*Leiomyomas* and *carcinoid* tumors are very rarely multiple enough to produce a polyposis pattern.
Neurofibromatosis (Fig. 35)	Multiple small-bowel neurofibromas have an eccentric distribution. They may mimic sessile or pedunculated polyps.	Café-au-lait pigmentation and cutaneous fibromas are characteristic.
Metastases	Multiple intraluminal or intramural filling defects characteristically have a target or bull's eye appearance.	The most frequent primary neoplasms are melanoma and carcinomas of the breast and lung. Other carcinomas and lymphoma may produce a similar pattern.

F. "Granularity" of the Small Bowel Mucosa

Disease	Radiographic Findings	Comments
Macroglobulinemia	A sand-like radiographic pattern in the small bowel mucosa represents enlarged intestinal villi. The folds are not thickened.	A plasma cell dyscrasia with large amounts of IgM in the serum, anemia, bleeding, lymphadenopathy, and hepatosplenomegaly.
Nodular lymphoid hyperplasia	The bowel mucosa is studded with innumerable tiny polypoid masses uniformly distributed throughout the involved segment, usually jejunum. Enlarged and distorted fold pattern suggests associated giardiasis.	In children and young adults, lymphoid hyperplasia of the terminal ileum is a normal finding. Elsewhere in adults, it is almost invariably associated with a late-onset *immunoglobulin deficiency*. *Giardiasis* is common.
Histoplasmosis	A sand-like covering superimposed on irregular distorted folds.	The lamina propria is infiltrated by histoplasma-laden macrophages creating the appearance of innumerable filling defects.
Intestinal lymphangiectasia Whipple's disease Yersinia enterocolitis (healing) Eosinophilic enteritis Mastocytosis	Sandlike pattern may occasionally be present in these conditions, but other radiographic features are more characteristic.	See above in this Table.

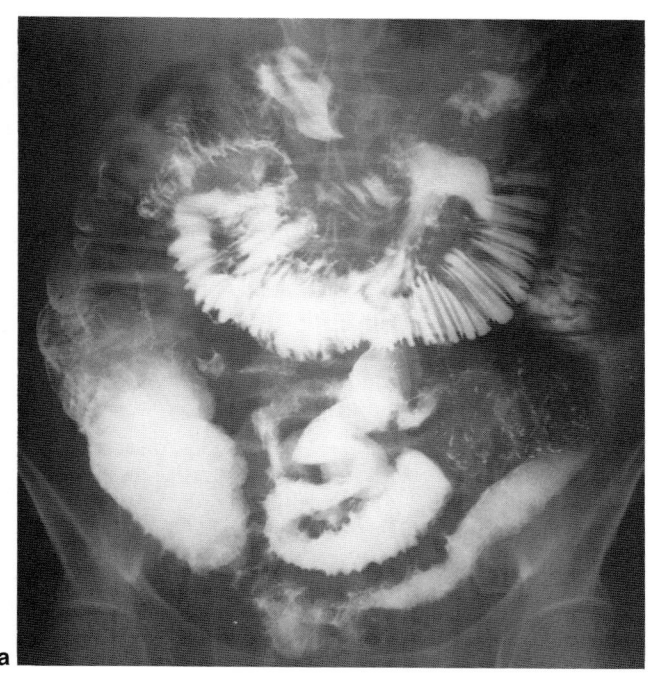

Figure **34a, b** **Radiation enteritis,** secondary to the therapy of a gynecologic tumor. **a** Thickening and irregularity of both small- and large-bowel mucosa; loss of normal mucosal patterns is most extensive close to the area of highest radiation dose. Thumbprinting is seen in the sigmoid and cecum, too. A fistulous tract is seen higher in the midabdomen from one loop of small bowel to another. **b** Smooth but thickened mucosal folds in the distal ileum in another patient with a similar history.

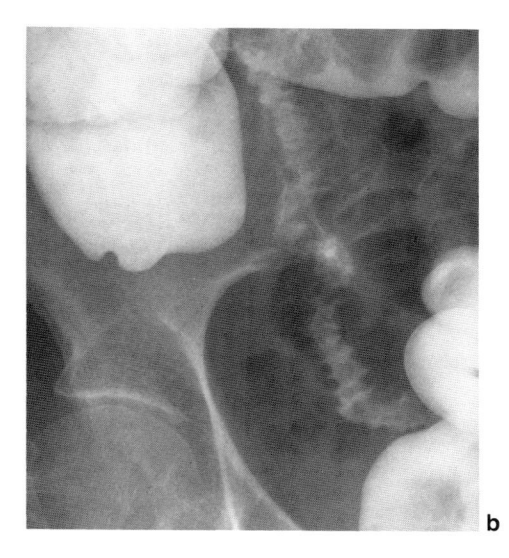

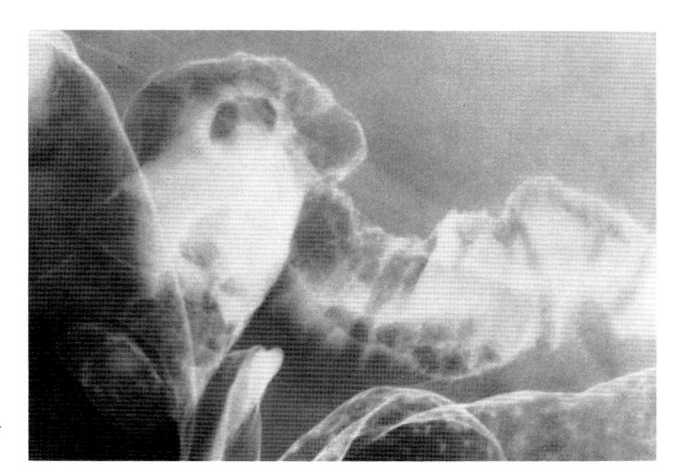

Figure **35** Multiple polypoid filling defects in the distal ileum ▶ in a patient with **neurofibromatosis.**

Table 4 (Cont.)   **Abnormal Mucosal Pattern in the Small Bowel**

Disease	Radiographic Findings	Comments
G. Small-Bowel Dilatation with Normal Folds		
Mechanical obstruction Adynamic ileus (Fig. 36)	Increased caliber of the small bowel above the obstruction (or throughout in ileus). Increased fluid causes haziness, poor coating, and flocculation of barium suspension, but valvulae conniventes are normal.	For more detailed discussion of bowel obstructions, see Chapter 1, p. 2. In *chronic idiopathic intestinal pseudoobstruction,* radiographic and clinical signs of mechanical obstruction are intermittently present without an organic lesion.
Vagotomy Drugs	Prolonged transit time and dilatation of the small bowel with normal folds.	Drugs that cause decreased smooth muscle activity include atropine, morphine, L-dopa and barbiturates.
Sprue (Figs. 37, 38)	The barium in the dilated small bowel has a coarse, granular, or hazy appearance due to increased bowel fluid. The contours of the jejunum are smooth, unindented due to atrophy and effacement of mucosal folds ("moulage sign"). Segmentation or flocculation of barium are unreliable signs of malabsorption.	Adult nontropical sprue (celiac disease), tropical sprue (infectious), and celiac disease of children are clinically and radiographically similar. The degree of bowel dilatation is related to the severity of the disease. Diffuse intestinal lymphoma may complicate long-standing sprue and cause thickening and distortion of mucosal folds.
Scleroderma Dermatomyositis (Fig. 39)	Dilated small bowel with normal-sized folds that are closely packed together. Extremely prolonged transit time. Dilatation is most prominent in the duodenum. Large broad-necked pseudosacculations in the antimesenteric border of the bowel are also characteristic. They are caused by mesenteric fibrosis which also pulls folds asymmetrically together.	Skin changes, joint symptoms, or the appearance of Raynaud's phenomenon usually precede changes in the small bowel. Scleroderma and dermatomyositis produce identical small bowel changes. These two entities can be differentiated from sprue by the absence of hypersecretion, and by the presence of pronounced duodenal dilatation and markedly delayed barium transit time.
Lactase deficiency	A conventional small-bowel examination is normal but the addition of lactose into the barium suspension results in dilatation of the small bowel, increased bowel secretions, and rapid transit.	A common enzyme defect resulting in watery diarrhea and abdominal discomfort soon after ingestion of milk products.
Ischemic bowel disease	Delayed intestinal transit and dilatation of bowel with increased intraluminal fluid.	Thickening of mucosal folds is commonly seen in acute conditions, but in chronic conditions (atherosclerosis, connective tissue diseases, massive amyloidosis) the fold pattern may remain normal despite bowel dilatation.
Chagas' disease	Small-bowel dilatation with normal folds.	Damage to visceral neurons may be the underlying cause. *Diabetes complicated by hypokalemia* may rarely be associated with small-bowel dilatation.

Abnormal Mucosal Pattern in the Gastrointestinal Tract 125

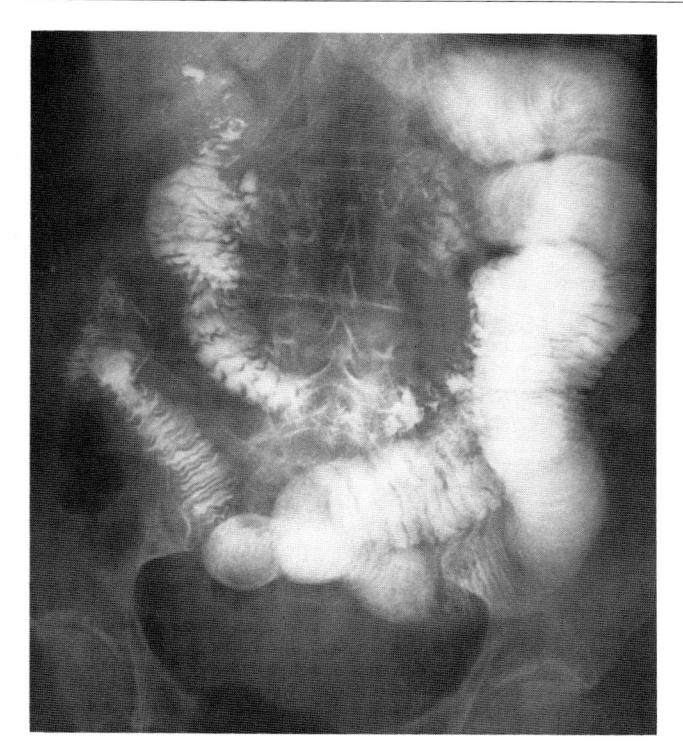

Figure 36 **Gallstone ileus.** Increased caliber of the small bowel above the impacted stone, and increased secretions but the valvulae conniventes are normal.

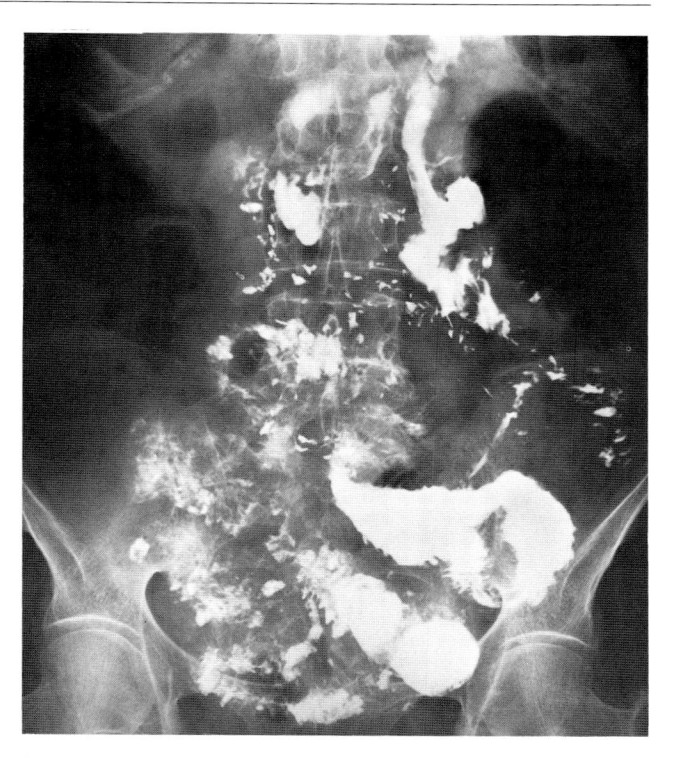

Figure 37 **Sprue.** Tubular appearance of several bowel segments with effaced mucosal folds are seen (moulage sign). Fragmentation and flocculation of the barium, and an increased amount of fluid in the bowel lumen are also present.

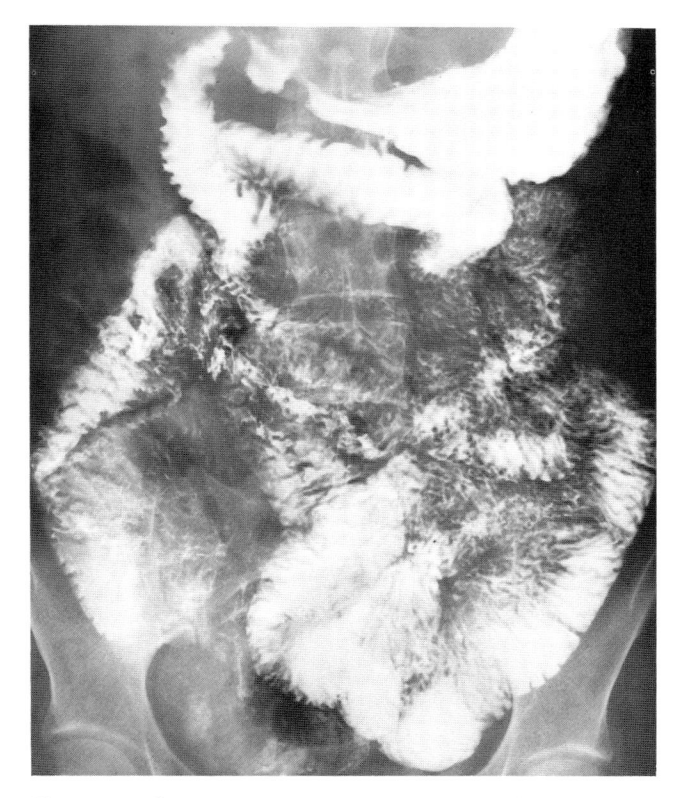

Figure 38 **Sprue.** In the absence of flocculation and moulage, with the modern barium suspensions, the small-bowel loops appear dilated, have slightly thickened folds, and increased fluid content that causes dilution of the contrast medium.

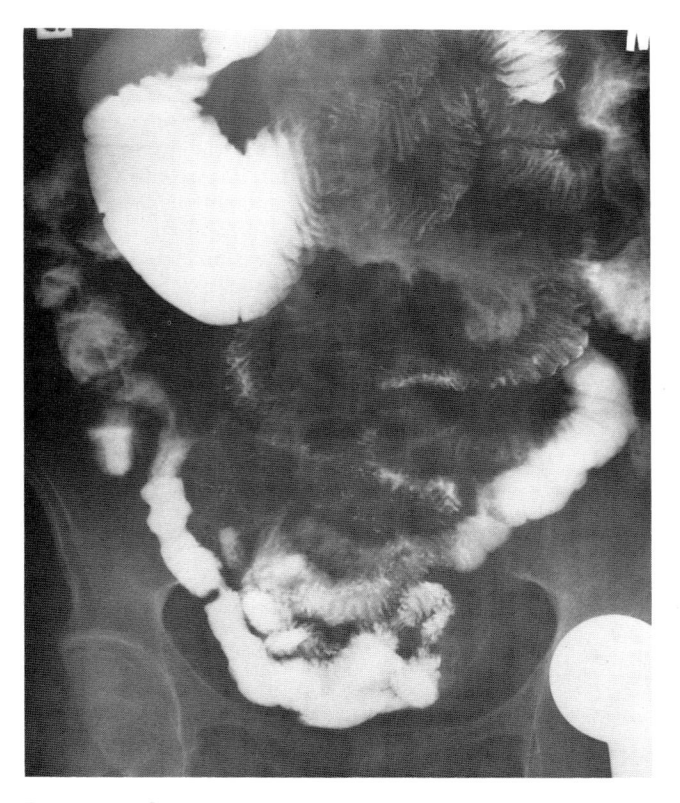

Figure 39 **Scleroderma.** Dilated small-bowel loops, especially the duodenum. Normal-sized folds. Prolonged transit time.

Table 5 Abnormal Mucosal Pattern in the Colon and Rectum

Disease	Radiographic Findings	Comments
Ulcerative colitis (Fig. 40)	The appearance and sequence of mucosal changes depend on duration and severity: Fine granularity of the mucosa in double contrast or haziness in single contrast (hyperemia and edema) Stippled mucosal pattern in double contrast, serration or spiculation in single contrast (superficial ulcers), which should be differentiated from transient pseudospicules (innominate lines) Larger marginal ulcerations symmetrically around the circumference of the bowel wall, ("collar-button" ulcers) Denuded flat mucosa, possibly with pseudopolyps. Filiform polyposis may occur, seen as thin, straight filling defects Shortening and rigidity of the colon ("lead-pipe" configuration) combined with mucosal atrophy Loss of haustral markings alone is an unreliable sign. Involvement of rectosigmoid is characteristic. Inflammatory changes may occur in the terminal ileum (*"backwash ileitis"*).	A majority of patients have mild disease with only distal colonic involvement. Acute fulminating disease is often complicated by perforation or *toxic megacolon* (see Chapter 1, p. 14), chronic by carcinoma of the colon. Extracolonic manifestations include *arthritis, spondylitis, pericholangitis, liver disease,* and *thrombotic complications.* Even biopsy is not fully diagnostic in some cases, since features of Crohn's disease or nonspecific ulcerating colonic disease may coexist.
Crohn's colitis (Figs. 41, 42)	Mucosal alterations usually appear in the following sequence: Punctate collections of barium with a halo of edema (aphthoid ulcers) surrounded by normal mucosa or small, irregular nodules Deeper, irregular ulcers surrounding mounds of edematous mucosa (cobblestone appearance), Penetrating asymmetric ulcers form long tracts parallel to the longitudinal axis of the colon or fistulas to adjacent organs, Stricture formation, Segmental involvement of the colon with extensive inflammatory changes in the terminal ileum, asymmetric ulceration, fistulas, sinus tracts, and mesenteric thickening are characteristic. Filiform polyposis may occur.	Symptoms such as diarrhea, pain, and weight loss are often more severe than in ulcerative colitis. Extraintestinal complications similar to ulcerative colitis are less frequent. Increased incidence of biliary and renal stones results from ileal disease. Aphthoid ulcers can also occur in other forms of colonic inflammation, e.g., amebic colitis, tuberculosis, yersinia colitis, and Behçet's syndrome.

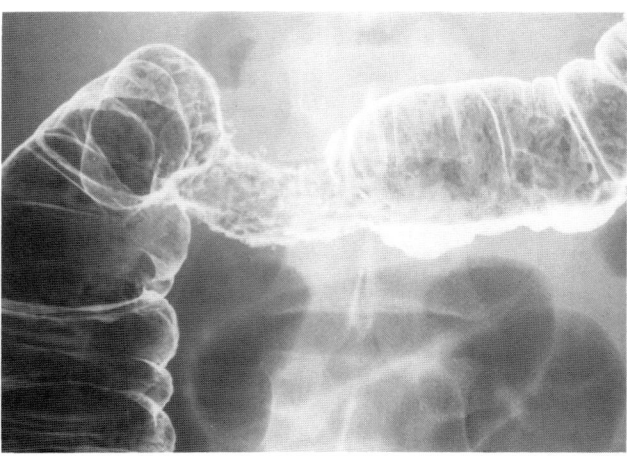

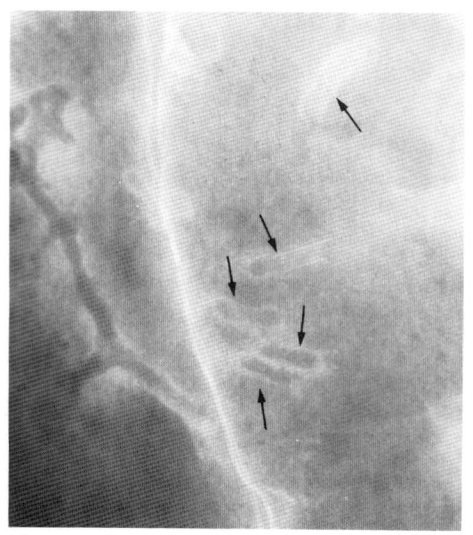

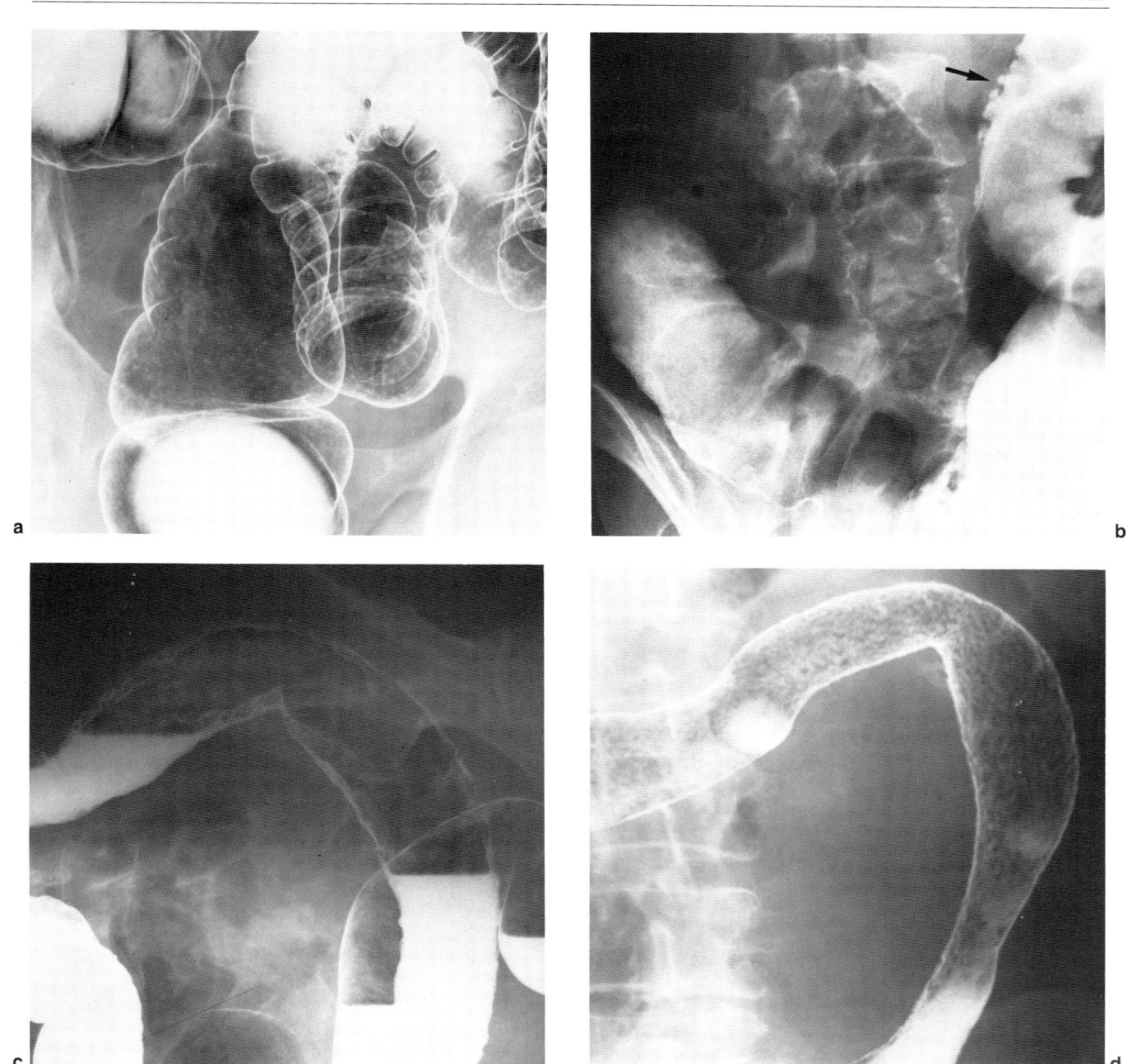

Figure 40a—d **Mucosal changes in ulcerative colitis: a** Stippled mucosal pattern representing superficial ulcers. **b** Larger marginal ulcerations, including collar button ulcers (arrow). **c** Denuded flat mucosa with numerous pseudopolyps. **d** Short, rigid colon with a mottled surface pattern.

◀ Figure 41 **Crohn's colitis.** Segmental narrowing of the proximal transverse colon, with irregular nodules and ulcers.

◀ Figure 42 Multiple **filiform polyps** (arrows) in the colon of a colitis patient.

Table 5 (Cont.) Abnormal Mucosal Pattern in the Colon and Rectum

Disease	Radiographic Findings	Comments
Ischemic colitis (Fig. 43)	Mucosal changes depend on the phase of the disease: Serrated margin and fine superficial ulcerations are the earliest findings and may simulate ulcerative colitis. "Thumbprinting", pseudopolyposis and deep ulcers occur later in most cases. Eventually the changes may disappear, develop into a stricture or proceed into infarction that may be evident by the presence of gas in the bowel wall and in the portal system. The splenic flexure and the sigmoid area are common locations.	Abrupt onset of abdominal pain and rectal bleeding with diarrhea is a common presentation. A history of prior cardiovascular disease is frequent. Mucosal findings may be indistinguishable from ulcerative or Crohn's colitis, but typical history, short clinical course, and the location of changes are helpful. Ulcerating nodularity with pseudopolyps may occur proximal to colonic obstruction. They may be caused by *ischemia secondary to distension of the bowel wall.*
Amebiasis (Fig. 44)	Colonic mucosal changes are similar to ulcerative or Crohn's colitis. Segmental involvement of the colon as in Crohn's colitis is common. The cecum is affected in 90% of cases and may have a cone-shaped appearance.	Clinical symptoms have a wide spectrum. Hepatic abscess develops in about one-third of cases of amebic dysentery. Concomitant ileal disease favors Crohn's colitis rather than amebiasis. Stool specimens are usually diagnostic.
Schistosomiasis	The colonic mucosa is edematous and spiculated simulating ulcerative colitis. Small ulcers, spasm, disturbed motility, and loss of haustral pattern are common. Later characteristic multiple 1–2 cm filling defects develop representing granulomas. The descending and sigmoid colon are most frequently involved.	The parasite penetrates colonic wall and causes an inflammatory reaction. Detection of ova in freshly passed stools is diagnostic. Very rarely *strongyloidiasis* causes severe ulcerating colitis.
Trichuriasis	Granular mucosal pattern throughout the colon with flocculation of barium and multiple small filling defects.	The pattern is similar to mucoviscidosis. Only found in the tropics and subtropics.
Shigellosis (basillary dysentery)	Shallow, ragged ulcers encircle the colon, which shows mucosal edema and exudation. Barium enema cannot usually be tolerated, but if successful, it shows deep "collar button" ulcerations and intense spasm. The changes may be segmental or generalized.	Incubation period after ingestion of the organisms is usually 2–3 days or more, after which profuse diarrhea begins. The radiographic patterns of salmonellosis and shigellosis may be similar, but involvement of the ileum favors salmonellosis.
Salmonellosis (typhoid fever)	Barium enema is rarely performed due to short course. Small ulcerations and edematous thickening of folds may be seen. Unlike in shigellosis, terminal ileum is usually involved.	Incubation period is often as short as 12 hours, recovery takes place within 4–5 days.
Tuberculous colitis (Fig. 45)	Radiographic findings closely simulate Crohn's disease. Cecum and distal ileum are most commonly affected.	If caused by *Mycobacterium tuberculosis*, coexistent pulmonary tuberculosis is often demonstrated radiographically. In tuberculous colitis caused by *Mycobacterium bovis*, pulmonary tuberculosis is usually absent.
Gonorrheal proctitis	Barium enema is usually normal. Mucosal edema or ulceration of the rectum occurs rarely.	Most patients with rectal gonorrhea are asymptomatic and diagnosed by staining and culture of purulent exudates.
Staphylococcal enterocolitis	Radiographic features of generalized ulcerating colitis may be seen in severe cases.	Usually secondary to administration of broad spectrum antibiotics.
Yersinia enterocolitis	Multiple small colonic ulcerations similar to those seen in Crohn's colitis, associated with thick mucosal folds, nodular filling defects, or ulceration of the distal small bowel.	A relatively common cause of ileitis and colitis in children, which causes fever, diarrhea, or symptoms simulating appendicitis.
Campylobacter colitis	Similar to acute or early changes of ulcerative colitis, e.g., mucosal edema and superficial ulcerations.	An acute colitis simulating ulcerative colitis but has a self-limited course.

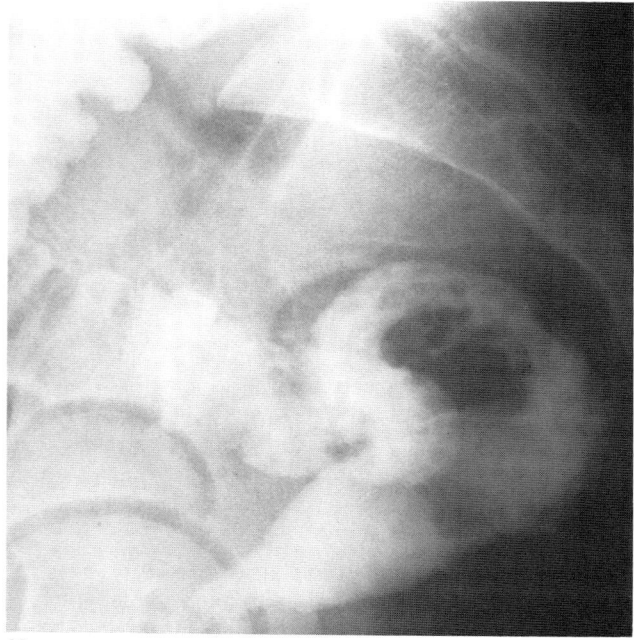

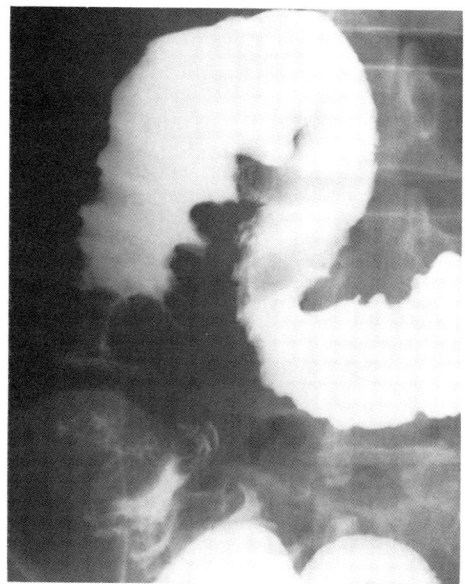

Figure **43 Ischemic colitis** (occlusion of the inferior mesenteric artery). Mucosal irregularities with early pseudopolyposis are seen in the sigmoid colon.

Figure **44 Amebic colitis.** A mass (ameboma) is present in the cecum. Ulcerations and thumbprinting are seen in the proximal colon.

Figure **45 Tuberculous colitis.** A long stricture is present in the cecum and ascending colon. Superficial mucosal changes are seen in a small area above the strictured segment. These changes are similar to Crohn's colitis.

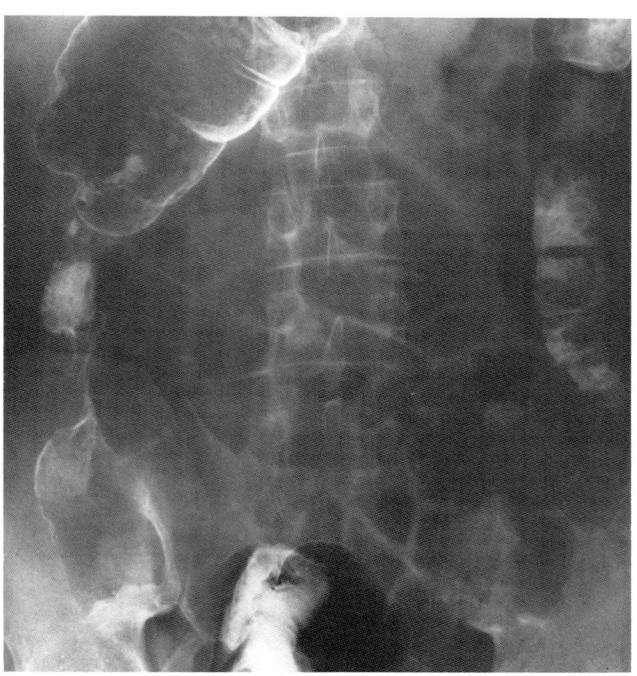

Table 5 (Cont.) Abnormal Mucosal Pattern in the Colon and Rectum

Disease	Radiographic Findings	Comments
Fungal colitis (candidiasis, histoplasmosis, actinomycosis, mucormycosis)	Irritable spastic colon with thick irregular mucosal folds, and occasionally ulcers.	These are rare causes of colitis in chronically ill patients. The fungal infection may be primary or spread from another site in the body.
Lymphogranuloma venereum	Spasm, irritability, mucosal edema, ulcers, fistulas, or sinus tracts are seen in the rectum. The rest of the colon is not involved.	Rectal involvement is common (25%), especially in women and homosexual men. As the disease progresses, rectal stricture develops.
Herpes zoster	Small ulcerations in a narrowed segment of colon. A pattern of raised polygonal "urticaria" plaques may also occur.	Herpes zoster is a rare cause of colonic ulcerations. Typical clinical history and skin lesions suggest the correct diagnosis.
Cytomegalovirus colitis	Mucosal ulceration, luminal narrowing, "thumbprinting," or even tumor-like defects in the cecum.	The most important cause of severe lower gastrointestinal tract bleeding in renal transplant recipients on immunosuppressive therapy and in AIDS patients.
Pseudomembranous colitis (Fig. 46)	Barium enema is contraindicated in severe cases. In mild or healing cases thickened colonic wall and haustral markings, irregular bowel wall due to pseudomembranes, and mucosal ulcerations simulating other ulcerating conditions are seen.	A spectrum of colonic inflammatory states usually complicating antibiotic therapy, sometimes surgery, uremia or large bowel obstruction. In the latter cases the course may be fulminant and fatal.
Radiation-induced colitis (Fig. 34, p. 123)	Spasticity and ulceration of colonic wall are most severe in the segments adjacent the irradiated organs. The anterior rectal wall is most commonly involved. Strictures and fistulas may develop.	Usually secondary to pelvic irradiation for carcinoma of the cervix, endometrium, ovary, bladder, or prostate. The course is usually benign and self-limited.
Caustic colitis	3 to 5 days after exposure, ulcerations and mucosal sloughing similar to other ulcerating lesions may be observed.	A rare complication of a cleansing enema that contains detergents and the fluid is trapped in the proximal colon. Subsides within 3 to 4 weeks.
Pancreatitis	Irregularity or ulcerations and pseudopolyps in the transverse colon and splenic flexure.	Due to spread of pancreatitis along the transverse mesocolon.
Amyloidosis	May occasionally present as ulcerating colitis indistinguishable from other causes.	May occur both in primary or secondary (connective tissue disorders, chronic infection) amyloidosis. Rectal biopsy is diagnostic.
Inorganic mercury poisoning	Ulcerating lesions in the colon are associated with acute renal damage.	
Behçet's syndrome	Diffuse mucosal thickening and ulceration or multiple discrete ulcers in otherwise normal colon may occur. Rectum is spared but terminal ileum may be involved. Ulcers tend to be larger than in Crohn's colitis and easily perforate.	Characterized by ulcerations in the buccal and genital mucosa and skin lesions.
Diverticulosis	Sac-like outpouchings with short necks often associated with a sawtooth pattern must be differentiated from ulcers and polyps.	Most common in the sigmoid colon. Ulcerative colitis or Crohn's disease may coexist and simulate diverticulitis.
Solitary rectal ulcer syndrome	Nodularity of rectal mucosa may be followed by ulcerations on the anterior or anterolateral rectum within 15 cm of the anal verge and near a valve of Houston.	Usually occurs in young patients with rectal bleeding. May be associated with rectal mucosal prolapse or pelvic muscle discoordination during defecation. May lead to rectal stricture and simulate inflammatory bowel disease or carcinoma.
Nonspecific benign ulceration of the colon	Usually single, in up to 20% multiple ulcerative lesions usually in the cecum or ascending colon. Most occur in the antimesenteric border, in contrast to diverticula. A mass-like effect simulating carcinoma is frequent.	A diagnosis of exclusion, rarely made before operation. No precise cause can be identified. Lesions in the ascending colon may mimic appendicitis, those of descending colon simulate diverticulitis or carcinoma.

Table 5 (Cont.) Abnormal Mucosal Pattern in the Colon and Rectum

Disease	Radiographic Findings	Comments
Nodular lymphoid hyperplasia	Nodular tiny (~ 2 mm) filling defects are evenly distributed throughout the colon simulating familial polyposis, pseudopolyposis of bowel inflammation, or nodular lymphoma. A fleck of barium in the center of the nodules (umbilication at the apex of the enlarged lymph follicles) is characteristic.	The filling defects in nodular lymphoid hyperplasia are sessile and uniform in size, whereas polyps in familiar polyposis vary in size and are often pedunculated. They are evenly distributed, and are smaller than the nodules of lymphoma.
Cystic fibrosis	Multiple poorly defined filling defects give the colonic mucosa a hyperplastic appearance simulating polyposis.	Caused by adherent collections of viscid mucus that are not removed by cleansing enema. *Trichuriasis* causes a similar appearance due to adherent whipworms and associated mucus.
Colonic urticaria (Fig. 47)	Large, round or polygonal, raised plaques in a grossly dilated (usually right) colon, representing submucosal edema.	An allergic reaction of the colonic mucosa to medication, with or without concomitant cutaneous lesions. The lesions regress once medication is withdrawn. Similar lesions may occur in *herpes zoster*.
Artifacts Foreign bodies	*Fecal material* adhered to the colonic mucosa is usually irregular and unevenly coated; barium tends to infiltrate into the mass and interpose between the mass and mucosa. *Radiolucent air bubbles* tend to appear as clusters of small bubbles adhered to a larger one. *Mucus strands* are seen as irregular branching defects and occasionally simulate filiform polyposis.	*Foreign bodies*, especially kernels of corn can simulate multiple polyps. Similar to other artifacts, they are usually freely movable and disappear in a repeat examination. *Sharp angulation* of the bowel may result in a long filling defect resembling the stalk of a polyp.

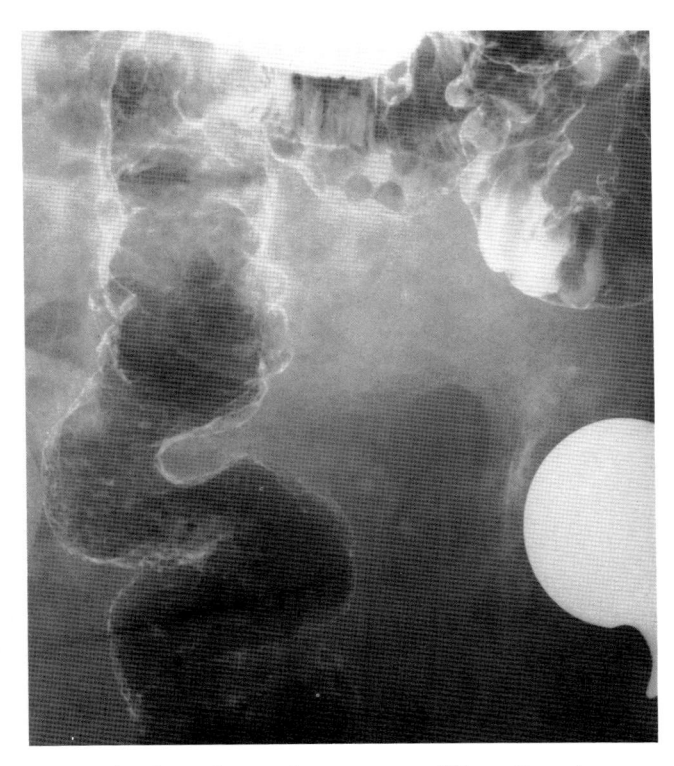

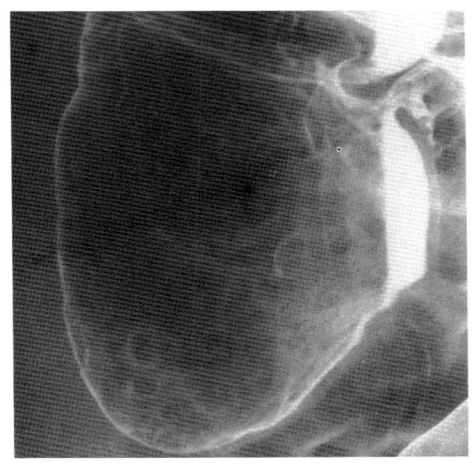

Figure **46 Pseudomembranous colitis.** Pseudomembranes are most obvious in the sigmoid colon, seen as multiple filling defects. Ulcerations are present in the rectal mucosa.

Figure **47** Raised plaques in the mucosa of the cecum which rapidly vanished and were considered to represent **colonic urticaria.**

Table 5 (Cont.) Abnormal Mucosal Pattern in the Colon and Rectum

Disease	Radiographic Findings	Comments
Lymphoma	Multiple irregular filling defects are a rare manifestation and usually associated with ileal changes.	A more common presentation of colonic lymphoma is a single, relatively large lesion, which may occasionally infiltrate over a long segment of the colon.
Leukemia	In lymphocytic leukemia diffuse mucosal or submucosal interlacing filling defects of the colon may occur. In myelogenous leukemia diffuse plaques, nodules, or masses are sometimes seen.	Usually asymptomatic but may cause necrotizing enterocolitis, hemorrhage, or perforation.
Metastases	Spiculations of the bowel contour as in ulcerative colitis. Mucosal thickening, nodular masses, or multiple eccentric strictures can simulate Crohn's disease.	Hematogenous metastases from breast, lung, stomach, ovary, pancreas, uterus, or melanoma may cause this pattern, which clinically usually manifests as bloody diarrhea. Multiple primary carcinomas of the colon occur in 1%.
Familial polyposis (Fig. 48)	Myriad of small (less than 1 cm) polyps (adenomas) may blanket the whole colon or spare the right colon. May look like a poorly cleansed colon. Other parts of the gastrointestinal tract are usually spared.	An inherited autosomal dominant condition arising around puberty and clinically manifesting usually at third or fourth decade. Virtually all develop carcinoma of the colon or rectum. *Disseminated gastrointestinal polyposis* may be a variant of familial polyposis. *Turcot syndrome* refers to multiple adenomatous polyps of the colon associated with gliomas which occur in the second decade.
Gardner's syndrome	The colonic lesions are indistinguishable from the pattern of familial polyposis.	Associated with bony overgrowth or osteomas of the skull, keloid formation, soft tissue tumor, sebaceous cysts, and a 100% risk of colorectal carcinoma.
Peutz–Jeghers syndrome	Polyps (hamartomas) are primarily present in the small bowel, but multiple polyps occur in colon and rectum.	An inherited autosomal dominant disorder which manifests during childhood or adolescence. Excessive melanin deposits on the lips and buccal mucosa are characteristic. A slightly increased risk of intestinal carcinoma or ovarian tumor exists.

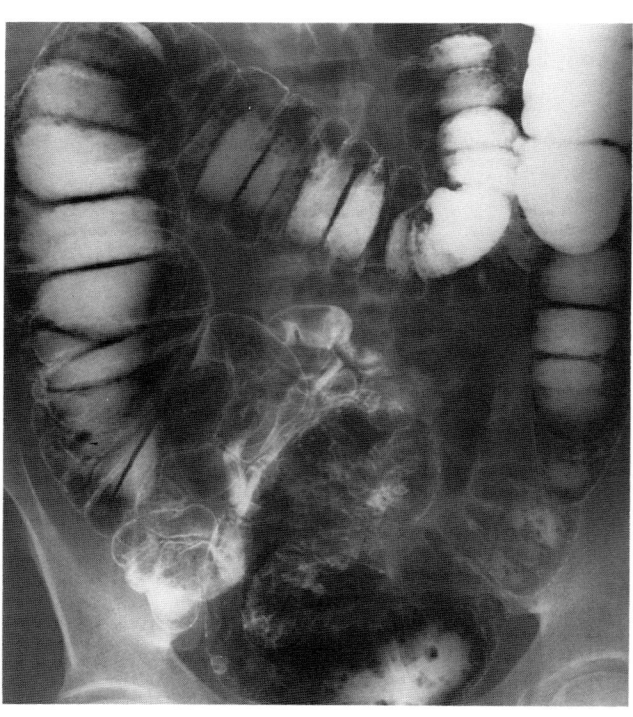

Figure **48 Familial polyposis.** A great number of small polyps cover the colonic mucosa. The distal ileum is normal. The pattern mimics a poorly cleansed colon.

Table 5 (Cont.) Abnormal Mucosal Pattern in the Colon and Rectum

Disease	Radiographic Findings	Comments
Multiple hamartoma syndrome (Cowden's disease)	Single or multiple polyps may be present in the colon.	Circumoral papillomatosis and nodular gingival hyperplasia are characteristic.
Juvenile polyposis syndromes (juvenile polyposis coli, generalized gastrointestinal juvenile polyposis)	Multiple hamartomatous polyps of the colon usually found in childhood. Polyps may be present also in the stomach and small bowel.	*Canada–Cronkhite syndrome* presents in later life with multiple hamartomatous polyps and malabsorption. The syndrome is characterized by alopecia, nail dystrophy, and hyperpigmentation, and may be lethal soon after diagnosis.
Neurofibromatosis of the colon	Multiple diffuse intraluminal or intramural nodules tend to be larger than in the hereditary polyposis syndromes, and have a characteristic eccentric distribution; the nodules being located entirely on the mesenteric side.	Characteristic skin lesions (café-au-lait spots and cutaneous fibromas) are diagnostic.
Colonic lipomatosis	Multiple filling defects are seen usually in the right colon without mucosal ulcerations.	Histologic verification is required.
Multiple colonic hemangiomas	Intraluminal or intramural filling defects in the colon.	Can be diagnosed radiographically only if phleboliths are associated with the lesions.
Hemorrhoids	Rectal filling defects may simulate polyps or are seen as linear shadows of enlarged veins.	Hemorrhoids often remain undetected in the barium enema examination. They should be differentiated from the normal rectal columns of Morgagni.
Pneumatosis intestinalis (Fig. 49)	Intramural gas collections may simulate broad-based polyps but are more radiolucent.	
Colitis cystica profunda	Multiple irregular filling defects simulate adenomatous polyps. They occur usually in the pelvic colon and rectum.	Mucous subepithelial cysts are frequently associated with proctitis or colitis. A rare condition called *colitis cystica superficialis* is associated with pellagra. Minute cysts are diffusely distributed throughout the colon.

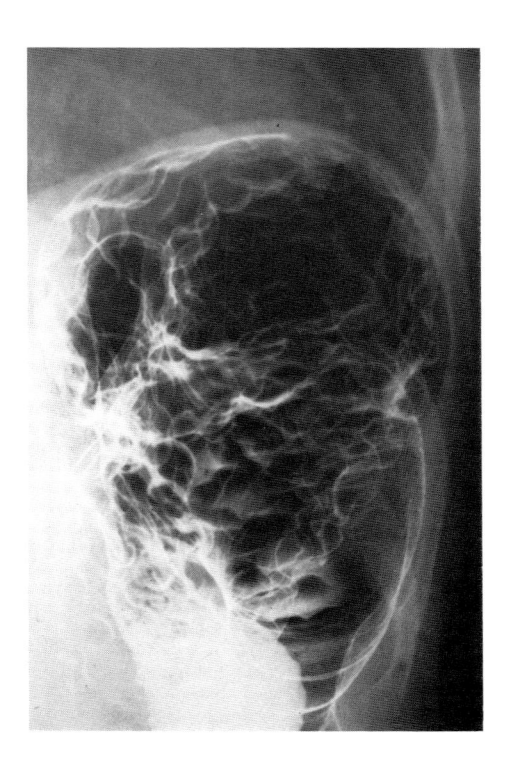

Figure **49** **Pneumatosis intestinalis.** Intramural gas collections in the splenic flexure simulate broad-based polyps but are radiolucent.

Chapter 6 Narrowing in the Gastrointestinal Tract

An acquired circumferential narrowing in the gastrointestinal tract is generally caused either by edema, inflammation or hemorrhage with eventual scar formation, or by tumor encasement. Other conditions that may occasionally produce a stenosis include congenital lesions (e.g., webs or congenital strictures), localized spasm or hypertrophy, especially of a sphincter (e.g., esophageal sphincter or pylorus), or the torsion or kinking of a freely mobile bowel segment (e.g., volvulus or herniation).

Radiologic differential diagnosis between benign and malignant stenosis is usually difficult and in the majority of cases requires a biopsy for an unequivocal diagnosis. A discrete, irregular, and asymmetric narrowing with associated ulcerations or a well-demarcated filling defect with overhanging edges strongly suggest a malignant lesion. A smooth concentric stenosis with tapering margins generally favors a benign condition, but many malignancies can present radiographically in similar fashion.

The differential diagnosis of stenotic lesions in the gastrointestinal tract are discussed in Tables **1** to **5.**

Table 1　Narrowing of the Esophagus

Disease	Radiographic Findings	Comments
Web (congenital or acquired) (Fig. 1)	Single or less commonly multiple, band-like concentric or eccentric narrowing, preferentially located in the cervical esophagus. Congenital webs always originate from the anterior wall.	Usually incidental finding without clinical symptoms. *Plummer–Vinson* syndrome: Iron deficiency anemia and acquired esophageal webs that may cause dysphagia. Certain skin diseases (e.g., *epidermolysis bullosa* and *benign mucous membrane pemphigoid*) may also be associated with esophageal webs.
Cartilagenous ring (tracheobronchial rest)	Short stricture-like narrowing in the distal esophagus. Characteristic are tiny fistulas that extend from the narrowed segment and may fill with barium.	Usually diagnosed in infancy, but occasionally in adults with long history of dysphagia. Other *congenital strictures* cannot be differentiated from acquired lesions.
Schatzki's ring (lower esophageal ring) (Fig. 2)	Smooth concentric narrowing at the junction between esophageal and gastric mucosa. Only seen in conjunction with a sliding hiatal hernia when the ring is located above the diaphragm.	Symptoms related to the ring (intermittent dysphagia or occasionally total obstruction) are only found when the ring diameter is less than 12 mm.
Carcinoma (primary) (Fig. 3)	Annular constriction often with overhanging margins, irregular lumen, and destroyed or ulcerated mucosa. These findings indicate an advanced stage of the disease. Preferred location is middle and lower esophagus in this order. More than one carcinoma might occasionally be present.	Usually in patients over 40 years of age with much higher incidence in men than women, often with both heavy smoking and drinking history.
Metastases (Fig. 4)	By direct invasion from carcinoma in adjacent organs or lymph nodes. Narrowing may be relatively smooth and often symmetric (especially from mediastinal metastases of a bronchogenic or breast carcinoma) or irregular and often ulcerated simulating a primary lesion (e.g., by direct extension of a cardia carcinoma into the distal esophagus or by invasion of a larynx, pharynx, or thyroid carcinoma into the cervical esophagus).	
Lymphoma (Fig. 5)	Involvement occurs by direct extension of gastric lymphoma, presenting often as a nodular, nonobstructive narrowing that may be difficult to differentiate from a gastric carcinoma progressing to the distal esophagus, or by enlarged, lymphomatous nodes encircling the esophagus and causing a relatively smooth narrowing.	Lymphomatous rather than metastatic carcinomatous involvement is likely in patients below 40 years of age.
Infectious esophagitis (Fig. 6)	Smooth, usually symmetric and often long strictures with tapering at both ends are characteristic and develop in the healing phase.	Candida and herpes simplex or zoster esophagitis develop usually in compromised hosts or AIDS patients. Tuberculosis, histoplasmosis, and syphilis are rare.
Crohn's disease and eosinophilic gastroenteritis	Rare causes of an esophageal stricture.	Esophageal involvement invariably associated in both conditions with manifestation of the disease in other parts of the gastrointestinal tract.

Narrowing in the Gastrointestinal Tract   137

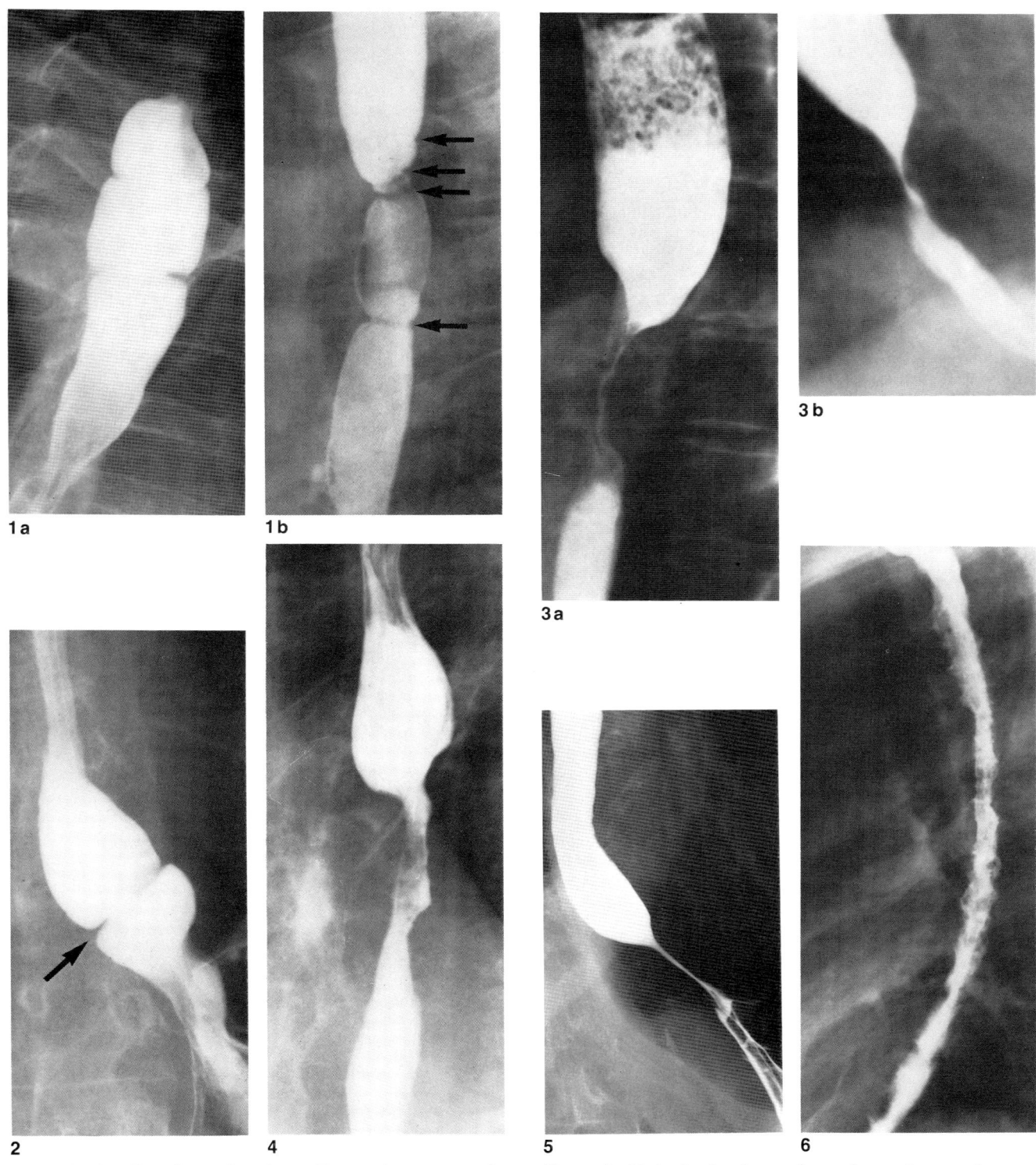

Figure **1a,b Esophageal webs. a** Two webs are seen in Plummer–Vinson syndrome in the upper esophagus. **b** Four concentric webs of unknown etiology are seen in the mid-esophagus (arrows).

Figure **2 Schatzki's ring in hiatal hernia.** A smooth concentric and symptomatic narrowing with a diameter of 1 cm is seen in a small sliding hiatal hernia (arrow).

Figure **3a,b Esophageal carcinomas. a** A slightly irregular and eccentric stricture is seen in the middle esophagus. **b** A smooth concentric stenosis is seen in the lower esophagus that is indistinguishable from a benign structure.

Figure **4 Metastasis from bronchogenic carcinoma.** Extrinsic narrowing of the mid-thoracic esophagus without apparent mucosal abnormalities is seen. Although the described findings suggest extrinsic metastatic involvement, a primary esophageal carcinoma may present in similar fashion.

Figure **5 Lymphoma.** The smooth stricture-like narrowing of the distal esophagus and cardia was caused by a large encircling lymphomatous mass.

Figure **6 Infectious esophagitis** caused by candida. Narrowing of the entire esophagus with mucosal abnormalities is seen. In this case the disease is still active and has not yet progressed to stricture formation.

Table 1 (Cont.) Narrowing of the Esophagus

Disease	Radiographic Findings	Comments
Reflux esophagitis (Fig. 7)	Often somewhat asymmetric and slightly irregular narrowing of the distal esophagus with funnel-shaped proximal end and absent mucosal pattern. A hiatal hernia is usually associated. A marginal ulcer at the gastroesophageal junction (peptic esophagitis) may be present and cause severe spasm and inflammation.	Changes caused by spasm and inflammation often cannot be differentiated from fibrotic healing, except that the two former are reversible, whereas the latter is not.
Barrett's esophagus (Fig. 8)	Smooth but often asymmetric stricture in the midesophagus resulting from a healed (Barrett's) ulcer.	Barrett's esophagus consists of islets of gastric mucosa in the esophagus away from the cardia with tendency to produce a peptic ulcer.
Intramural pseudodiverticulosis	Multiple cystic pouches of 1–3 mm are found in a short segment, or occasionally the entire length, of the esophagus. A stricture, usually of the mid-esophagus, is associated in about two-thirds of patients.	Dysphagia of long duration is often present.
Corrosive (caustic) esophagitis (Fig. 9)	Long smooth strictures involving the lower and often middle esophagus.	Strictures may appear as early as 2 weeks after ingestion of a caustic liquid.
Mediastinitis (infectious, abscess-forming, or sclerosing)	Concentric or eccentric, usually smooth narrowing of various lengths at different locations of the intrathoracic esophagus.	May be the sequela of a perforated or ruptured esophagus (e.g., post-instrumentation, trauma, or severe vomiting – *Boerhaave's syndrome:* complete tear of all layers of the esophageal wall above the gastroesophageal junction).
Hematoma	Both intramural or paraesophageal bleeding and subsequent fibrosis may produce a smooth narrowing at various levels.	In bleeding disorders, posttraumatic, post-instrumentation, and rarely in the *Mallory–Weiss* syndrome (hematemesis secondary to repeated vomiting caused by mucosal tear usually originating just below the gastroesophageal junction that may extend into the esophagus).
Iatrogenic strictures	Smooth, benign-appearing strictures may develop after repair of hiatal hernia or gastric surgery that permits bile to reflux into the esophagus, after prolonged nasogastric intubation and irradiation.	*Prolonged nasogastric intubation* predisposes to both gastroesophageal reflux (by preventing hiatal closure) and mucosal ischemia (by tube compression). Strictures may also develop after endoscopic obliteration of esophageal varices.
Motility disorders	Achalasia and prolonged lumen-obliterating contractions may simulate smooth organic strictures.	*Secondary contractions* spread simultaneously upwards and downwards from the middle and lower esophagus and produce radiographically a temporary hour glass deformity. See also Chapter 4, page 83.

7a 7b 8 9

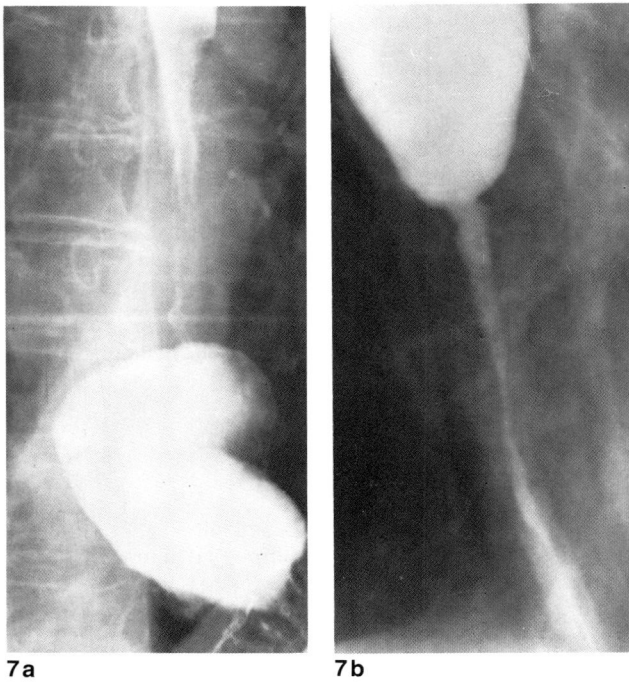

Figure **7a, b Reflux or peptic esophagitis. a** A slightly asymmetric and somewhat irregular narrowing of the distal esophagus is seen in conjunction with a hiatal hernia. **b** A stricture in the distal esophagus has formed secondary to peptic esophagitis. The ulcer in the gastroesophageal junction is no longer seen.

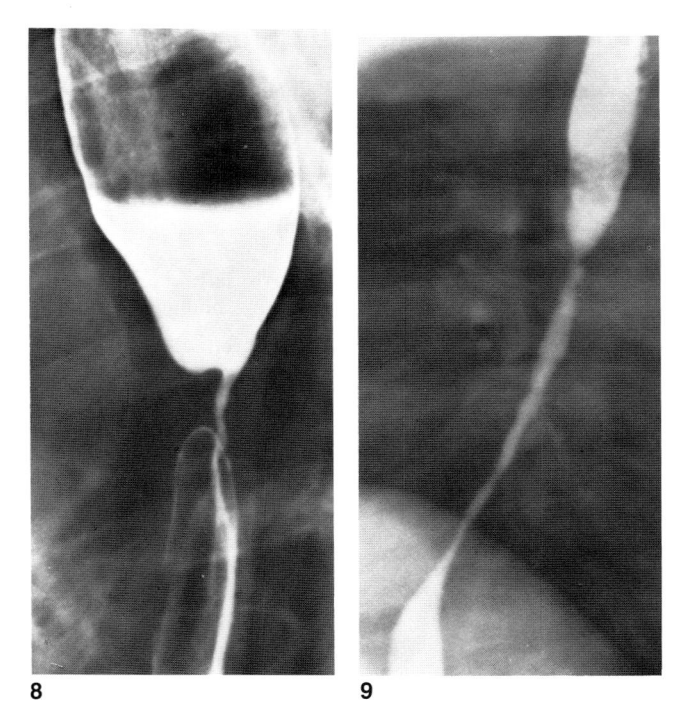

Figure **8 Barrett's esophagus.** A short and smooth but eccentric stricture is seen in the midesophagus after healing of a Barrett's ulcer.

Figure **9 Corrosive esophagitis.** A long and relatively smooth stricture has formed in the distal esophagus several weeks after ingestion of a caustic agent.

Table 2 Narrowing of the Stomach (Linitis Plastica Appearance)

Disease	Radiographic Findings	Comments
Carcinoma (scirrhous) (Fig. 10)	Part or entire stomach is shrunken into a rigid tubular stricture without peristaltic contractions. Rugal folds are generally flattened or totally obliterated and the mucosal pattern is often effaced. Involvement originates usually near pylorus and progresses slowly upwards, the fundus being least involved.	*Linitis plastica* ("water bottle stomach") refers to all conditions in which the stomach appears as narrowed rigid tube. By far the most common cause is scirrhous carcinoma of the stomach. The condition is caused by a desmoplastic response stimulated by tumor invasion.
Metastases (Fig. 11)	Circumferential stenosis to complete linitis plastica appearance may be caused by direct invasion from pancreatic and less common transverse colon carcinoma. Hematogenous metastases (e.g., from carcinoma of breast or lung) can also diffusely infiltrate the stomach wall and produce a similar radiographic appearance.	Tumor invasion from transverse colon carcinoma occurs via gastrocolic ligament.
Lymphoma (Fig. 12)	Irregular narrowing usually beginning in the antrum. Abnormal but usually not effaced mucosal pattern, often with small ulcerations. Contrary to carcinoma some flexibility of the stomach wall and residual peristalsis are usually maintained.	Besides the ileum, primary lymphoma affects most often the stomach and is usually of the non-Hodgkin variety. Secondary gastric involvement is more common and occurs with both Hodgkin's and non-Hodgkin's lymphoma. *Pseudolymphoma* may present also as constricting gastric lesion, that is often associated with a large ulcer crater.

Narrowing in the Gastrointestinal Tract 141

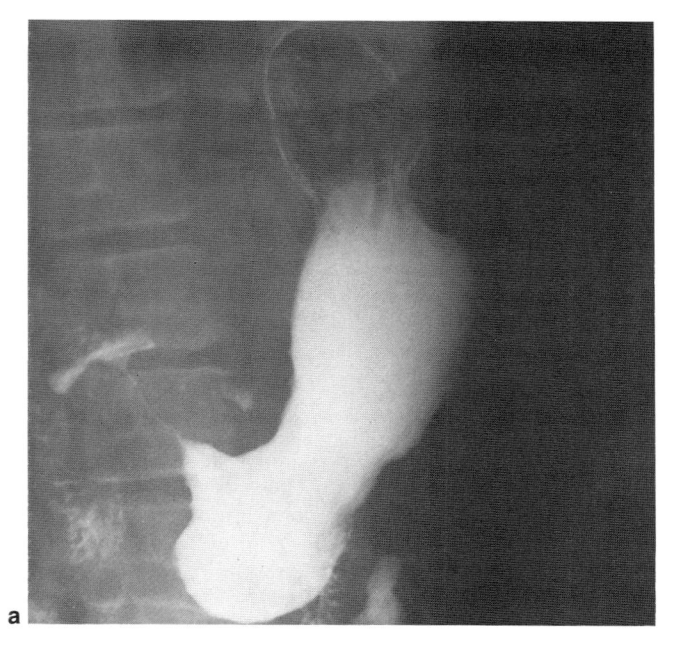

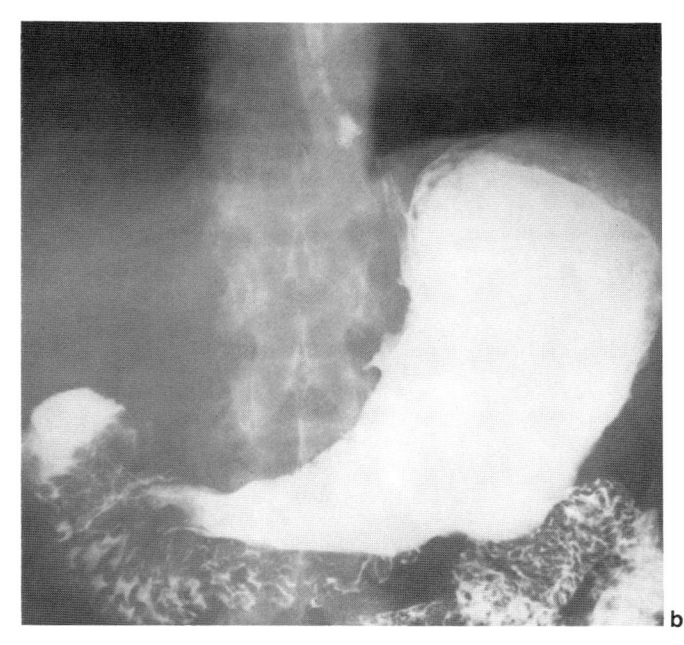

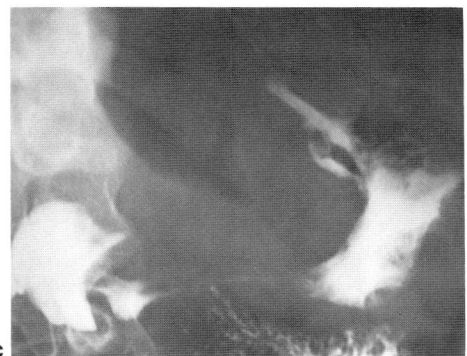

Figure **10a–c Gastric carcinoma (scirrhous) producing a linitis plastica appearance.** In all three cases the carcinoma originated near the pylorus and progressed to a varying degree upward. The involved part of the stomach presents as a rigid tubular stricture without peristaltic contractions and with completely effaced mucosal pattern. **a** Antrum and lower part of the body are involved. **b** Entire stomach is involved and has water bottle appearance. Note also the malignant-appearing flat ulcer on the lesser curvature. **c** Shrinkage of the entire stomach is seen in this most advanced case.

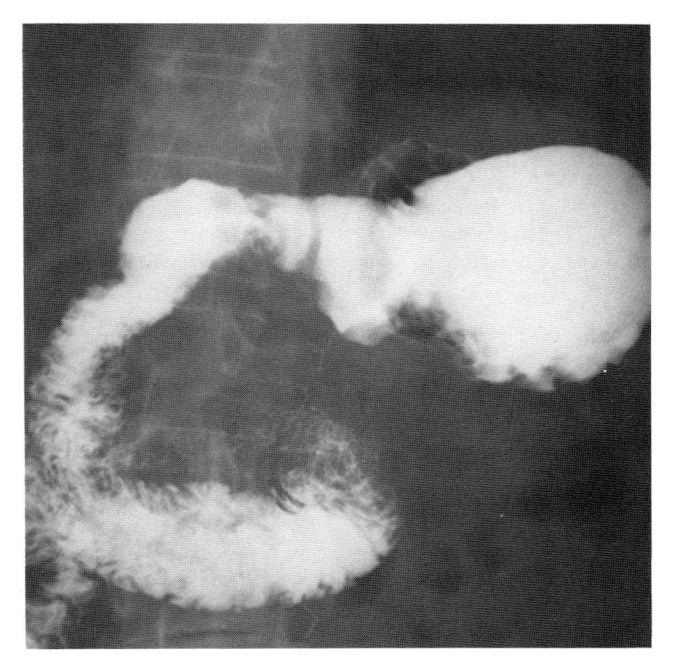

Figure **11 Pancreatic carcinoma invading the stomach.** Circumferential involvement of the antrum is seen but the greater curvature is much more severely affected than the lesser curvature. Note also the widening and infiltration of the duodenal sweep.

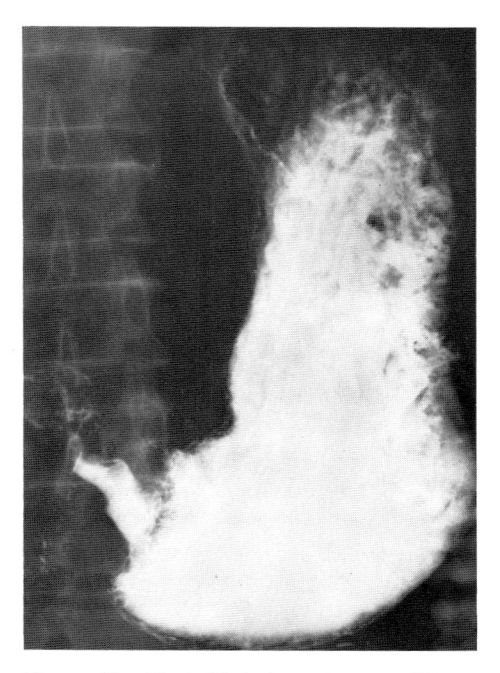

Figure **12 Hodgkin's lymphoma with secondary gastric involvement.** Irregular narrowing of the antrum with destroyed mucosal pattern is seen. Note also the lymphomatous involvement of the greater curvature with nodular lesions some of which demonstrate central ulcerations.

Table 2 (Cont.) Narrowing of the Stomach (Linitis Plastica Appearance)

Disease	Radiographic Findings	Comments
Exogastric mass (Fig. 13)	Extrinsic compression of the lesser curvature may produce a markedly narrowed stomach that is otherwise normal.	For example, with severe hepatomegaly or large pancreatic pseudocyst.
Peptic ulcer disease (Fig. 14)	Antral rigidity and narrowing can be seen with a distal gastric ulcer and is caused by either intense spasm in the acute stage or fibrosis in a chronic stage. An ulcer may radiographically not be demonstrable in either condition. Fibrotic healing of an ulcer in the body of the stomach may result in characteristic hourglass deformity.	An inflammatory antral process leading to submucosal fibrosis is occasionally termed *"stenosing antral gastritis"* and indistinguishable from healed ulcer disease.
Phlegmonous gastritis	Irregular narrowing in the antrum extending to the body, often with both effaced mucosal folds in one area and thickened in another. Gas-producing organism may produce intramural air bubbles, that are diagnostic.	Rare bacterial infection of the stomach with high mortality rate. Presents clinically with severe, acute abdominal symptoms (pain, nausea, and vomiting). Purulent emesis is rare but diagnostic when present.
Granulomatous gastritis (tuberculosis, sarcoidosis, syphilis)	Concentric narrowing, preferentially of the antrum, often with erosions and ulcerations.	Rare manifestations of these diseases.
Crohn's disease	Smooth, concentrically narrowed and relatively rigid antrum flaring into a normal gastric body and fundus (ram's horn sign). Duodenal involvement is almost always associated. Ulcerations and fissures are often present. Gastric outlet obstruction is a relatively common complication.	Concomitant involvement of gastric antrum, duodenal bulb and proximal sweep may simulate partial gastrectomy and Billroth I anastomosis ("pseudo-Billroth I").
Eosinophilic gastritis (Fig. 15)	Irregular narrowing of the antrum often associated with contiguous spread of the disease into duodenum and small bowel (eosinophilic gastroenteritis).	Benign self-limited condition that is often clinically and radiographically confused with Crohn's disease.
Corrosive (caustic) gastritis (Fig. 16)	Rigid and smooth stricture of the stomach with predilection for the antrum.	Develops within a few weeks after ingestion of corrosive agent (e.g. acids, alkalis, ferrous, sulfites).
Radiation gastritis	Rigid narrowing of the gastric lumen in the field of previous irradiation may develop in the healing phase.	A fractionated therapeutic dose in excess of 45 Gy is usually required.
Hepatic arterial chemotherapy	Narrowing of the antrum and proximal duodenum, often associated with ulcerations. Involvement corresponds to blood supply of gastroduodenal artery.	Caused by inadequate catheter placement with a high blood concentration of chemotherapeutic agent reaching gastroduodenal artery. May resolve after discontinuation of hepatic artery perfusion.
Gastroplasty (gastric stapling)	Narrowing of an otherwise normal stomach and presence of metallic suture material.	This surgical procedure is performed for weight reduction in morbid obesity.
Amyloidosis	Rare cause of rigid narrowing particularly of the antrum.	In systemic primary and secondary amyloidosis with manifestations of the disease in other organs.
Volvulus (Fig. 17)	Organoaxial volvulus: Stomach rotates upward around its long axis (line connecting cardia with pylorus). Mesenteroaxial volvulus: Stomach rotates around a line connecting the middle of the lesser curvature with the middle of the greater curvature. Characteristic findings include inversion of the stomach with greater curvature above lesser curvature, cardia and pylorus at the same level, and downward pointing of pylorus and duodenum.	Usually associated with diaphragmatic hernias, eventration or paralysis of the diaphragm. May be asymptomatic when neither vascular compromise nor outlet obstruction is present.

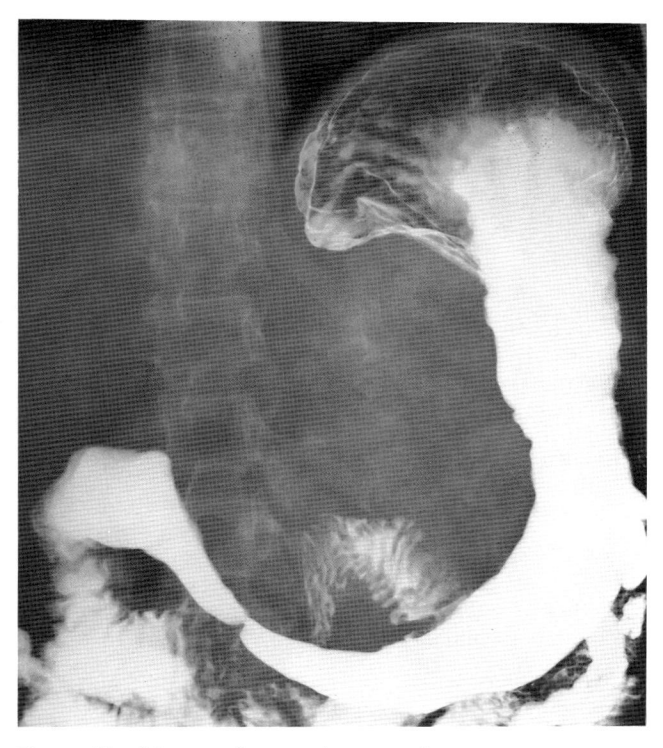

Figure 13 **Metastatic ovarian carcinoma.** A large and diffusely calcified mass involving both the left liver lobe and the lesser omentum causes extensive narrowing and elongation of the stomach.

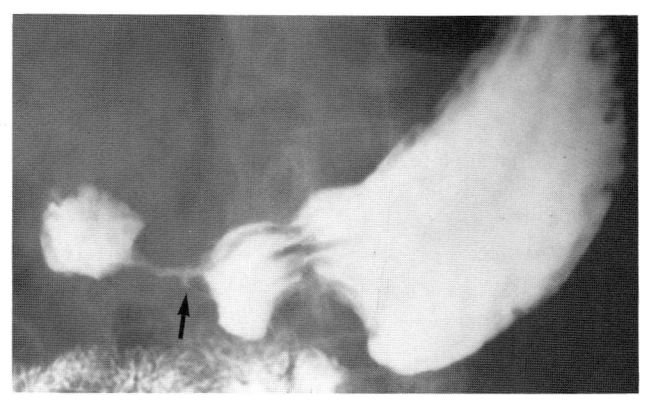

Figure 14 **Peptic ulcer disease.** Circumferential narrowing of the antrum with a small ulcer niche (arrow) is seen. Note also the normal peristaltic indentation on the greater curvature just proximal to the involved antrum that helps to differentiate this condition from a scirrhous carcinoma.

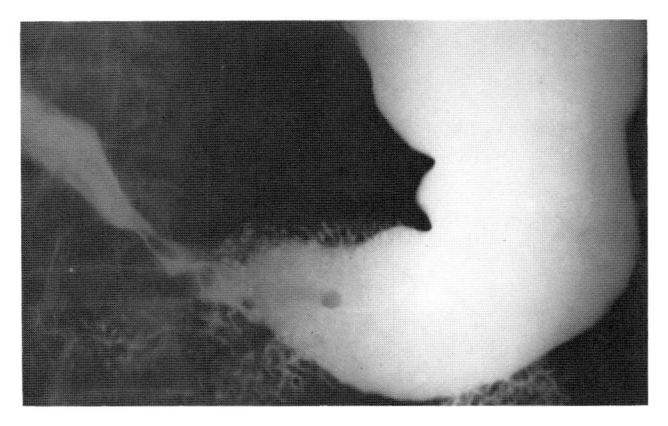

Figure 15 **Eosinophilic gastritis.** An irregular narrowing of the antrum with mucosal abnormalities and small polypoid filling defects is seen.

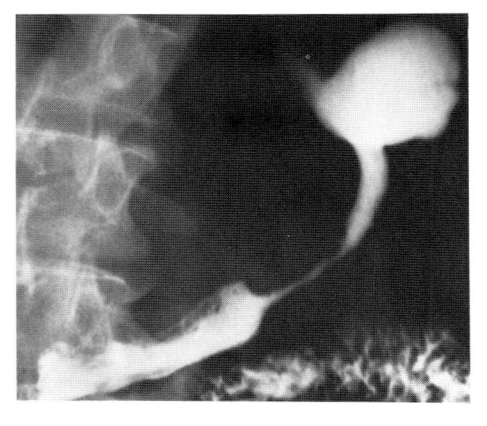

Figure 16 **Corrosive gastritis.** Extensive narrowing of the body and antrum with relative sparing of the fundus is seen.

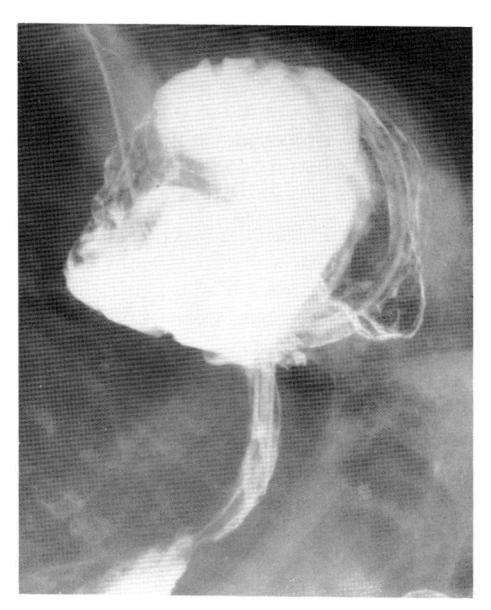

Figure 17 **Gastric volvulus.** An organoaxial volvulus of the stomach that is partially herniated through the diaphragm is seen.

Table 3 Narrowing of the Duodenum

Disease	Radiographic Findings	Comments
Double bubble sign in infants with complete or high-grade duodenal obliteration.	Presence of gas in the small and large bowel indicates that the duodenal obstruction is incomplete.	Represents a localized dilatation of the common bile duct.
Webs (duodenal diaphragms)	Membrane-like structures, preferentially located in the second portion of duodenum, which may cause varying degrees of obstruction.	These diaphragms are congenital and usually diagnosed in infancy and childhood.
Annular pancreas (Fig. 18)	Extrinsic narrowing of the second portion of the duodenum from the lateral side and above the level of the ampulla. The mucosa is intact unless duodenal ulceration develops, which is not uncommon in adults with symptomatic annular pancreas.	Annular pancreas may first be diagnosed in adulthood. Obstruction, even in infancy, is almost always incomplete.
Midgut volvulus (Fig. 19)	Duodenal obstruction associated with spiraling of small bowel and inferiorly and to the right displaced duodenojejunal junction (ligament of Treitz) is diagnostic. Cecum is located in midabdomen or on the left side, indicating incomplete rotation of the gut.	Only found with incomplete rotation of the gut, resulting in a narrow mesenteric attachment of the small bowel. Usually diagnosed in childhood.
Ladd's bands (congenital duodenal or peritoneal bands)	Extrinsic duodenal narrowing of anterior wall of the second or third portion of the duodenum.	May cause partial or intermittent obstruction. Symptoms often increase in upright and decrease in supine position.
Duodenal duplication cyst	Intramural or extrinsic fluid-containing mass of spherical or tubular shape that may encroach the duodenum.	Usually asymptomatic, but may rarely cause a high-grade duodenal obstruction.
Choledochal cyst (Fig. 20)	Extrinsic narrowing and widening of the duodenal sweep, when the choledochal cyst occurs near the ampulla of Vater.	Represents a localized dilatation of the common bile duct.
Carcinoma of the duodenum (primary) (Fig. 21)	Constricting narrowing with nodular mucosal destruction, ulcerations, and often overhanging edges. Preferentially located at or distally to the ampulla of Vater.	Clinical symptoms include obstruction and bleeding. Obstructive jaundice is present with periampullary location.
Pancreatic carcinoma (Fig. 22)	Narrowing of usually the second portion and rarely the third and fourth portion of the duodenum occurs in advanced stages. Mucosal destruction usually but not always present.	Two thirds of pancreatic carcinoma originate in the head, the rest of the body, and tail, in this order.
Metastases and lymphoma (Fig. 23)	Narrowing preferentially located in the distal half of the second portion and the third portion of the duodenum. An abnormal mucosal pattern with nodular lesions and ulcerations may be associated.	Caused by neoplastic aortic and pancreaticoduodenal lymph node involvement. A *retroperitoneal sarcoma* can rarely produce similar changes.
Postbulbar ulcer disease (Fig. 24)	Postbulbar ulcers, usually located on the medial wall of the second portion of the duodenum may cause concentric narrowing and obstruction of the duodenum. Abnormal mucosa and demonstration of an ulcer differentiate this condition from an annular pancreas.	Duodenal narrowing and obstruction is caused in the acute stage by spasm and in the chronic stage by a fibrotic stricture.
Crohn's disease	One or several areas of usually concentric narrowing associated with mucosal effacement, nodularity, and ulcerations. Stomach is almost always involved, also.	Similar findings are seen in *tuberculosis, strongyloidiasis, nontropical sprue* (healing phase after ulceration) and *eosinophilic gastroenteritis*. All these conditions are, similar to Crohn's disease, also associated with manifestations of the disease in other parts of the gastrointestinal tract.

Narrowing in the Gastrointestinal Tract   145

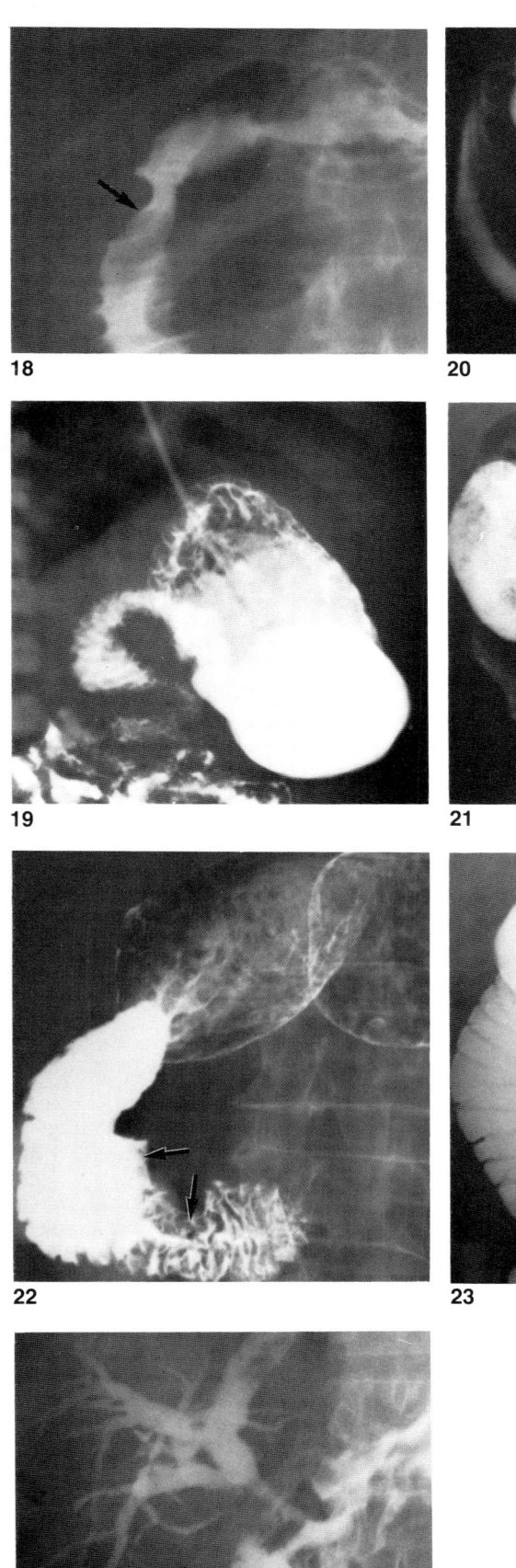

Figure 18 Annular pancreas. Extrinsic narrowing of the second portion of the duodenum from the lateral side is seen (arrow).

Figure 19 Midgut volvulus. Duodenal obstruction and spiraling of the jejunum are characteristic.

Figure 20 Choledochal cyst. Widening of the duodenal sweep with marked extrinsic compression of the duodenum is seen.

Figure 21 Duodenal carcinoma. Irregular narrowing of the duodenal sweep that is not widened is associated with complete mucosal destruction.

Figure 22 Pancreatic carcinoma. Complete obstruction of the third portion of the duodenum with an extrinsic mass defect on the second and third portion of the duodenum (arrows) is seen. Note also the marked prestenotic dilatation.

Figure 23 Non-Hodgkin's lymphoma. Extrinsic defects on the medial aspect of the distal half of the second portion of the duodenum and narrowing with partial obstruction of the third portion of the duodenum are caused by enlarged aortic and parapancreatic lymph nodes.

Figure 24 Postbulbar ulcer disease. A concentric narrowing of the upper descending duodenum is seen. Note also the barium reflux into the biliary system that may be caused by ulcer perforation into a bile duct or incompetence of Oddi's sphincter secondary to scarring.

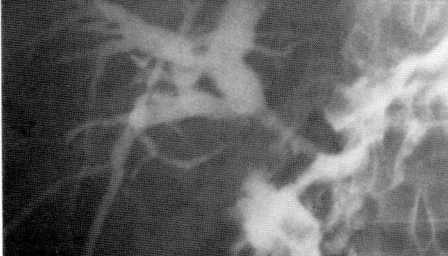

Table 3 (Cont.) Narrowing of the Duodenum

Disease	Radiographic Findings	Comments
Pancreatitis or pancreatic pseudocyst (Fig. 25)	Spasm in the acute stage and fibrosis in the chronic stage may cause narrowing of the second or occasionally, when the mesenteric root is mostly involved, the third portion of the duodenum. Mucosal thickening and spiculation can be seen, but there is no mucosal destruction as in pancreatic cancer. Duodenal narrowing may also result from extensive compression by a pancreatic pseudocyst.	Similar radiographic findings can occasionally be found with *cholecystitis*, but are usually located in the proximal half of the second portion of the duodenum.
Superior mesenteric artery syndrome	Extrinsic anterior narrowing and obstruction of the third portion of the duodenum where it crosses the spine. The duodenal mucosa is intact. Characteristically, the finding is more pronounced in supine position and partially to completely relieved in prone or lateral decubitus position.	In thin patients, hyperlordosis lumbalis, prolonged immobilization, decreased peristalsis, thickened mesenteric root (e. g., by inflammation or tumor), and abdominal aortic aneurysm.
Hematoma (Fig. 26)	Compression of second and third portion of the duodenum by hematoma or subsequent fibrosis.	Hematoma might be intramural or retroperitoneal secondary to trauma, anticoagulation therapy, bleeding diathesis, or bleeding aortic aneurysm.
Iatrogenic strictures	Relatively smooth narrowing of the second or third portion of the duodenum.	Following retroperitoneal surgery (e. g. repair of aortic aneurysm, insertion of prosthetic aortic graft) or pancreaticoduodenal surgery and radiation therapy.

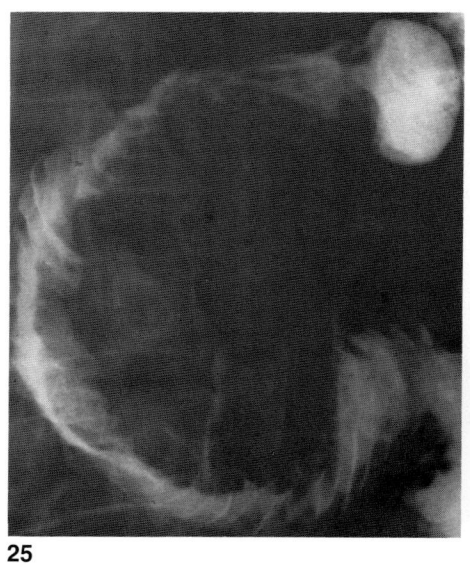

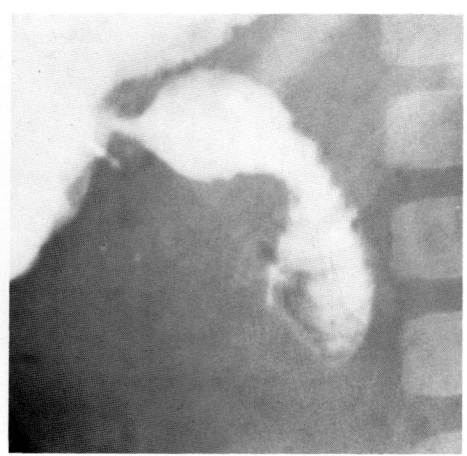

Figure **25 Pancreatitis with pancreatic pseudocyst.** Marked widening of the duodenal sweep with extrinsic narrowing is seen. Note also the mucosal spiculation.

Figure **26 Hematoma.** Duodenal obstruction between the second and third portion of the duodenum is seen.

Table 4 Narrowing of the Jejunum or Ileum

Disease	Radiographic Findings	Comments
Congenital atresia and stenosis	Minimal to complete obstruction of jejunum or ileum.	Usually diagnosed in infancy or childhood. Atresia is a more severe variant in the newborn associated with *meconium ileus* (evident as scattered abdominal calcifications). The associated microcolon (thin and ribbon-like) is most pronounced in low ileal atresia and progressively less with a more proximal location. Meconium ileus is also found in *cystic fibrosis*.
Carcinoid (Fig. 27)	Narrowing and angulation of adjacent, preferentially ileal loops, which are fixed and separated from each other. Mucosa of involved segments is irregularly thickened and transversely elongated or destroyed. One or several small filling defects may be seen but are usually not conspicuous.	This presentation is caused by a carcinoid that has locally infiltrated the mesentery and lymph nodes.
Carcinoma	Localized narrowing preferentially of the jejunum with destroyed and ulcerated mucosa.	Obstruction and pain most common clinical presentation.
Metastases (Fig. 28)	Usually multiple areas of narrowed and fixed loops. Tethering of the mucosa and transverse stretching of mucosal folds often combined with extrinsic or less commonly intrinsic mass lesions, which may undergo ulcerations. May resemble carcinoids or primary carcinoma, but multiple sites of involvement with varying presentations suggest metastases.	Common primary tumors that metastasize to the mesentery and small bowel include carcinomas originating in the gastrointestinal tract, pancreas, urogenital tract, lung, breast, and skin (melanoma).

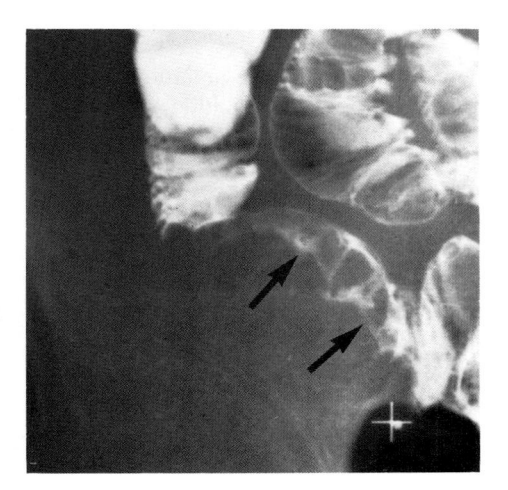

Figure 27 **Carcinoid.** Localized narrowing and angulation of an ileal loop by a mainly extraluminally growing mass (arrow) is seen.

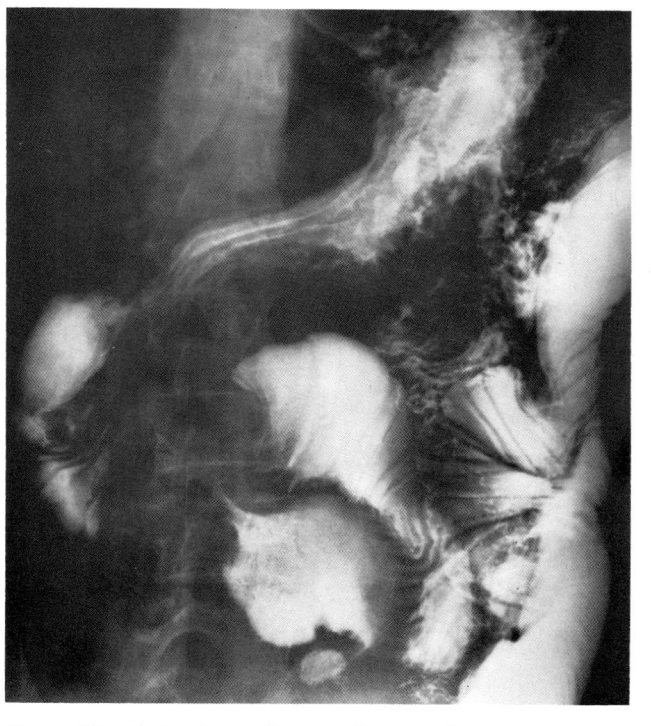

Figure 28 **Metastases from colon carcinoma.** Extensive metastatic disease is present involving the greater curvature of the stomach, duodenum, and small bowel loops that are fixed and narrowed at many locations by either extrinsic tumor infiltration or concentric constriction with prestenotic dilatation. Note also the mucosal tethering and destruction in many areas.

Table 4 (Cont.) Narrowing of the Jejunum or Ileum

Disease	Radiographic Findings	Comments
Lymphoma (Fig. 29)	Narrowing of usually multiple small bowel segments by either extrinsic compression or infiltration of the bowel wall. Irregular, thickened folds with small nodular defects and ulcerations are often present. Loops draped around mesenteric masses are fixed and demonstrate mucosal tethering. Obstruction occurs only in advanced disease. Differentiation from metastases is often impossible.	Primary and secondary involvement of the small bowel is much more common with non-Hodgkin's lymphoma than Hodgkin's disease.
Inflammation of adjacent structures	Localized narrowing of neighboring small bowel that may demonstrate a normal or edematous mucosal pattern, by spasm in the acute and stricture formation in the chronic stage.	For example, in pancreatitis, appendicitis, diverticulitis, intraperitoneal abscess formation.
Tuberculosis (Fig. 30)	Findings similar to Crohn's disease, but with greater tendency for stricture formation and higher incidence of associated cecal and ascending colon involvement.	Rare. Not necessarily associated with pulmonary tuberculosis.
Parasitic infections (giardiasis, strongyloidiasis)	Limited to duodenum and jejunum where the lumen is often narrowed by severe spasm and the mucosa thickened and irregular.	Clinical symptoms of malabsorption are only found with severe infestations.
Crohn's disease (Fig. 31)	Development of one or several stenotic segments with obstruction is common and most frequently seen in the terminal ileum but can involve any part of the gastrointestinal tract. In the acute stage, marked ulceration with severe spasm produces "string" sign evident as narrowed, poorly delineated bowel segment with effaced mucosal pattern resembling a frayed cotton string. In a more chronic stage, pipelike narrowing of varying lengths and often separated by normal segments ("skip" lesions) are seen, caused by thickening and fibrosis of the bowel wall. Irregular strictures can be seen in advanced fibrotic stage. Thickened mucosa with ulcerations ("cobblestone" pattern), perforation, fistula, and abscess formations are commonly associated features.	Small-bowel obstruction is a common complication in severe Crohn's disease.
Retractile mesenteritis	Narrowing, separation, and angulation of small-bowel loops by an apparent mesenteric mass.	A poorly understood, rare condition characterized by fibrosis, inflammation, and fatty infiltration of the mesentery. Related entities include *isolated lipodystrophy* and *lipogranuloma* of the mesentery, *nodular panniculitis* and *Weber–Christian disease*.
Adhesions (Fig. 32)	Extrinsic or concentric narrowing of a short segment with obstruction, which may be intermittent by kinking or compression of bowel loops at the site of previous surgery or inflammation.	Most common cause of small-bowel obstruction. Usually caused by previous surgery or peritonitis.
Anastomotic stricture	Localized, relatively smooth narrowing at anastomotic site caused initially by edema and hematoma and later by fibrotic stricture formation.	Must be differentiated from local recurrency, which is often irregular and may be associated with a growing mass lesion.

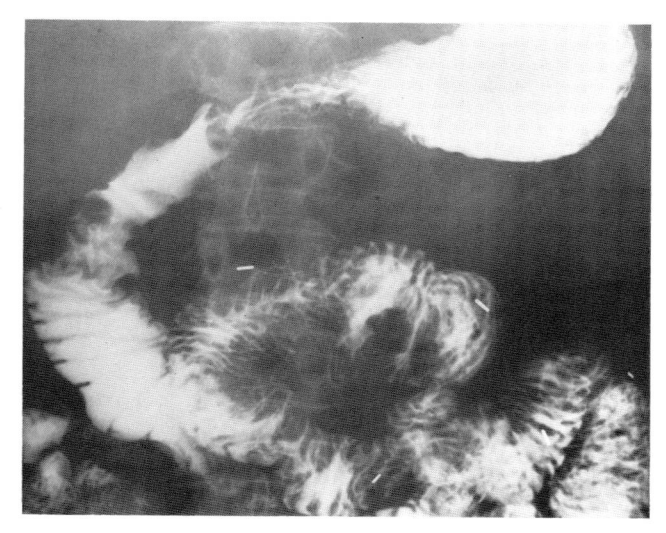

Figure 29 **Non-Hodgkin's lymphoma.** A jejunal loop draped around a mesenteric mass with mucosal tethering is seen. Note also the circumferential narrowing of the duodenum with destroyed mucosal pattern and nodular defects.

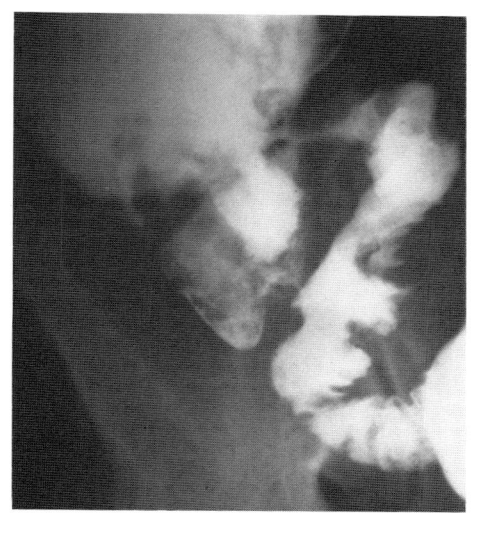

Figure 30 **Tuberculosis.** An abnormal terminal ileum with destroyed mucosal pattern, ulcerations, and several areas of localized narrowing is seen. Note also the narrowed ("cone-shaped") cecum.

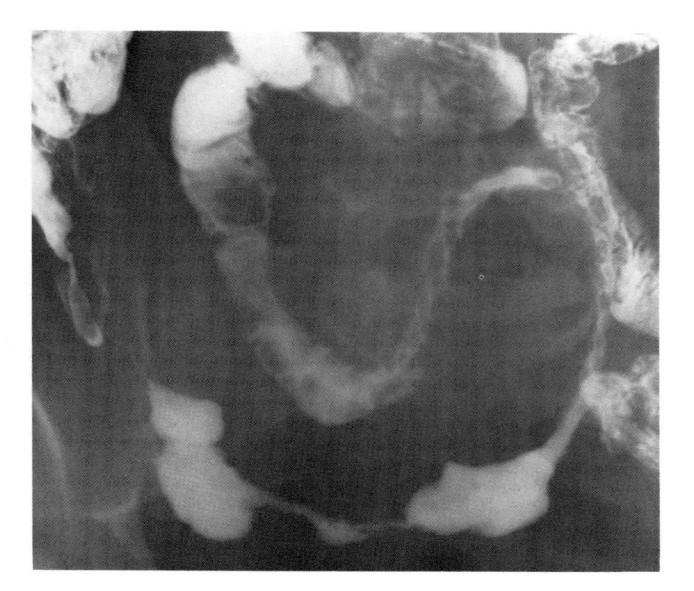

Figure 31 **Crohn's disease.** Several strictures separated by normally distended bowel segments ("skip" lesions) are seen.

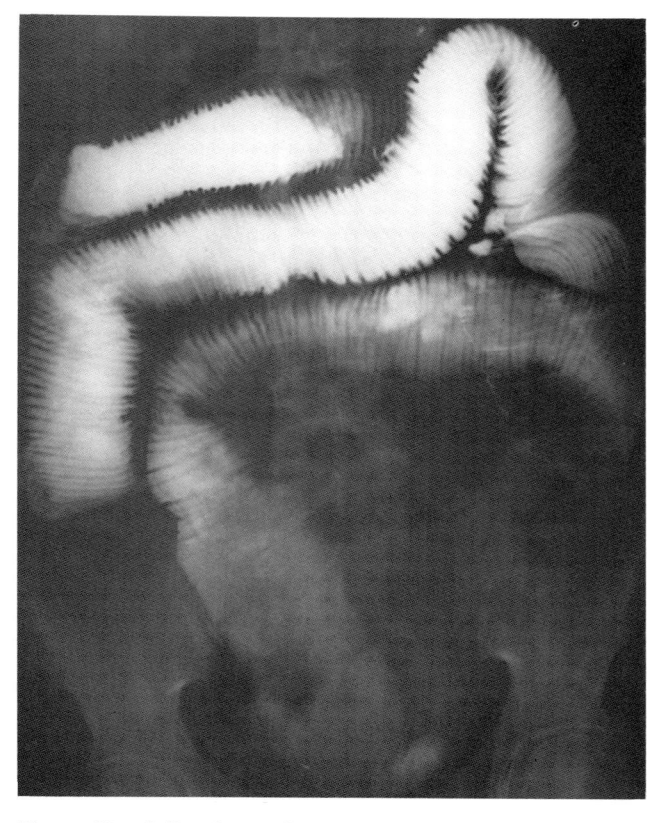

Figure 32 **Adhesions.** Small-bowel obstruction is caused by postoperative adhesions in the pelvis. Note the markedly dilated, prestenotic small-bowel loops with circular but not thickened folds.

Table 4 (Cont.) Narrowing of the Jejunum or Ileum

Disease	Radiographic Findings	Comments
Radiation therapy	One or several stenotic segments of varying lengths in field of irradiation.	Narrowing may be caused by submucosal edema and spasm in the acute stage, where mucosal thickening and shallow ulcerations might be associated, followed by fibrosis in the chronic stage.
Ischemic bowel disease	Narrowing of the involved segment by edema and spasm in the acute stage, with thickened folds and marginal filling defects ("scalloping" or "thumbprinting"). With incipient healing, the mesenteric border becomes flattened and rigid and the antimesenteric border plicated forming multiple sacculations or pseudodiverticula. With progressive fibrosis the involved segment becomes tubular with smooth surface and finally forms a stricture up to 10 cm in length.	Usually in elderly patients with cardiac failure. Similar radiographic findings are seen in *collagen diseases, thromboangiitis obliterans,* and *Henoch-Schönlein syndrome.*
Hernias (external and internal) (Figs. 33, 34)	Narrowing of the herniated bowel loops at characteristic locations with or without vascular compromise that may be evident as mucosal edema. In internal hernias, the trapped bowel loops are packed together into a small confined space and are clearly separated from the remaining small bowel.	External hernias (inguinal, femoral umbilical, incisional) are the second most common cause of small-bowel obstruction after adhesions. Internal hernias result from congenital abnormalities or surgical defects within the mesentery. In left paraduodenal hernias (most common internal hernia) and herniation through the foramen of Winslow, the trapped bowel loops are located in the left upper quadrant.
Volvulus	Twisted small-bowel segment with obstruction and vascular compromise.	Rare cause of obstruction in the adult. Associated with defective fixation of the mesentery permitting abnormal rotation or adhesions acting as pivot for small bowel segments to rotate about.

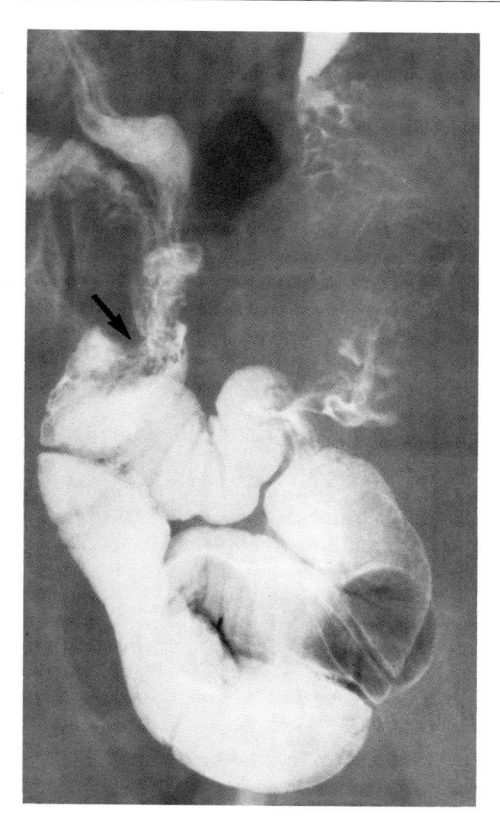

Figure 33 **Inguinal hernia.** Narrowing of the afferent and efferent ileal loop at the entry into the hernial sac (arrow) while the herniated ileal loops are distended, indicating partial obstruction.

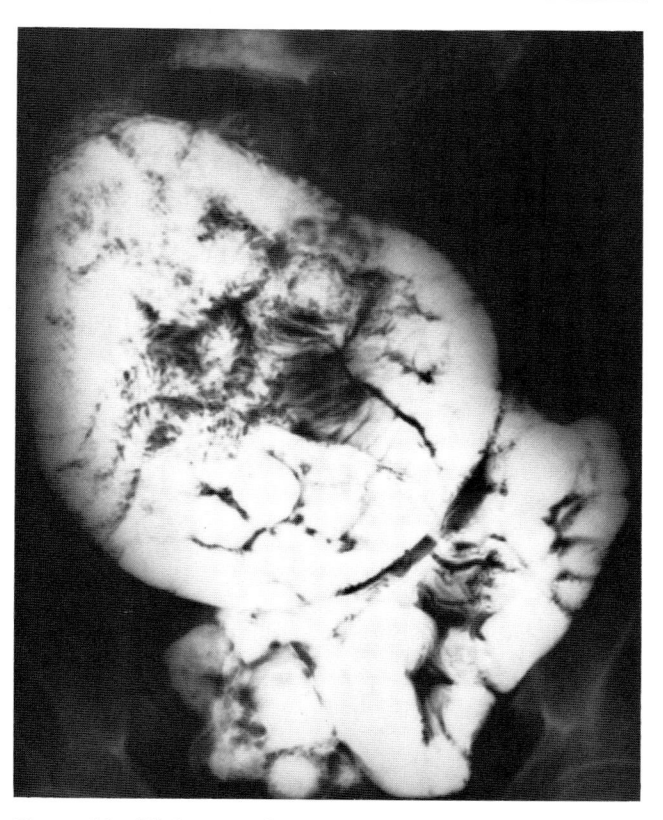

Figure 34 **Right paraduodenal hernia.** Jejunal loops are bunched together on the right side of the abdomen. Right paraduodenal hernias are associated with incomplete intestinal rotation with the duodenojejunal junction being located in a low right paramedian position.

Table 5 Narrowing of the Colon and Rectum

Disease	Radiographic Findings	Comments
Microcolon in neonates	Thin, unused colon associated with complete low small-bowel or proximal colonic obstruction. In both distal colonic and rectal atresia and imperforate anus, the colon proximal to the point of obstruction is dilated.	In meconium ileus (e.g., in cystic fibrosis), ileal and colonic atresia. If the obstruction is higher in the jejunum or duodenum, then the colon is normal in size.
Hirschsprung's disease (aganglionosis)	Rectum and distal sigmoid only mildly narrowed with abrupt transition to grossly dilated remaining colon.	Occasionally first diagnosed in late childhood and early adulthood. The narrowed, relatively normal-appearing distal segment is the pathologic part with absence of ganglion cells in the myenteric plexus. Hirschsprung's disease rarely involves other segments of the colon or even the entire colon. *Meconium plug syndrome* (local inspissation of meconium) and *imperforate anus* also produce low colonic obstruction and have to be differentiated in the neonatal period from Hirschsprung's disease.
Transient localized spasm (Fig. 35)	Concentric transient localized narrowing with normal mucosal pattern. Spasm is usually relieved with intravenous glucagon.	Occurs anywhere in the colon, but particularly common in the transverse, descending, and sigmoid colon, where the so-called *colonic sphincters* are located.
Endometriosis	Constricting narrowing with intact mucosa measuring up to several centimeters in length, usually involving the rectosigmoid. Irregular or pleated folds and polypoid filling defects can occasionally be associated.	Limited to women in child-bearing age. This form is seen when the endometrial implant induces a desmoplastic reaction and hyperplasia of the smooth muscle.
Carcinoid	Rarely present in cecum and ascending colon as circumferential colonic narrowing with destroyed but usually not ulcerated mucosal pattern, simulating adenocarcinoma.	Carcinoids of the colon often occur at a younger age than primary adenocarcinomas.
Carcinoma (Fig. 36)	Concentric narrowing is a common presentation of primary adenocarcinoma producing "apple-core" or "napkin-ring" lesions. The abrupt transition from normal bowel to the annular tumor with destroyed and often ulcerated mucosa and the production of a "tumor shelf" with "overhanging edges" are characteristic. Longer stenotic segments (up to 12 cm) with tapered ends and gradual transition to normal colon are seen in the relatively rare scirrhous carcinoma.	Annular carcinomas originate from flat tumor plaques (saddle lesions) that involve originally only part of the circumference of the colonic wall. Approximately 75% of colon carcinomas occur in the rectosigmoid area. Clinical symptoms are often late and nonspecific (change in bowel habits, anemia, rectal bleeding). Scirrhous carcinomas have a very poor prognosis. The luminal narrowing is caused by an intense desmoplastic reaction in the bowel wall.
Metastases (Fig. 37)	Besides extrinsic compression and fungating, often ulcerating intraluminal masses, a smooth or irregular stenosis, and an annular constricture are common presentations. In contrast to primary carcinoma, however, the ends are often more tapered without a pronounced "tumor shelf" and "overhanging edges" appearance.	By direct invasion from neighboring organs (prostate, uterus, ovary, kidney, pancreas, stomach), intraperitoneal seeding, and hematogenous (e.g., from carcinoma of breast, lung, and melanoma) or lymphangitic spread.
Lymphoma	Localized narrowing of the colon (especially the cecum) by constricting and infiltrating lesion with mucosal destruction is a rare presentation. Extrinsic compression and narrowing by large mesenteric lymph node masses may also occur.	This manifestation is virtually limited to non-Hodgkin's lymphomas.

Narrowing in the Gastrointestinal Tract 153

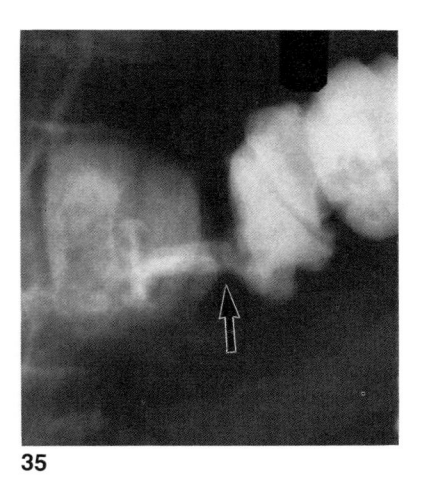

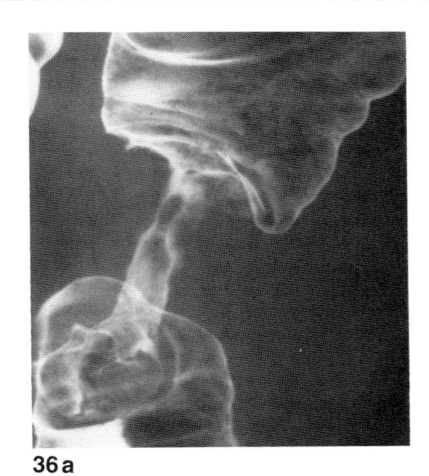

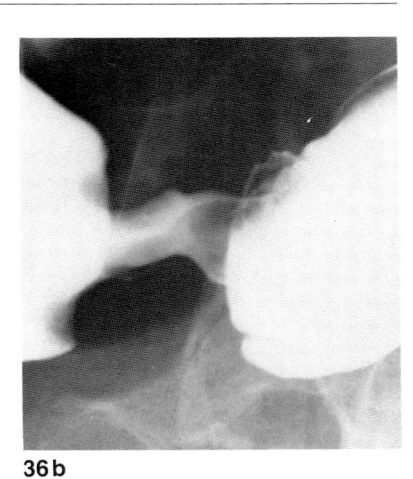

Figure **35 Transient localized spasm of the colon.** An area of localized concentric narrowing with intact mucosa is seen in the transverse colon.

Figure **36a, b Colon carcinoma.** A localized narrowing producing an "apple-core" or "napkin-ring" lesion is seen **a** in the descending colon and **b** in the sigmoid colon. Note the abrupt transition from normal bowel to the annular tumor with destroyed mucosa producing a "tumor shelf" with "overhanging edges."

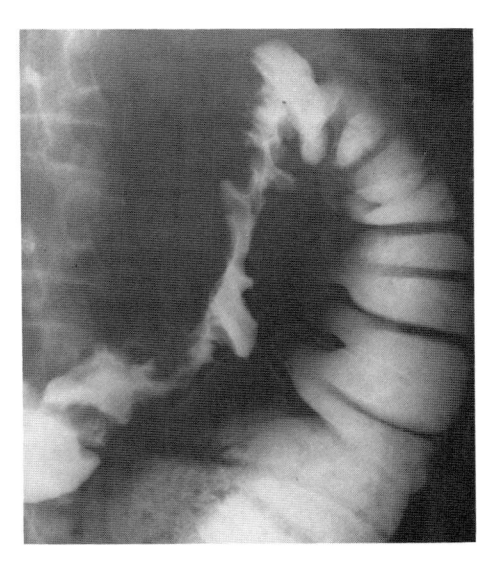

Figure **37 Colonic metastasis from carcinoma of the stomach.** An irregular narrowing of the transverse colon with destroyed mucosa and ulceration is seen. Although there is no pronounced "tumor shelf" production with "over-hanging edges," this lesion cannot be differentiated from a primary colon carcinoma on the basis of its radiographic appearance alone.

Table 5 (Cont.) Narrowing of the Colon and Rectum

Disease	Radiographic Findings	Comments
Diverticulitis (Fig. 38)	Narrowing of the involved segment (usually the sigmoid) by spasm in the acute and fibrosis in the chronic stage. An extrinsic filling defect caused by paracolic abscess secondary to a perforated diverticulum may be seen. Contrast extravasation from a diverticulum, evident as tiny collection at a tip of a diverticulum or rarely as filling of an abscess, is diagnostic. Diverticula adjacent to an abscess are spastic and often draped around it.	Incidence of colonic *diverticulosis* increases with age. In this condition large numbers of diverticula may shorten the involved segment and produce a "saw-tooth" appearance by the thickened circular muscle. This condition is occasionally referred to as "spastic diverticulosis", but its clinical relevancy is controversial. Diverticulitis is a relatively rare complication of diverticulosis in which the diverticular perforations resulted in the development of peridiverticular abscesses.
Extracolonic inflammatory process (Fig. 39)	Localized narrowing by spasm and edema or less commonly, at a later stage, by adhesions and stricture formation.	Caused by adjacent abscess or inflammation (e.g., pancreatitis: narrowing of the distal transverse colon and splenic flexure; cholecystitis: narrowing of the hepatic flexure; appendicitis: narrowing of the cecum). These diseases may also present as a localized ileus instead of a localized spasm in the adjacent colon (see Table 5, page 102).
Bacillary dysentery (shigellosis)	Narrowing of the colon by spasm associated with mucosal edema and superficial ulcerations. May progress to rigid, tubular stenosis with loss of haustration. Preferential location is the rectosigmoid area.	Acute or chronic (with periodic episodes of exacerbation and remission) inflammatory disease of the colon. May resemble clinically and radiographically ulcerative colitis. *Typhoid fever* and *Yersinia enterocolica* infection can produce inflammatory changes in the terminal ileum with narrowing and irregularity of the cecum.
Tuberculosis (see Fig. 30, p. 149)	Shortening and narrowing of the cecum ("cone-shaped") is most common manifestation. Involvement of terminal ileum is usually associated with cecal involvement. Segmental narrowing with irregular contours and ulcerations can occur in the remaining colon.	Pulmonary tuberculosis is not invariably associated.
Amebiasis	Cecum is concentrically narrowed and appears cone-shaped, whereas the terminal ileum is usually normal, in contrast to Crohn's disease or tuberculosis. Ileocecal valve is usually thickened and fixed in open position, permitting free reflux into the terminal ileum. Segmental lesions with superficial ulcerations and localized spasm may progress to fibrotic, rather long strictures, which are often multiple and most commonly located in the transverse and sigmoid colon and both flexures. Amebomas may present occasionally as annular constricting mass lesions.	The cecum is involved in 90% of chronic amebiasis. The diagnosis is made by the demonstration of *Entamoeba histolytica* in stool and rectal biopsy.
Fungal disease	Narrowing of the cecum or less commonly the colon, associated with inflammatory mass, often simulates primary adenocarcinoma.	*Actinomycosis* may mimic an appendiceal abscess. *South American blastomycosis* involving terminal ileum and cecum may be mistaken for Crohn's disease.
Schistosomiasis	Narrowing of the sigmoid colon or, less commonly, any other segment by progressive fibrosis occurs especially, when the disease originally presented as granulomatous process with extensive pericolonic infiltration. An initial presentation with multiple 1–2 cm polypoid granulomas, however, progresses only rarely to stricture formation.	Chronic debilitating disease that may involve multiple organs and affects over 200 million people in the tropics and subtropics. *Strongyloides stercoralis* can occasionally produce colonic strictures following ulcerating colitis. *Anisakiasis* (ascaris-like nematode) can produce severely inflamed and narrowed terminal ileum, cecum, and ascending colon in people eating raw fish.

Table 5 (Cont.) Narrowing of the Colon and Rectum

Disease	Radiographic Findings	Comments
Lymphogranuloma venereum (Fig. 40)	Short or long tubular rectal stricture of varying length, beginning just above the anus and extending in some cases to the sigmoid, which may be involved also. Ulcerations, fistulas, and perirectal abscesses are commonly associated.	Viral venereal disease particularly common in sexually promiscuous individuals and in the tropics. Presents initially as herpetiform lesion on the external genitalia 2 weeks after infection. *Herpes zoster* may produce short segments of colonic narrowing with small ulcerations. *Cytomegalovirus* infection may produce colonic ulcers, edema and narrowing, especially in immunosuppressed renal transplant recipients.
Nonspecific benign ulcer disease	Stricture formation can be a late sequela, especially in the cecum and rectum.	In the rectum the entity is termed *solitary rectal ulcer syndrome* and must be differentiated from lymphogranuloma venereum.

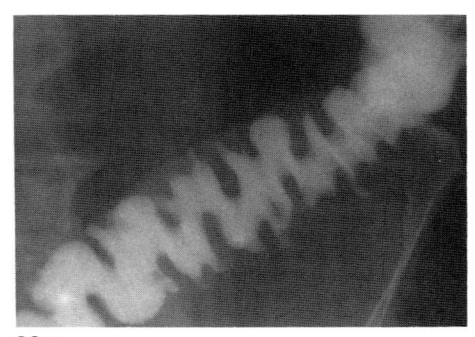

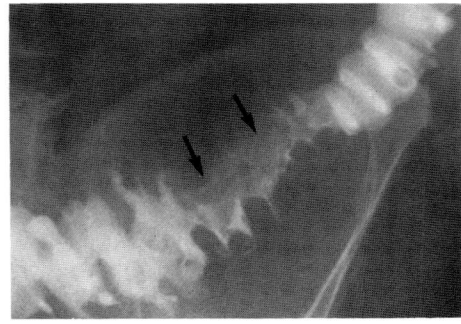

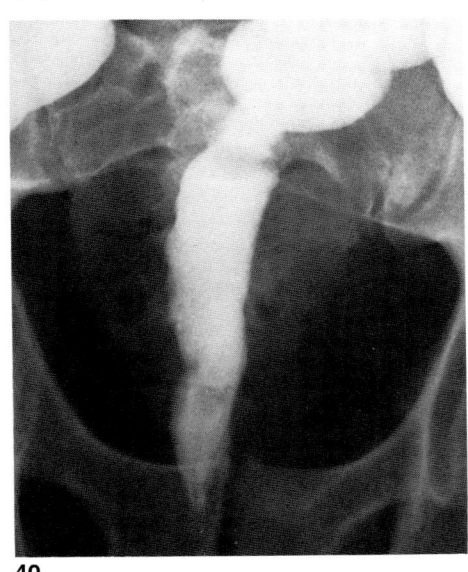

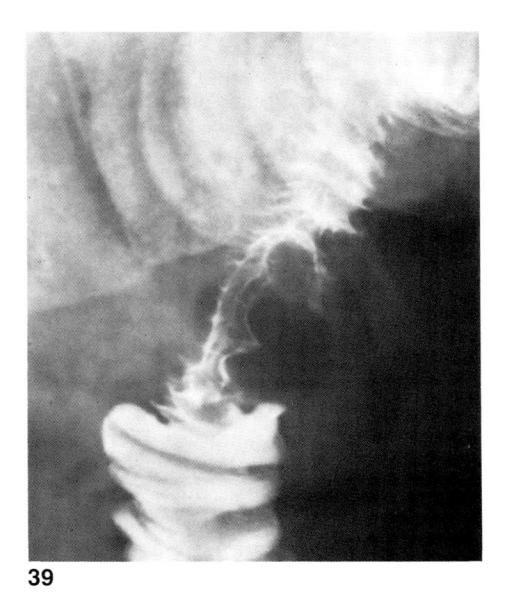

Figure **38a, b Diverticulosis progressing to diverticulitis** in a two-year interval. **a** A shortened sigmoid colon with "saw-tooth" appearance is seen that is caused by thickened and spastic circular muscle in the presence of numerous diverticula. This appearance is occasionally also referred to as "spastic diverticulosis." **b** Two years later, diverticulitis has developed. Narrowing of the involved segment by spasm and abscess formation (arrows) is now seen, besides thin mucosal spiculations.

Figure **39 Pancreatitis with secondary involvement of the descending colon.** Concentric narrowing of the inflamed part of the descending colon by spasm and edema is seen. Note that in contrast to a carcinoma the mucosal pattern in the narrowed segment is intact but edematous. Together with the fine mucosal spiculations, this suggests an inflammatory rather than neoplastic nature of the abnormality.

Figure **40 Lymphogranuloma venereum.** Narrowing of the entire rectum beginning just above the anus is seen.

Table 5 (Cont.) Narrowing of the Colon and Rectum

Disease	Radiographic Findings	Comments
Ulcerative colitis (Fig. 41)	Foreshortening of the colon with depression of flexures, narrowing of the lumen, and absent haustral pattern with relatively smooth surface are characteristic for chronic stage ("lead-pipe" colon). Localized concentric strictures of varying length with relatively smooth contours and tapering margins are seen in different stages of the disease and rarely cause obstruction. Carcinomas complicating ulcerative colitis develop preferentially in the distal half of the colon, may be multicentric in 20% of cases, and are often very difficult to differentiate from a benign stricture, since they present often as a narrowed 2–6 cm segment with tapered ends, but the narrowed lumen is usually somewhat eccentric and the contours tend to be irregular.	Incidence of colon carcinoma is approximately 20 times higher in ulcerative colitis than normal population. Risk of developing carcinoma is particularly high with universal colitis and increases with duration of the disease. Rarely a carcinoma develops during the first 10 years after onset of the disease.
Crohn's colitis (Fig. 42)	Solitary or multiple stenotic segments are often already encountered in an early stage of the disease when other more characteristic findings are also present ("cobblestone" pattern, skip lesions and fistulas). In the chronic stage, a "lead-pipe" colon identical to ulcerative colitis and localized benign strictures, which occasionally may be eccentric and difficult to differentiate from a carcinoma, are often seen.	The incidence of colon carcinomas in Crohn's colitis is higher than in the normal population, but this association is less striking than in ulcerative colitis. Carcinomas complicating Crohn's colitis present usually as fungating mass lesions in the proximal colon and are therefore relatively easily recognized.
Ischemic colitis (Fig. 43)	Besides "thumbprinting," annular constricting lesions simulating carcinoma may be seen in acute phase. During healing, flattening of the mesenteric border combined with pleating of the antimesenteric margin may produce multiple sacculations or pseudodiverticula. Progressive fibrosis may finally result in tubular narrowing and smooth stricture formation. Preferentially located in the splenic flexure, descending and sigmoid colon.	Usually in elderly patients with cardiac failure. A similar sequence of events (from "thumbprinting", to smooth stricture formation) may occasionally also be seen with intramural bleeding of different etiologies. Acute ischemic colitis reverts to normal radiographic appearance when adequate collateral circulation is established. This occurs invariably in the rare so-called *"evanescent ischemic colitis"* of adolescents and young adults, in which no apparent underlying cause is found.
Cathartic colon	Foreshortened tubular colon with loss of haustration similar to burned-out ulcerative colitis. In contrast to the latter, the right side is usually more severely involved and often shows constant areas of concentric narrowing, whereas the rectum and sigmoid appear often normal.	In patients with history of life long constipation and habitual use of irritant cathartics for 15 years and longer.
Caustic colitis	Tubular narrowing to severe stricture formation begin within one month after enemas with caustic agents.	For example, following detergent enema.
Pseudomembranous colitis	Healing may occasionally result in a tubular colon without haustral markings. Strictures can develop very rarely.	Complete healing without any radiographic sequelae occurs usually after discontinuation of the offending antibiotic.

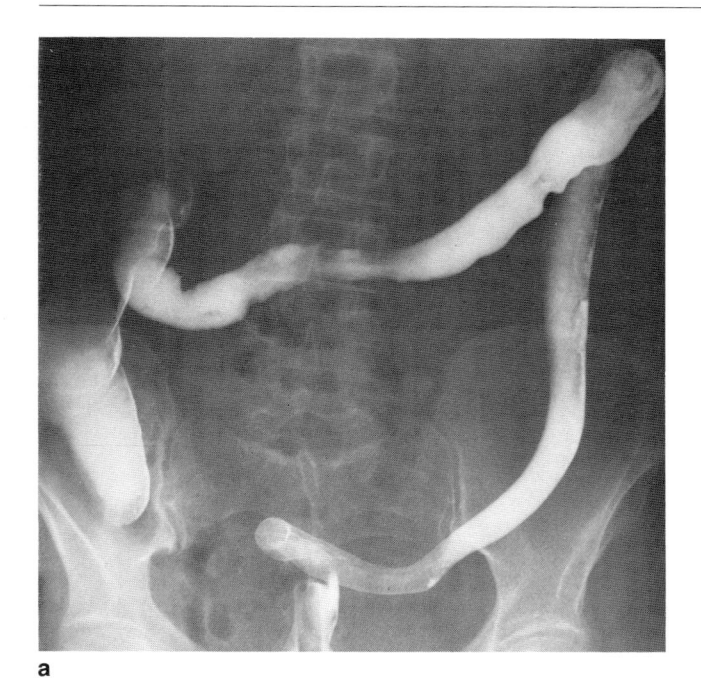

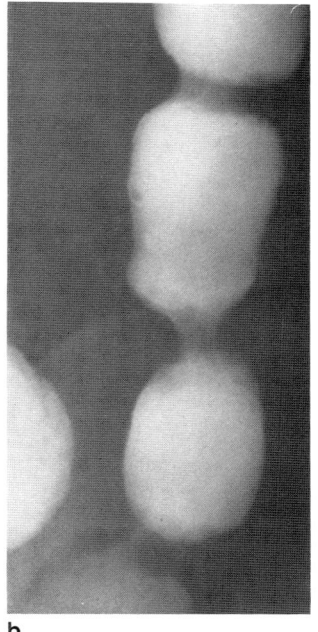

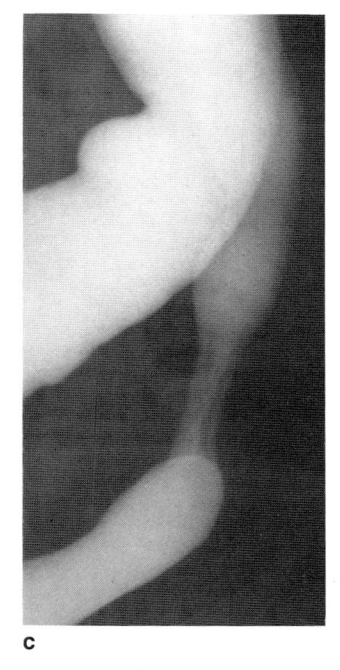

Narrowing in the Gastrointestinal Tract 157

Figure **41a–c Ulcerative colitis in three different patients. a** "Lead-pipe" colon. Foreshortening and narrowing of the entire colon with more severe involvement of the left side, absent haustral markings, and depression of the flexures is characteristic for the chronic stage. **b** Three areas of benign concentric narrowing are seen in the descending colon of this patient with chronic ulcerative colitis. **c** Carcinoma in chronic ulcerative colitis, presenting as benign-appearing stricture of the descending colon, although the lumen stricture is slightly eccentric.

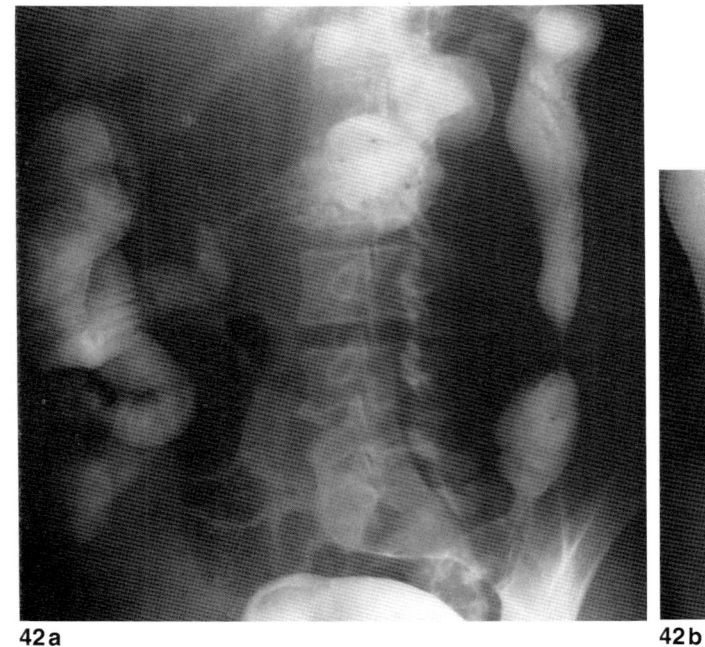

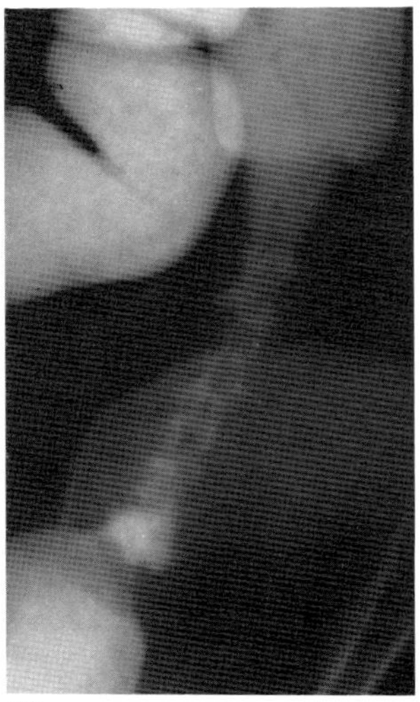

Figure **42a, b Crohn's colitis** in a patient with ileocolostomy performed four years earlier for colon carcinoma. **a** Several benign stenotic segments are seen in the remaining distal half of the colon with the two most severe strictures being located at the anastomotic side between ileum and transverse colon and in the descending colon. Note also the abnormal mucosal pattern in both ileum and colon with relative sparing of the rectosigmoid. **b** The carcinoma had originally presented as a fungating mass in the ascending colon in this patient with a long history of Crohn's disease.

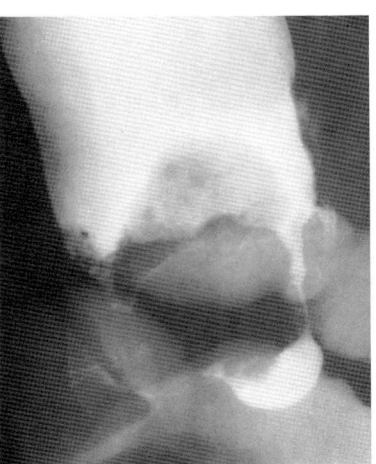

Figure **43 Ischemic colitis.** A constricting lesion with "thumbprinting" is seen in the descending colon.

Table 5 (Cont.) Narrowing of the Colon and Rectum

Disease	Radiographic Findings	Comments
Radiation therapy (Fig. 44)	Segmental narrowing of varying lengths in the field of previous irradiation, most commonly found in the sigmoid and rectum. Narrowing is caused by spasm in the acute stage and associated with mucosal edema, serrations, and ulcerations, whereas a smooth tubular stricture is found in the chronic fibrotic stage.	Fibrotic tubular strictures develop 6 to 24 months after irradiation with a dose in excess of 40 Gy.
Anastomotic stricture	Localized, smooth narrowing with at least limited distensibility at anastomotic site is caused by edema and hematoma in the immediate postoperative period and may progress to a fibrotic stricture.	Must be differentiated from a local recurrency where the stricture is often irregular, nondistensible and progressively worsening.
Adhesions	Short smooth stenotic areas with intact mucosa.	Secondary to abdominal surgery or inflammation.
Pelvic lipomatosis (Fig. 45)	Narrowing and vertical elongation of the rectum and sigmoid with intact mucosa and distensible wall. The increased pelvic radiolucency caused by the excessive fat deposition may already be appreciated by conventional radiography; otherwise CT is diagnostic.	Benign condition with increased deposition of normal adipose tissue in the pelvis. A similar narrowing of the rectosigmoid may occasionally be seen with *retractile mesenteritis*, which more commonly involves the small bowel.
Pelvic fibrosis	Narrowing of the rectum and/or sigmoid.	After pelvic surgery, trauma, inflammation, irradiation, and edema (e. g. chronic obstruction of the inferior vena cava).
Pelvic carcinomatosis and lymphoma	Narrowing of the rectum and/or sigmoid with or without tumor infiltration.	Metastases from urogenital or intestinal malignancies.
Pelvic mass	Extrinsic narrowing and often elongation of the rectum and/or sigmoid.	Ovarian cyst, enlarged uterus, neurogenic and sacral lesions (retrorectal), hematoma (pelvic fractures), abscess, urinoma and lymphocele.
Amyloidosis	Rare cause of rigid narrowing with effacement of haustral markings preferentially in the rectosigmoid area.	May mimic chronic ulcerative colitis.
Volvulus (cecal and sigmoid) (Fig. 46)	The tapered contrast column at the level of obstruction has characteristically the appearance of a "bird's beak."	Plain film findings may already be diagnostic. See Figs. **26** and **27**, page 101.
Hernias (Fig. 47)	Localized narrowing and obstruction of displaced transverse or sigmoid colon, often complicated by strangulation.	Inguinal, femoral, umbilical, diaphragmatic, incisional as well as internal hernias (e.g., through the foramen of Winslow) occur.

Narrowing in the Gastrointestinal Tract   159

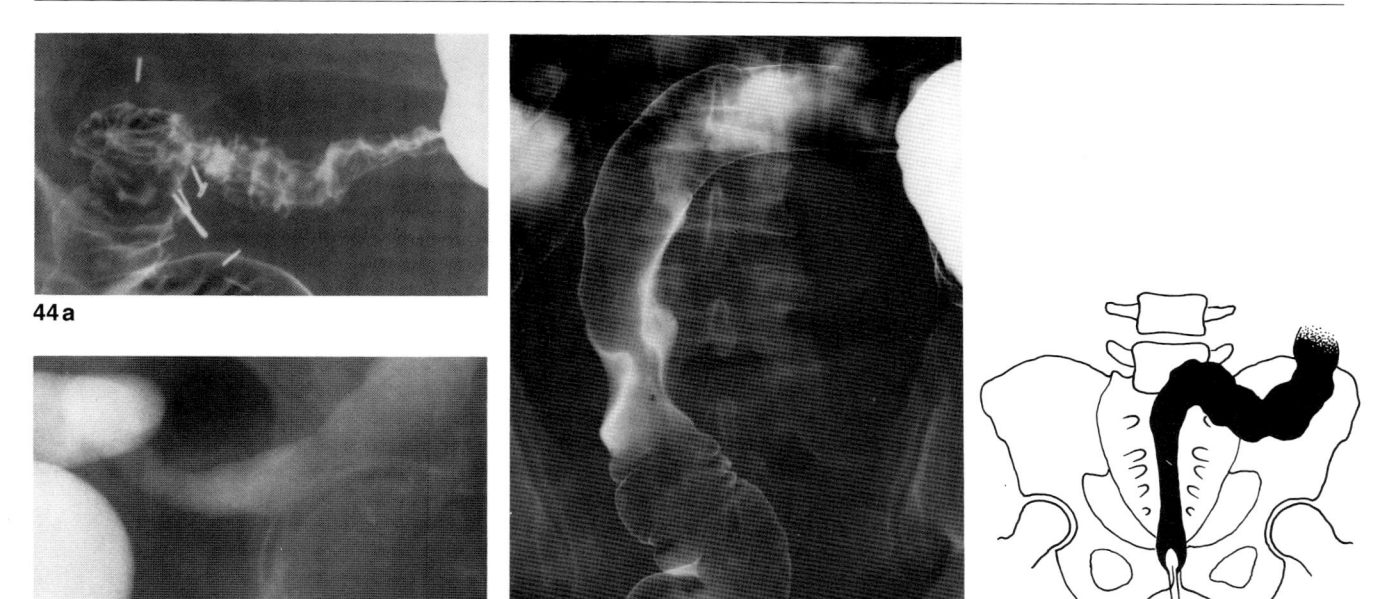

Figure **44a, b**   **Radiation colitis, a** in the acute and **b** in the chronic phase. A localized narrowing of the sigmoid colon is seen in both phases. Mucosal abnormalities including ulcerations are associated in the acute stage, whereas a tubular stricture is seen in the chronic stage.

Figure **45a, b**   **Pelvic lipomatosis.** Narrowing and vertical elongation of the rectum and distal sigmoid with intact mucosa and distensible wall is characteristic.

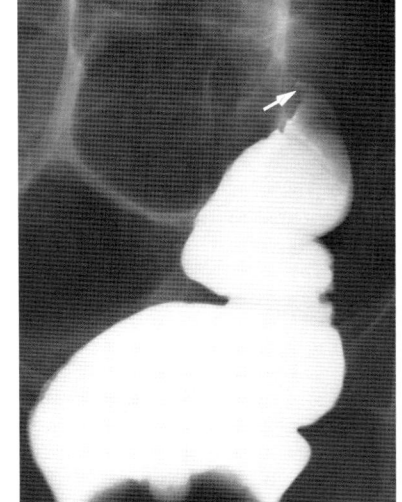

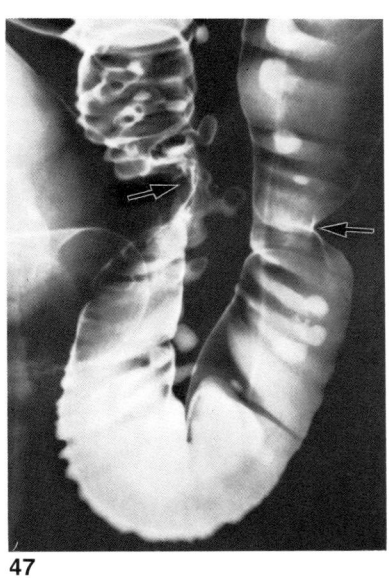

Figure **46**   **Sigmoid volvulus.** A tapered edge of the obstructed contrast column pointing toward the site of torsion ("bird's beak") is characteristic (arrow).

Figure **47**   **Inguinal hernia.** Localized extrinsic compression of the afferent and efferent loop of sigmoid colon at the site of entry into the hernial sac is seen (arrows). Note also the multiple diverticula.

Chapter 7 Filling Defects in the Gastrointestinal Tract

In the gastrointestinal tract, space-occupying lesions are visualized during barium examinations as filling defects. A variety of normal and pathologic structures can produce a filling defect in the gastrointestinal tract, although neoplasms are the most common cause. They may originate from the mucosa, the remaining bowel wall, or an adjacent organ. Depending on the site of origin, intrinsic and extrinsic mass lesions can be differentiated radiographically.

An *intrinsic lesion* is characterized by the fact that the larger portion of the mass projects into the lumen of the bowel. Using this definition, any lesion with a stalk obviously falls into this category. Lesions in which the barium column forms an acute angle between the mass and bowel wall, when viewed in profile, are also intrinsic (Fig. **1**). If such a lesion involves the entire circumference of the bowel, acute angles ("shouldering") may be seen on both sides of the lumen. Most intrinsic lesions originate from the mucosa, but occasionally an intramural lesion (e.g., a leiomyoma of the bowel wall) may produce radiographic features characteristic of an intrinsic or polypoid mass.

When the barium column forms an obtuse angle between the lesion and bowel wall in profile projection, the tumor can be either intrinsic or extrinsic. An infiltrating carcinoma presenting as a plaque would be an example of an intrinsic lesion that can present radiographically in this way. A similar filling defect can be produced by an *extrinsic mass*, but in this case only a small segment of the mass protrudes into the lumen, while the larger portion of it is located outside the bowel lumen (Fig. **1**). Assuming the extrinsic mass has a more or less globular shape, the radiographically visualized tumor segment is always smaller than the part of the lesion projecting outside the lumen. Assessment of the size of the extraluminal component may be the only clue to help differentiate between an intrinsic and extrinsic lesion when both form an obtuse angle with the bowel wall.

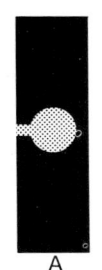

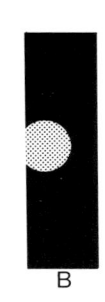

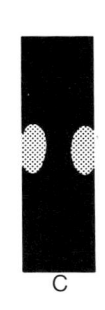

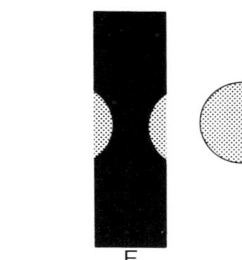

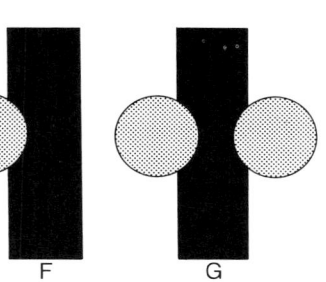

Figure 1 **Differentiation between intrinsic** (A to E) **and extrinsic** (F and G) **lesions.** Radiographic signs of an intrinsic lesion include the demonstration of a pedicle (A) or the demonstration of an acute angle between lesion and bowel wall (B and C). An obtuse angle between lesion and bowel is not diagnostic, since it can be found with both intrinsic (D and E) and extrinsic (F and G) lesions, both producing the same radiographic profile. However, with extrinsic lesions a larger extraluminal component is invariably present, as shown in F and G.

Extrinsic filling defects in the gastrointestinal tract can be caused by normal, or more commonly by pathologically altered organs in the immediate vicinity. In the esophagus, this includes the spine, thyroid, trachea, left main bronchus, aorta, heart, lymph nodes, and other tissue structures of the posterior mediastinum (Fig. 2). Displacement of an esophageal segment, however, is not only caused by *extrinsic compression,* but may at times also result from *retraction* produced by a scarring process. This occurs, for example, in apical pleuropulmonary fibrosis.

Differentiation between *benign* and *malignant* mass lesions can be difficult. Rigidity of the involved bowel segment, a destroyed mucosal pattern, and ulcerations associated with a mass strongly suggest a malignancy. A soft and pliable or pedunculated mass lesion with a normal mucosal pattern favors a benign process. Tumor size is an unreliable criterion for differentiating between benign and malignant lesions, although polypoid lesions measuring less than 10 mm in diameter are likely to be benign. On the other hand, an increase in the size of a mass on follow-up examination is highly likely to indicate a malignant process. The growth rate of gastrointestinal malignancies can occasionally be very slow, with tumor-doubling times exceeding three years. One has to keep in mind that an increase in diameter of only 26% is required to double the volume of a spherical lesion.

In air contrast studies, differentiation between a *polypoid lesion* and a *diverticulum* may be difficult when the lesion is seen face-on in a double-contrast examination. In these conditions, a sharp inner border of barium around the lesions is characteristic for a polypoid lesion, whereas in a diverticulum the outer border is sharply defined (Fig. 3).

The differential diagnosis of filling defects in the gastrointestinal tract is discussed in Tables **1** to **5.**

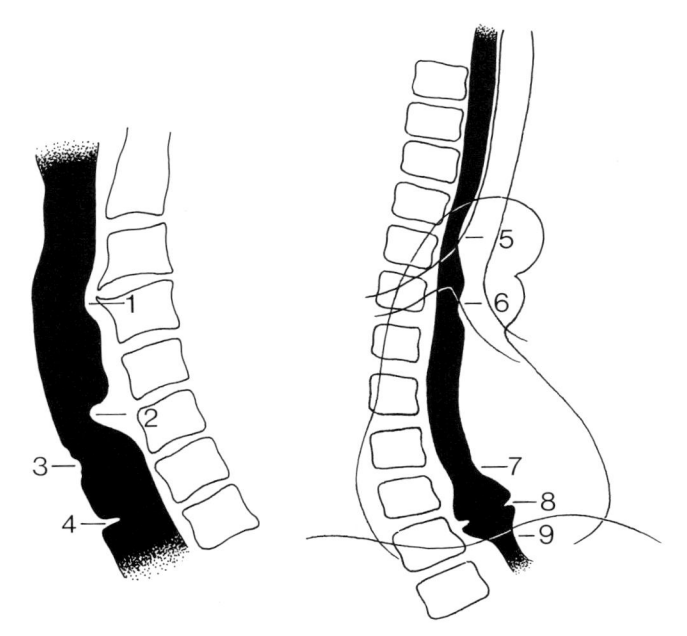

Figure **2 Normal and pathologic filling defects in the esophagus.** (**a**) Lateral cervical esophagus and (**b**) left posterior oblique thoracic esophagus.
1 Posterior defect caused by osteophytes.
2 Intermittent posterior defect at the C5/C6 disk level by cricopharyngeus muscle.
3 Anterior impression at the C6 level caused by pharyngeal venous plexus.
4 Esophageal web arising characteristically from the anterior wall.
5 Left anterior impression caused by aortic arch.
6 Anterior impression caused by left main bronchus.
7 Junction between tubular esophagus and phrenic ampulla (vestibule).
8 Lower esophageal or Schatzki's ring.
9 Narrowing caused by diaphragmatic hiatus.

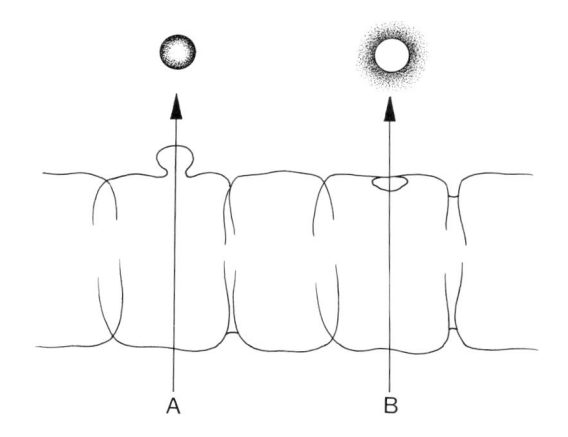

Figure **3 Differentiation between diverticulum** (A) **and polyp** (B) when viewed face-on in double-contrast examinations. A diverticulum has a sharp outer border and a fuzzy inner border (A), whereas a polyp has a sharp inner border and a fuzzy outer border (B).

Table 1 Filling Defects in the Esophagus

Disease	Radiographic Findings	Comments
Normal structures:		
Cricopharyngeal muscle (Fig. 2)	Intermittent posterior filling defect at the pharyngoesophageal junction (at the C5/C6 disk level.	*Cricopharyngeal achalasia:* functional disturbance with dysphagia caused by failure of this muscle to relax. Produces a persistent filling defect radiographically. Idiopathic, or associated with a variety of neuromuscular disorders and partial pharyngectomy. Hypertrophy of the cricopharyngeus may also occur after laryngectomy with the development of esophageal speech.
Pharyngeal venous plexus	Occasional shallow anterior impression at the level of C6.	
Left main bronchus (Fig. 2)	Anterior impression below aortic arch.	
Vascular structures:		
Aortic arch (Fig. 2)	Left anterior impression best demonstrated in right anterior oblique projection.	Extrinsic filling defect much more pronounced with anteriosclerotic or aneurysmatic aortic arch.
Arteriosclerosis or aneurysm of descending aorta	Displacement of esophagus varies, but is often anterior.	
Right aortic arch	Type 1: characteristic right anterior impression. Type 2: characteristic large posterior defect in esophagus.	Type 1: mirror-image branching, commonly associated with congenital heart disease. Type 2: Posterior right aortic arch. Most common type, not associated with congenital heart disease. Associated aberrant left subclavian artery and left ligamentum arteriosum may form complete vascular ring.
Double aortic arch	Large posterior defect caused by junction of both arches and small and higher anterior defect produced by trachea pressed against esophagus. Right and left lateral impression corresponds to each arch.	May cause dysphagia and dyspnea by compression.
Aberrant right subclavian artery	Posterior defect with characteristic appearance. In frontal projection the esophageal defect is oblique, begins at the upper border of the aortic arch, and ascends from left to right at an angle of 70 degrees.	Usually an incidental finding, but may occasionally cause dysphagia.
Aberrant left pulmonary artery	Anterior indentation of esophagus at level of carina by left pulmonary artery arising from right pulmonary artery.	Signs of respiratory obstruction and infection may be present.
Left atrial enlargement	Localized compression and displacement of esophagus posteriorly and to the right below carina.	Mitral valve disease is by far the most common cause of isolated left atrial enlargement. When the left ventricle is also enlarged, the esophagus is displaced posteriorly along the entire length of its contact with the heart.

Table 1 (Cont.) Filling Defects in the Esophagus

Disease	Radiographic Findings	Comments
Cysts (intramural and mediastinal) (Fig. 4)	Smooth round extrinsic or, less commonly, intrinsic filling defects.	Rare. Besides congenital or duplication cysts, retention cysts originating in the esophageal glands occur. For further differentiation see Table 3, page 172.
Benign esophageal tumors (Fig. 5, 6)	Smoothly outlined intramural lesions that bulge into the esophageal lumen or may be pedunculated. *Leiomyomas* are usually found in the lower third of the esophagus and may occasionally ulcerate.	Rare and usually asymptomatic. Besides leiomyomas (most common), *lipomas, angiomas, neurogenic tumors, granular cell myoblastomas, polyps* (fibromuscular or inflammatory), *papillomas,* and *villous adenomas* are found.
Thyroid enlargement or tumor	Significant extrinsic displacement of both the trachea and the cervical or paratracheal esophagus occurs even with a relatively small goiter. Thyroid carcinomas may invade the esophagus, causing an abnormal mucosal pattern.	All thyroid mass lesions, which do not infiltrate into the surrounding structures, move up and down with the larynx during swallowing. Fluoroscopy is virtually diagnostic.
Carcinoma of the esophagus (Fig. 7)	An irregular circumferential lesion with destroyed or ulcerated mucosa, overhanging edges and abrupt transition to normal tissue is the most common presentation. A fungating mass with superficial ulceration is less frequently found. Early spread into mediastinal tissue occurs, possibly because of lack of serosal membrane on the esophagus.	The majority are squamous cell carcinomas. Adenocarcinomas, verrucous carcinomas (exophytic or warty tumors that rarely metastasize), primary melanomas, and metastases are rare intrinsic esophageal malignancies of epithelial origin.
Carcinoma of the stomach (Fig. 8)	Irregular mass in the distal esophagus.	Caused by gastric carcinoma of the cardia extending upward.
Leiomyosarcoma (Fig. 9)	Extrinsic or intrinsic bulky mass lesions with a smooth or irregular outline. Ulcerations occur frequently.	*Carcinosarcomas* and *pseudosarcomas* are other rare tumors that present as large intrinsic mass lesions with irregular outline.
Lymphoma	One or several extrinsic filling defects caused by mediastinal lymphadenopathy are the most common presentation. Infiltration of the esophagus from mediastinal lymph nodes or stomach producing irregular filling defects can occur. Primary lymphoma of the esophagus is extremely rare.	Occurs with Hodgkin's and non-Hodgkin's lymphoma.

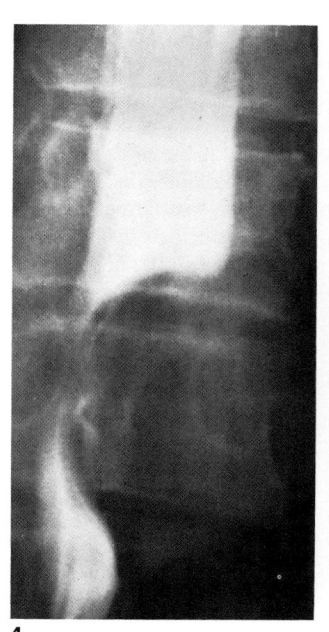

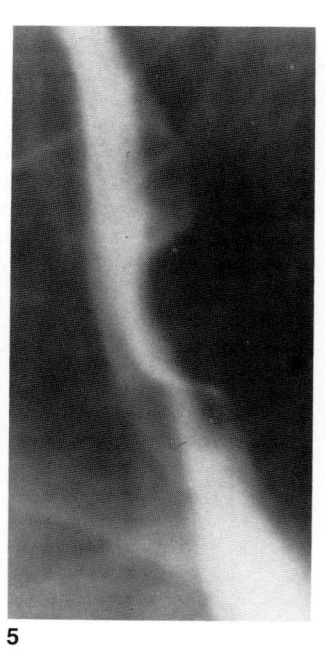

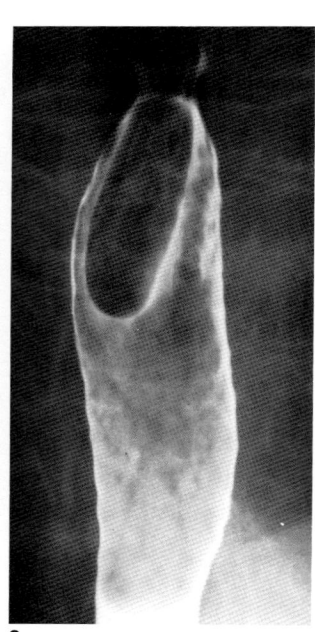

Figure 4 **Intramural esophageal cyst.** A smooth filling defect is seen.

Figure 5 **Leiomyoma.** A smooth semicircular defect is seen.

Figure 6 **Lipoma.** A smooth, oval deformable mass is seen in the upper esophagus.

Filling Defects in the Gastrointestinal Tract   165

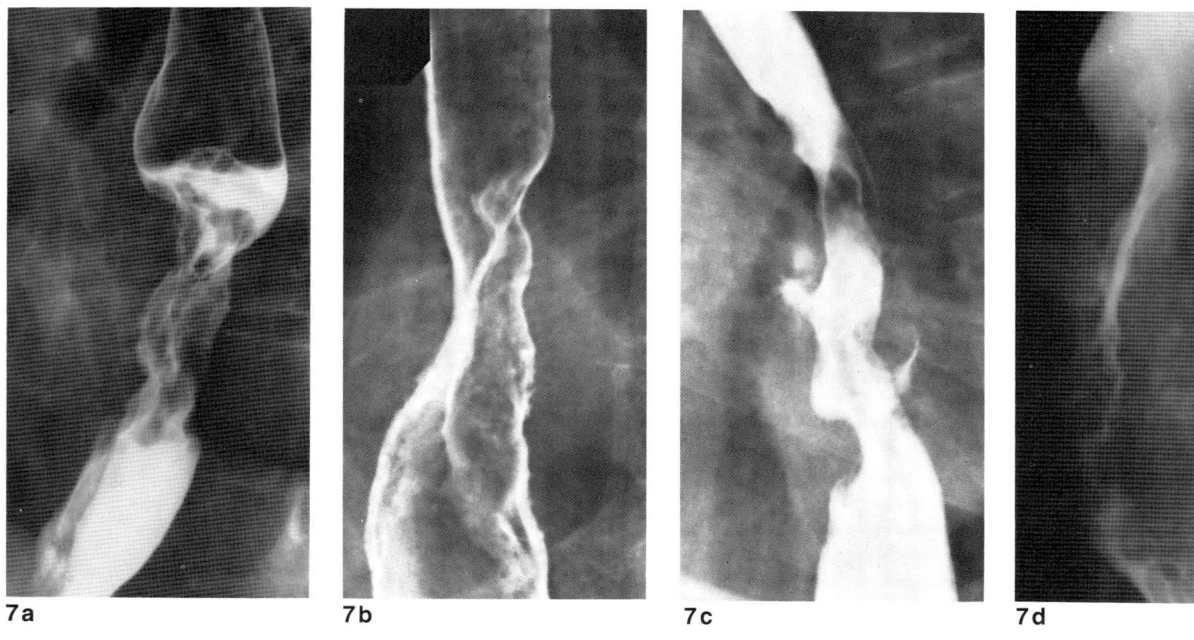

7a   7b   7c   7d

Figure 7 **Esophageal carcinoma** presenting **a** as a circumferential lesion with destroyed mucosa, **b** as a plaque-like lesion, **c** as an ulcerating mass, or **d** as an intraluminal mass with overhanging edges.

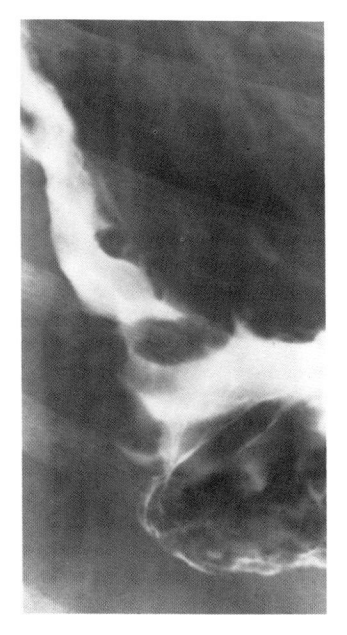

Figure 8 **Carcinoma of the stomach** invading the distal esophagus. An irregular mass is seen in the distal esophagus.

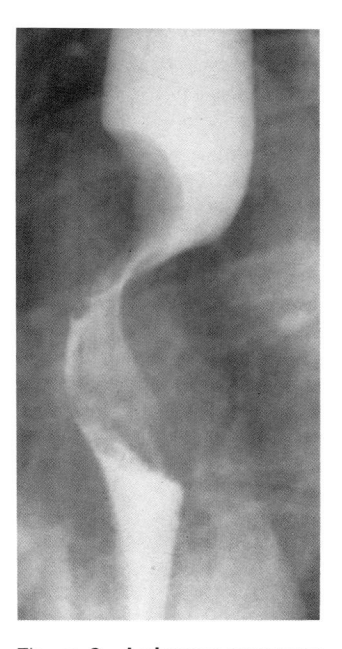

Figure 9 **Leiomyosarcoma.** A large spiraling mass with mainly extrinsic tumor component is seen.

Table 1 (Cont.) Filling Defects in the Esophagus

Disease	Radiographic Findings	Comments
Mediastinal tumors	Extrinsic filling defects caused by tumors or lymphadenopathy of the posterior mediastinum.	Common. *Metastases* (e.g., from bronchogenic carcinoma) and lymphoma may cause dysphagia at a relatively early stage. Primary mediastinal tumors are much less common and may cause considerable displacement without causing dysphagia. For further differentiation see Table 3, page 172.
Infectious esophagitis (Fig. 6, p. 140)	Multiple small round or oval defects are occasionally seen, and are usually associated with a shaggy mucosa and fine ulcerations.	Usually caused by candidiasis and rarely by herpes in compromised hosts and AIDS patients.
Mediastinal abscess (Fig. 22b, p. 171)	Localized extrinsic mass that may contain air.	Usually due to esophageal rupture, which is diagnosed by extravasation of ingested contrast material.
Granulomatous mediastinitis	Anterior esophageal compression by enlarged paratracheal lymph node, which may be calcified.	Patient usually asymptomatic. *Tuberculosis, histoplasmosis,* and *sarcoidosis* are the most common etiologies. *Sclerosing mediastinitis* may rarely produce a filling defect similar to a carcinoma.
Mediastinal hematoma	Extrinsic compression of the esophagus, usually in the upper mediastinum.	Trauma, surgery, aortic dissection.
Varices (Fig. 10)	Round or oval filling defects predominantly in the distal esophagus, often resembling beads of a rosary. Normal peristalsis and change in appearance between esophageal dilatation and contraction, where they usually disappear, are diagnostic.	In *portal hypertension* caused by liver cirrhosis or Budd–Chiari syndrome (both associated with ascites) and abnormal liver functions) or splenoportal vein occlusion (usually no ascites and normal liver functions).
Food or foreign body	May simulate intraluminal mass, particularly when located in prestenotic segment (organic stenosis or persistent spasm).	*Air bubbles* coated with barium cause only transitory changes and can easily be differentiated.
Spondylosis and spondylitis	Osteophytes of the cervical spine may produce one or more smooth extrinsic defects in the posterior wall of the esophagus. Infectious spondylitis can present as a posterior fusiform mass with vertebral destruction. It usually originates from the cervical or lower thoracic spine.	Tuberculous and nontuberculous spondylitis.

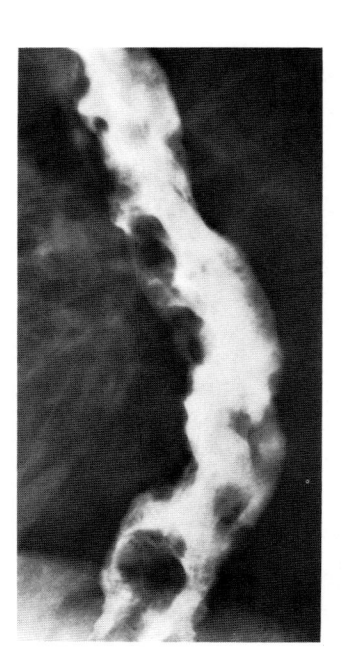

Figure **10** **Varices.** Large round and oval filling defects are seen in the distal esophagus. The absence of obstruction, normal peristalsis, and change in appearance between esophageal dilatation and contraction are characteristic.

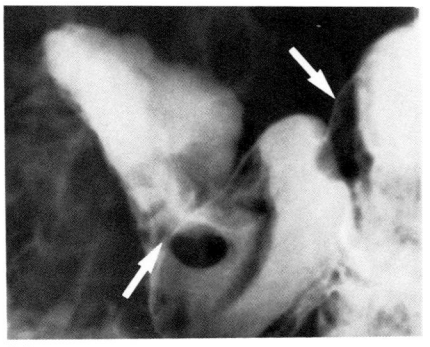

Table 2 Filling Defects in the Stomach

Disease	Radiographic Findings	Comments
Web (Fig. 11)	Circular membrane-like defect, usually located in antrum.	Rare congenital lesion.
Ectopic pancreas (aberrant) (Fig. 12)	Nodule measuring 1–4 cm in diameter and preferentially located in the antropyloric region. A central depression (umbilication) is characteristically present and can simulate an ulcer.	Heterotopic pancreatic tissue may occur anywhere in the gastrointestinal tract, but is most common in the stomach. Patient is normally asymptomatic.
Duplication cyst	Usually solitary 3–12 cm intramural lesion, preferentially on greater curvature. Alteration in configuration under external compression may indicate cystic nature of lesion.	Majority of duplication cysts are diagnosed in childhood.
Polyps and benign tumors (Figs. 13, 14)	Usually present as solitary and small submucosal nodules with intact mucosa. Ulcerations occur in *leiomyoma, neurogenic tumors,* and *lipomas*. Polyps, lipomas, and leiomyomas may be pedunculated. *Hyperplastic polyps* present as small (1 cm or less) and often multiple filling defects that are caused by excessive regenerative hyperplasia in an area of chronic gastritis, and must be differentiated from adenomatous polyps that are potentially malignant.	Any polypoid lesion larger than 2 cm is suspect of being malignant and should therefore be removed. Even histologically, it is often difficult to differentiate between benign and malignant leiomyomas and adenomatous polyps, respectively. The latter have a high incidence of malignancy and are often found in chronic atrophic gastritis. Multiple gastric polyps may also be seen in *familial polyposis* of the colon and in the *Canada-Cronkhite syndrome* (see Table 5, page 182). Multiple hamartomas presenting as small polypoid lesions are found in *Peutz–Jeghers, Canada–Cronkhite* and *Cowden's syndrome*. In all three conditions they are associated with hamartomas in other parts of the gastrointestinal tract (see Table 5, page 184).

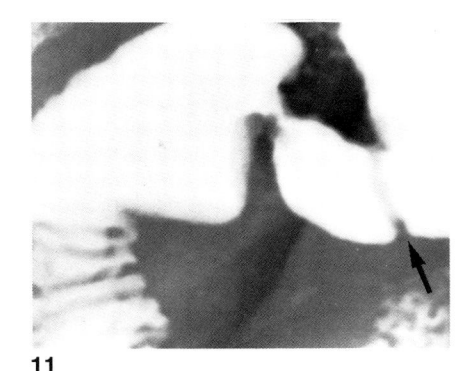

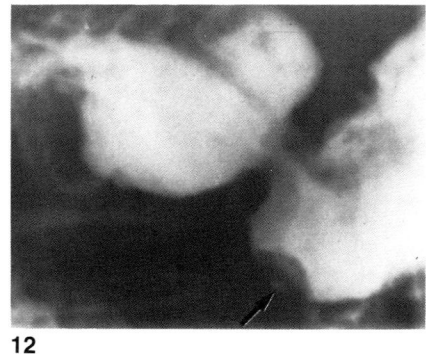

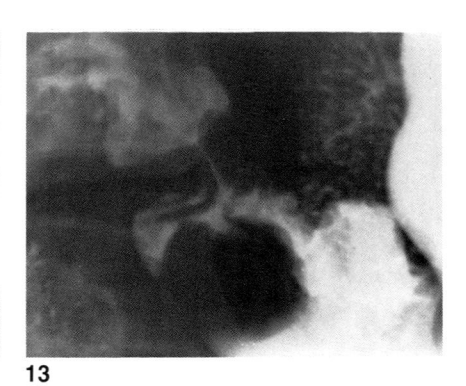

Figure 11 **Congenital antral web.** A circumferential membrane-like defect is seen in the antrum (arrow).

Figure 12 **Ectopic (aberrant) pancreas.** A small nodule with central umbilication (arrow) is seen on the greater curvature in the prepyloric region.

Figure 13 **Leiomyoma.** A nodular lesion is seen in the antrum.

Figure 14 **Adenomatous polyps.** Two round to ovoid filling defects with pedicles (arrows) are seen in the antrum.

Table 2 (Cont.) **Filling Defects in the Stomach**

Disease	Radiographic Findings	Comments
Villous adenoma (Fig. 15)	Usually a solitary, sessile mass of varying size. Because of the softness of the tumor, change in shape occurs with peristaltic contractions or external compression. Barium trapped between strands may produce a frond-like appearance.	Rare gastric tumor with relatively high incidence of malignancy.
Carcinoma (Fig. 16)	Ranging from polypoid lesions to large fungating masses with destroyed mucosal pattern (amputation of folds), ulcerations, and rigidity of the adjacent stomach wall are often present. May occur at any location, but slight preference for lesser curvature, especially near gastric incisura. Mucus-producing carcinomas may occasionally contain calcifications.	Other radiologic presentations of gastric carcinoma are the ulcerating form and the infiltrative (scirrhous) type.
Sarcoma (Fig. 17)	Intramural lesions with intraluminal component that varies greatly in size. Ranges from small circumscribed nodules to large exophytic masses, often with deep central ulceration. Calcifications are rarely present.	*Leiomyosarcoma* is the most common gastric sarcoma. *Neurogenic sarcomas*, *liposarcomas*, and *fibrosarcomas* are rare.
Lymphoma (Fig. 18)	Ranges from thickened folds with nodular lesions to large intrinsic or extrinsic masses. Ulcerations are relatively common.	Primary gastric lymphoma is usually of the non-Hodgkin's variety. When it presents as a localized gastric mass, it is radiographically indistinguishable from a *pseudolymphoma*. Secondary involvement of the stomach, occurs with both Hodgkin's and non-Hodgkin's lymphoma.
Metastases (hematogenous) (Fig. 19)	Rare. Usually multiple, sharply delineated filling defects, often with central ulcerations ("target lesions").	Metastases from melanoma are most common, followed by breast and lung carcinomas and rarely other malignancies.
Extrinsic mass (Fig. 20)	Extrinsic defects may be caused by normal or enlarged adjacent organs, inflammatory or neoplastic lesions. Gastric mucosa is characteristically normal unless it is infiltrated by a malignant lesion (e.g., carcinoma of pancreas infiltrating greater curvature and posterior wall of the stomach and simulating gastric carcinoma).	Extrinsic impression on anterior wall and lesser curvature is often caused by a normal or more often by an enlarged *liver*. In the distal antrum and pyloric region, an extrinsic defect may be caused by a *hypertrophic pylorus*. Extrinsic impression on the posterior wall and greater curvature can be caused by the *spleen, colon,* an enlarged retroperitoneal organ (especially *pancreas*, including pancreatic pseudocysts, *left kidney,* and *left adrenal*), or a pathologic *process* in the *lesser sac*. Intraperitoneal metastases may involve all surfaces of the stomach.

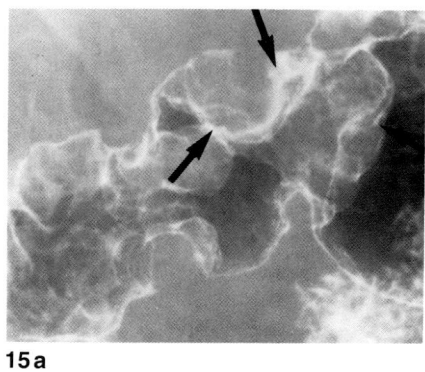

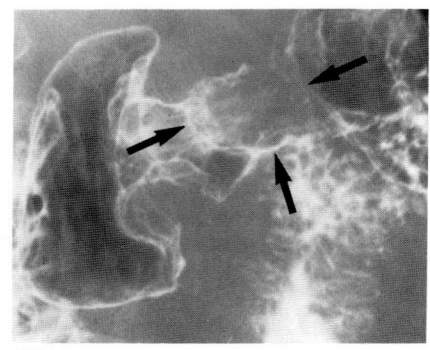

Figure **15a, b** **Villous adenoma** (histologically with early carcinomatous transformation). A sessile, soft mass (arrows) that changes shape with peristaltic contractions (note the difference between **a** and **b**) is seen in the antrum, but there is only minimal barium trapping between its villous strands.

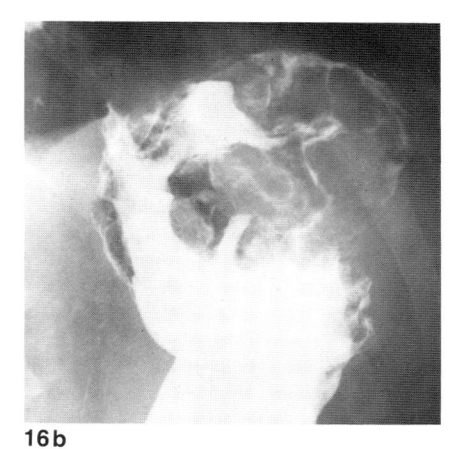

Figure 16a, b **Gastric carcinoma** in two different patients. (**a**) A mass originating from the lesser curvature that is completely rigid in this area, is seen. (**b**) A fungating mass with destroyed mucosal pattern and ulcerations is seen in the fundus.

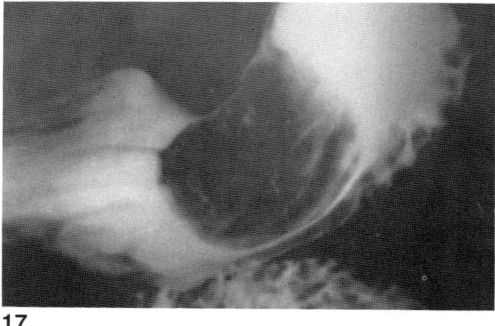

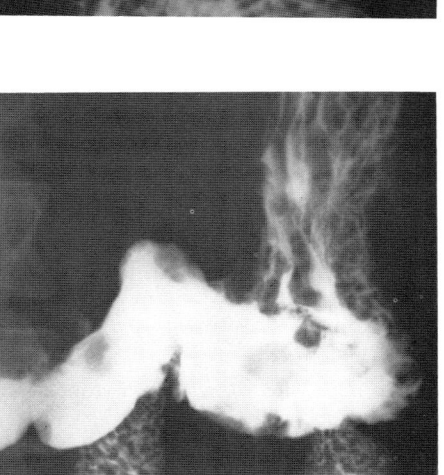

Figure 17 **Leiomyosarcoma.** A large mass lesion is present in the body of the stomach.

Figure 19 **Melanoma metastases.** Multiple nodular lesions some of which with central ulcerations ("target lesions") are seen in the body and antrum of the stomach.

Figure 18 **Non-Hodgkin's lymphoma.** A large mass lesion involving the fundus and body of the stomach is seen.

Figure 20a, b **Extrinsic mass lesions.** Extrinsic defects without mucosal involvement are seen **a** in the fundus, caused by an *accessory spleen* and **b** on the greater curvature, caused by *non-Hodgkin's lymphoma*. Note also the abnormal mucosal pattern in the distal duodenum and the ulceration in the duodenojejunal junction (arrow), which is caused by lymphomatous infiltration.

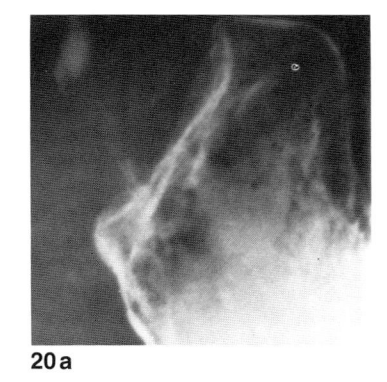

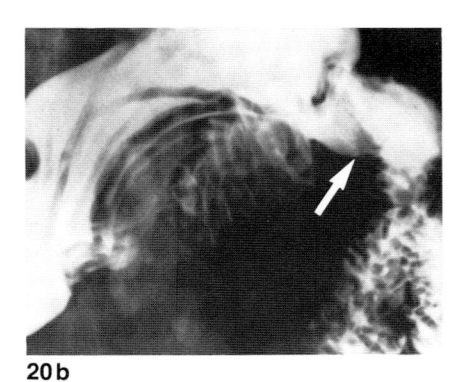

Table 2 (Cont.) **Filling Defects in the Stomach**

Disease	Radiographic Findings	Comments
Eosinophilic granuloma (inflammatory fibroelastic polyp) (Fig. 21)	Polypoid mass lesion measuring up to 9 cm in diameter. May be pedunculated. Almost always located in the gastric antrum. Ulceration is very rare.	This lesion is neither associated with peripheral eosinophilia nor food allergy and has nothing to do with the eosinophilic granuloma of the histocytosis X complex.
Ménétrier's disease (giant hypertrophic gastritis)	Multiple nodular filling defects caused by markedly enlarged gastric folds are seen, preferentially located in the fundus and along the greater curvature.	Ménétrier's disease is a protein-losing enteropathy. Similar nodular defects caused by enlarged gastric folds are occasionally seen in *Crohn's disease, eosinophilic gastritis, tuberculosis,* and *sarcoidosis.*
Peptic ulcer	Mucosal edema around ulcer may occasionally simulate an ulcerating tumor. A large indentation on the greater curvature opposite an ulcer on the lesser curvature should not be mistaken for a mass ("ulcer finger").	A double pylorus (short fistula connecting the prepyloric lesser curvature with the duodenal bulb secondary to peptic ulcer disease) may produce the appearance of an intraluminal prebulbar defect that is caused by the two pyloric channels surrounding the scar tissue in between.
Hematoma	Rare. Intramural mass of varying size.	Usually history of trauma or bleeding disorder.
Postoperative defect (Fig. 22)	Postoperative defects can measure up to 5 cm in areas of suturing. They may become less prominent or even disappear with time. *Fundoplication* deformities after hiatal hernia repair produce mass-like defects in the gastric fundus, caused by the invaginated esophagus.	A postoperative defect that increases in size on follow-up studies indicates complication (hematoma, abscess, etc.) or tumor recurrency.
Amyloidosis	Solitary or more commonly multiple, often ulcerated filling defects.	Usually associated with involvement of other parts of the gastrointestinal tract.
Varices (Fig. 23)	Multiple smooth lobulated filling defects preferentially located in the fundus. Occasionally, a single filling defect is caused by a large varix. Change in size and shape is characteristic. Usually associated with esophageal varices and splenomegaly.	Gastric varices not associated with esophageal varices occur in splenic vein occlusion (e.g., in pancreatitis or carcinoma of pancreas). The collateral flow passes in these cases from the short gastric veins via the left and right gastric veins to the portal vein.
Intussusception	Intraluminal, often polycyclic defect with characteristic circular and semicircular spring-like folds.	Occurs in resected stomach, or is caused by a pedunculated lesion.
Bezoar (Fig. 24)	Freely mobile, intraluminal mass with often characteristic mottled appearance, conforming to the shape of the stomach. May cause gastric dilatation and fill the entire lumen.	Phytobezoars are composed of plant products and trichobezoars of hair.
Foreign body, ingested food, blood clots	Single or multiple freely mobile filling defects of varying shape and size.	A *gallstone* passing either retrograde from the duodenum or through a cholecystogastric fistula can rarely produce an intraluminal filling defect.

Filling Defects in the Gastrointestinal Tract   171

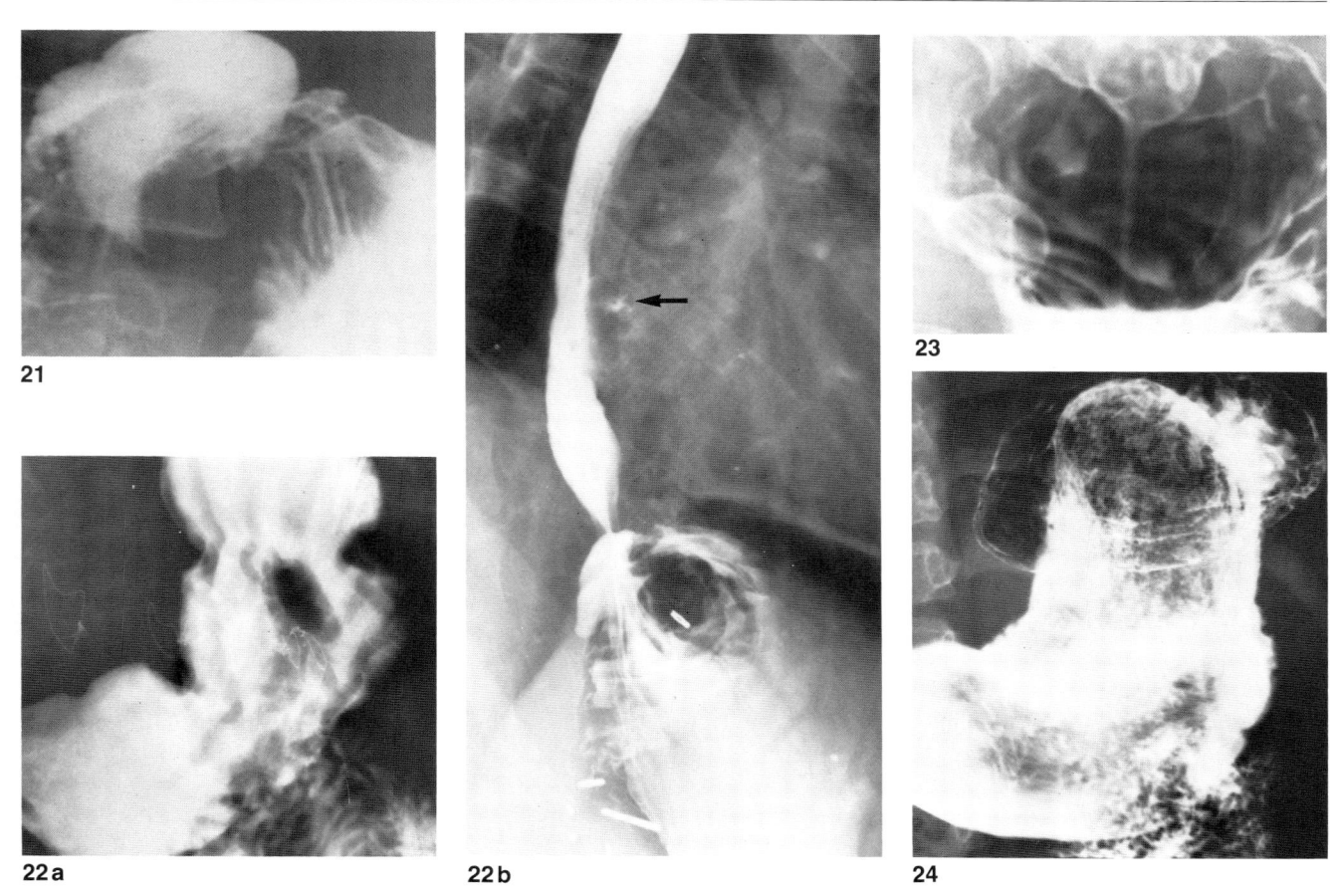

Figure 21 **Eosinophilic granuloma.** A large round mass lesion is seen in the antrum.

Figure 22a, b **Postoperative defects. a** An oval filling defect is seen in the body of the stomach. Note also the postoperative indentation on both the lesser and greater curvature at the same level. **b** Nissen fundoplication: a characteristic filling defect is seen in the cardia. Note also the small iatrogenic perforation (arrow) with abscess formation causing a gentle extrinsic compression in the lower esophagus.

Figure 23 **Gastric varices.** Smoothly lobulated nodular lesions are seen in the fundus.

Figure 24 **Trichobezoar.** A large mass with mottled appearance is seen in the stomach.

Table 3 Filling Defects in the Duodenum

Disease	Radiographic Findings	Comments
Web	Circumferential membrane-like filling defect usually located in the second portion of the duodenum. May cause varying degrees of obstruction.	Congenital abnormality.
Ectopic (aberrant) pancreas	Usually submucosal nodules, measuring 1 to 2 cm (rarely up to 4 cm). Central umbilication is characteristic and should not be confused with an ulcerating mass.	Aberrant pancreatic tissue in the gastrointestinal tract is found in 2% of all routine postmortems, most commonly located in stomach and duodenum.
Annular pancreas	Extrinsic ring-like or predominantly lateral defect on the superior part of the descending duodenum.	Often only diagnosed in adulthood, since no significant obstruction occurs in majority of cases.
Hypertrophy of Brunner's glands (Fig. 25)	Multiple diffuse or circumscribed small polypoid filling defects, measuring from a few millimeters ("cobblestone" pattern) to 1 cm in diameter. Preferential location is first portion of duodenum.	Often associated with peptic ulcer disease. Small *glandular adenomas* of *Brunner's glands* have also been described, but probably represent localized areas of hypertrophy rather than true neoplasms.
Nodular lymphoid hyperplasia (benign)	Innumerable tiny, 1–5 mm filling defects evenly distributed throughout the entire duodenum.	Usually an incidental finding but may be associated with hypogammaglobulinemia.
Heterotopic gastric mucosa	Multiple filling defects similar to benign lymphoid hyperplasia but more irregular and limited to the duodenal bulb.	Incidental finding. Compared to Brunner's gland hypertrophy, the filling defects are smaller and less uniform.
Duplication cyst	Intrinsic or extrinsic mass in first or second portion of duodenum. May become tubular in shape when communication with normal lumen occurs.	Very rare in the adult. May cause duodenal obstruction in infancy.
Choledochal cyst (Fig. 26)	Extrinsic mass on the inner aspect of the duodenal sweep, which might be widened and compressed, when the lesion is large enough.	Usually in girls under the age of 10, presenting with jaundice, right upper quadrant mass, and abdominal pain.
Intraluminal diverticulum (Fig. 27)	Rare form of duodenal diverticulum originating in the descending portion of the duodenum. The wall of the diverticulum may be seen as radiolucent line ("halo sign"). May be confused with communicating duplication cyst that is filled with barium.	
Polyps and benign tumors (Fig. 28)	Solitary or rarely multiple nodules that may be pedunculated. Central ulcerations can occur. Nodular lesions located in the bulb are usually benign.	May mimic ulcer symptoms and bleed. Histologically, *adenomas, leiomyomas, lipomas, neurinomas,* and others are found, but radiologic differentiation is usually not possible. Multiple hamartomatous polyps may be present in the *Peutz–Jeghers syndrome.* *Villous adenomas, carcinoids,* and *islet cell tumors* are potentially malignant lesions located preferentially in the first or second portion of the duodenum. Severe peptic ulcer disease or diarrhea is usually associated with carcinoids and islet cell tumors.
Duodenal carcinoma (Fig. 29)	Circumferential constricting lesion with mucosal destruction or polypoid mass, often with ulceration. Usually located distal to the papilla.	Most of the primary duodenal malignancies are adenocarcinomas, the rest sarcomas and lymphomas.

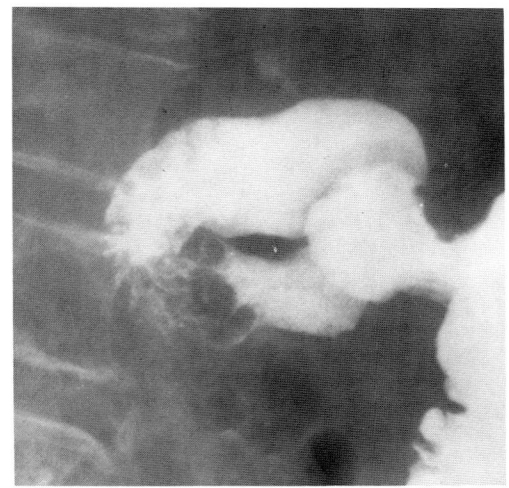

Filling Defects in the Gastrointestinal Tract 173

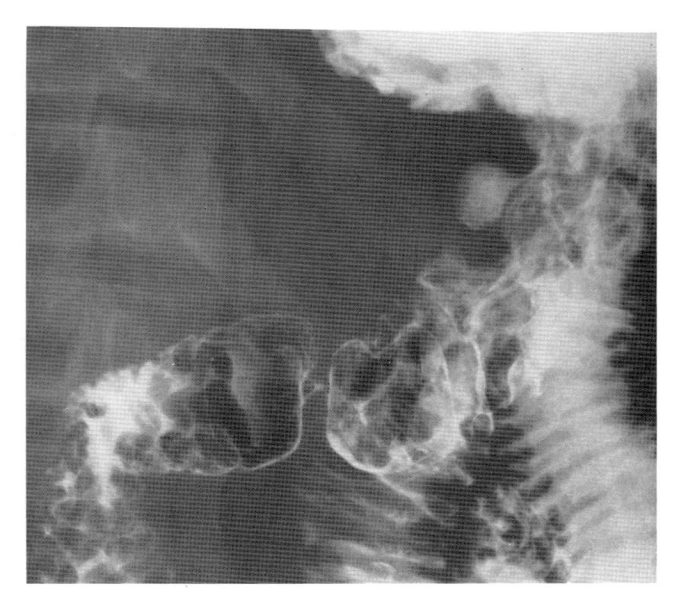

Figure 25 **Hypertrophy of Brunner's glands.** Multiple polypoid lesions measuring up to 1 cm are seen in the proximal duodenum, and are associated with a large peptic ulcer in the lesser curvature of the stomach.

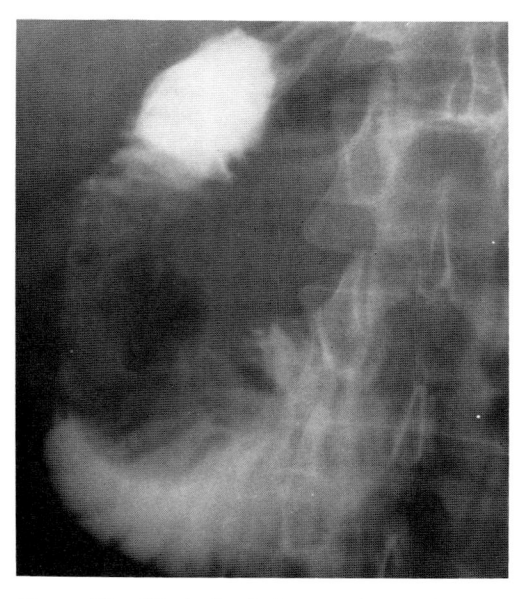

Figure 26 **Choledochal cyst.** An extrinsic filling defect is seen on the medial aspect of the second portion of the duodenum.

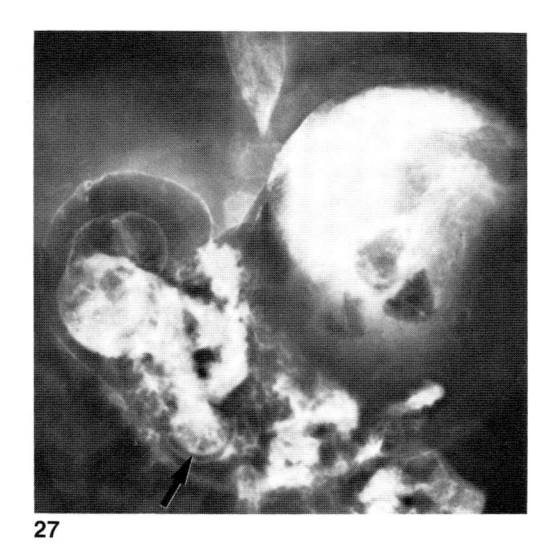

Figure 27 **Intraluminal duodenal diverticulum.** A barium-filled finger-like sac is seen in the second portion of the duodenum. Note the characteristic radiolucent band around its distal end (arrow) representing the wall of the diverticulum ("halo sign").

Figure 28 **Duodenal polyp.** A smooth ovoid filling defect with a large pedicle is seen in the second portion of the duodenum (arrow).

Figure 29 **Duodenal carcinoma.** An irregular filling defect with small ulcerations is seen in the duodenum.

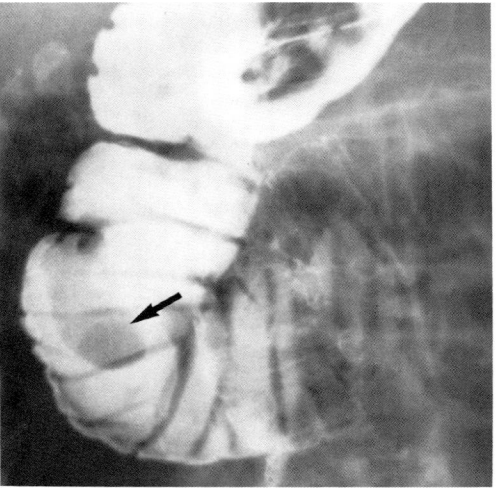

Table 3 (Cont.) Filling Defects in the Duodenum

Disease	Radiographic Findings	Comments
Metastases (Fig. 30)	Extrinsic compression with or without invasion of the duodenum by malignancy from an adjacent organ, with destruction, ulceration and mass formation. Intracanalicular and hematogenous metastases presenting as solitary or multiple nodular lesions are rare. Central ulceration in these metastases is quite characteristic (target lesions).	Found with carcinomas from neighboring organs such as the pancreas and biliary system, retroperitoneal malignancies, or by direct extension from the stomach (e.g. in lymphoma). Metastases presenting as target lesions originate usually from breast and lung carcinomas, melanoma or Kaposi's sarcoma.
Enlargement of the papilla of Vater (ampullary carcinoma, impacted gallstone) (Figs. 31, 32)	Extrinsic or intrinsic defect at medial border of second portion of duodenum.	Filling defects smaller than 1.5 cm are within normal limits. Somewhat larger filling defects are seen with inflammation (e.g., papillitis, pancreatitis, cholangitis) or edema (e.g., post iatrogenic manipulation or stone passage). Ampullary carcinomas and impacted gallstones are usually associated with obstructive jaundice.
Choledochocele	Filling defect at the medial border of the second portion of the duodenum.	Prolapse of the dilated cystic terminal portion of the common bile duct. It is usually only associated with obstructive jaundice when complicated by an impacted gallstone or secondary inflammatory changes.
Blood clots, food, foreign bodies, gallstones	Rare intraluminal, fully mobile filling defects of various size and shape. A gallstone eroded into the duodenum may rarely cause obstruction.	Reflux of barium into the biliary system supports the diagnosis of gallstone erosion into the duodenum.
Prolapsed gastric mucosa	Lobulated, mushroom-shaped filling defect at the base of the duodenal bulb with varying appearance during peristalsis.	Prolapse of redundant antral mucosa with peristaltic wave is usually an incidental finding of no clinical significance.
Prolapsed antral polyp (Fig. 33)	Usually a solitary round or oval filling defect at the base of the duodenal bulb.	Any polypoid gastric tumor may be the lead for a *gastric intussusception into the duodenum* (Fig. 34) causing symptoms of acute or chronic obstruction and incarceration.
Peptic ulcer	Surrounding edema and swelling may be prominent, simulating an intraluminal mass with central ulceration.	Inflammatory swelling most pronounced in fresh ulcers and in children.
Superior mesenteric artery syndrome	Characteristic extrinsic anterior impression of the third portion of the duodenum in supine position. Partial to complete relief in prone position.	In young, thin, asthenic or hyperlordotic individuals, in prolonged immobilization (e.g., body cast and after severe burns) and in persons with reduced duodenal peristaltic activity (e.g., scleroderma).
Varices	One or more filling defects, often simulating enlarged mucosal folds.	Varicose dilatation of pancreaticoduodenal veins is rare in portal hypertension.

Filling Defects in the Gastrointestinal Tract 175

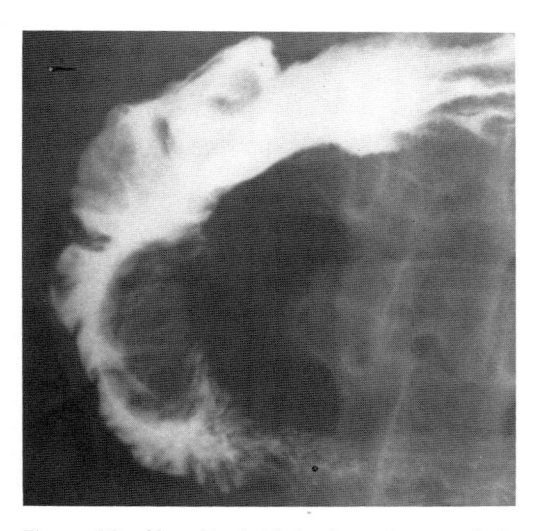

Figure 30 **Non-Hodgkin's lymphoma.** A large irregular mass indistinguishable from an ampullary carcinoma is seen in the medial aspect of the second portion of the duodenum. However, the correct diagnosis can be suggested by the nodular and ulcerative involvement of the proximal duodenum.

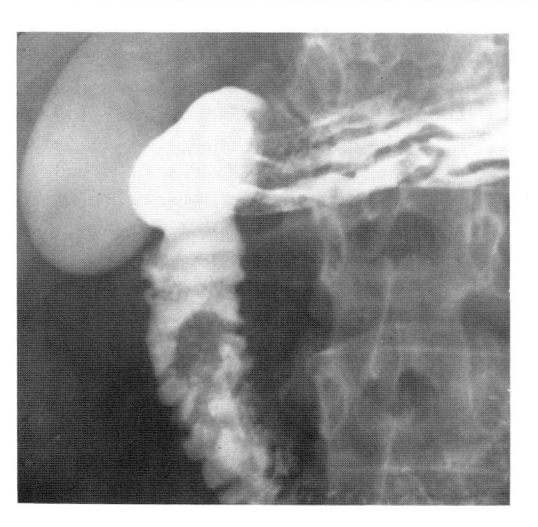

Figure 31 **Normal papilla of Vater.** An unusually large smooth filling defect is seen in the second portion of the duodenum. The gallbladder is opacified by oral cholecystography.

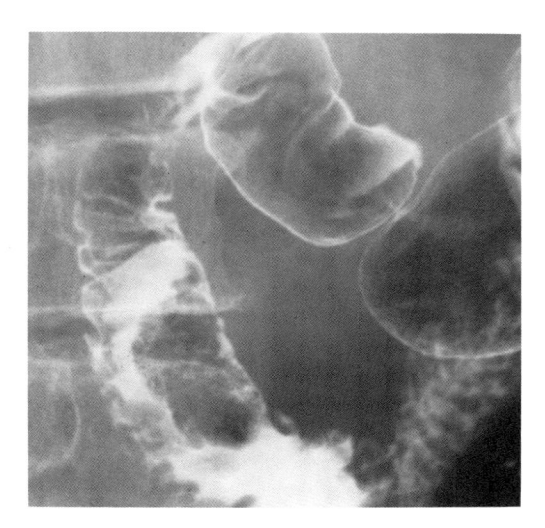

Figure 32 **Ampullary carcinoma.** An irregular filling defect is seen on the medial aspect of the second portion of the duodenum.

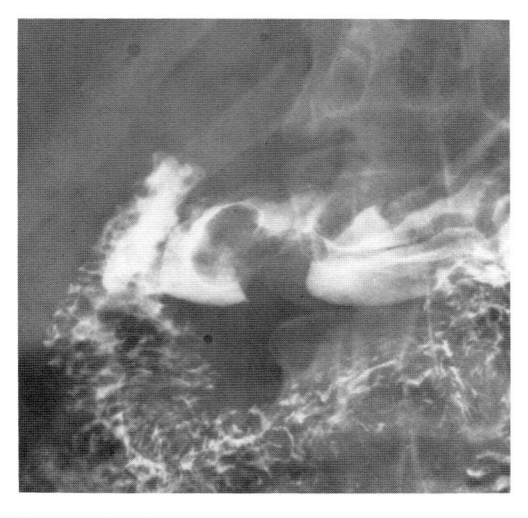

Figure 33 **Prolapsed antral polyp.** A smooth ovoid filling defect is seen in the duodenal bulb.

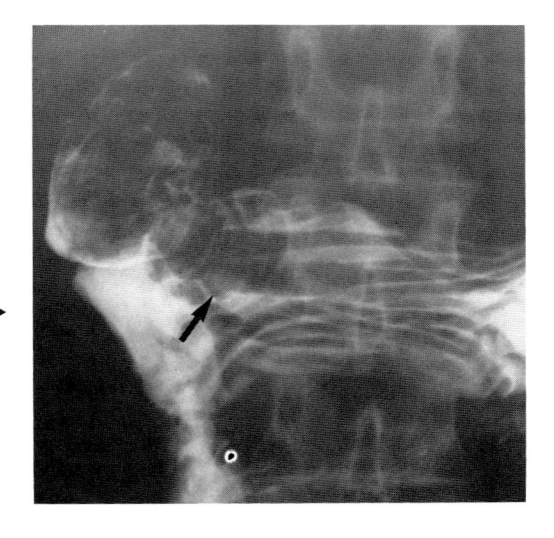

Figure 34 **Gastric intussusception** into duodenum caused by antral mass (non-Hodgkin's lymphoma). The intussuscepted antrum fills in the entire duodenal bulb, whereas the antral polyp is no longer recognizable. Note also the coil-spring appearance in the prepyloric part of the antrum caused by the intussusception (arrow). There is also an extrinsic defect on the greater curvature of the antrum caused by enlarged lymph nodes.

Table 3 (Cont.) Filling Defects in the Duodenum

Disease	Radiographic Findings	Comments
Hematoma (intramural or retroperitoneal) (Fig. 35)	Extrinsic filling defects commonly in the posterolateral aspect of the second and third portion of duodenum.	In bleeding disorders, posttraumatic or rarely spontaneous.
Postoperative defect	Extrinsic- or intrinsic-appearing defect in area of suturing.	A *stitch abscess* may produce a similar finding.
Pancreatic head enlargement (carcinoma, inflammation) (Fig. 36)	Widened duodenal loop with extrinsic impression of its inner border. Second portion may assume shape of inverted figure 3 ("inverted 3 sign"). Mucosal destruction, tumor invasion, and ulcerations suggest carcinoma; mucosal edema, calcifications, and pseudocysts (large extrinsic mass lesions in stomach or bowel) favor pancreatitis.	Elevated amylase levels are the most important clinical finding in *acute pancreatitis*, whereas *carcinoma of the head of the pancreas* is associated with jaundice in the great majority of cases. *Cystadenomas* and *cystadenocarcinomas* may occasionally widen the duodenal sweep (Fig. 37), although the majority of these tumors originate in the body and tail of the pancreas.
Gallbladder and dilated common bile duct (Fig. 37)	A physiologically distended gallbladder may cause an extrinsic defect on the anterolateral aspect of the junction between the first and second portions of the duodenum. An extrinsic impression of tubular shape on the posterior wall of the duodenal bulb may be caused by an abnormally dilated common bile duct.	Although an extrinsic duodenal impression is already seen with a normal gallbladder, larger defects can be found with pathologically altered gallbladders (e.g., hydrops, pericholecystic abscess, carcinoma).
Hepatic mass	Extrinsic posterolateral filling defect on the first and second portions of the duodenum.	Hepatic cyst, abscess, benign and malignant tumors, or focal hypertrophy (e.g., of the caudate lobe) may cause an extrinsic duodenal filling defects.
Subhepatic abscess	Extrinsic lateral filling defect on the second portion of the duodenum.	For example, postsurgical or secondary to ruptured gallbladder in acute cholecystitis.
Colon	Anterolateral filling defect in the fourth portion of the duodenum.	May be caused by fecal material or a mass in the transverse colon.
Retroperitoneal mass (Figs. 38, 39)	Extrinsic defects in the second and adjacent third portions of the duodenum, either on the posterolateral wall (e.g., enlarged right kidney or adrenal) or on the posteromedial wall (e.g., retroperitoneal lymphadenopathy, sarcoma, abscess, and aortic aneurysm).	Retroperitoneal mass lesions causing filling defects on the posteromedial wall of the second portion of the duodenum are radiographically similar to the findings in pancreatic head enlargement.

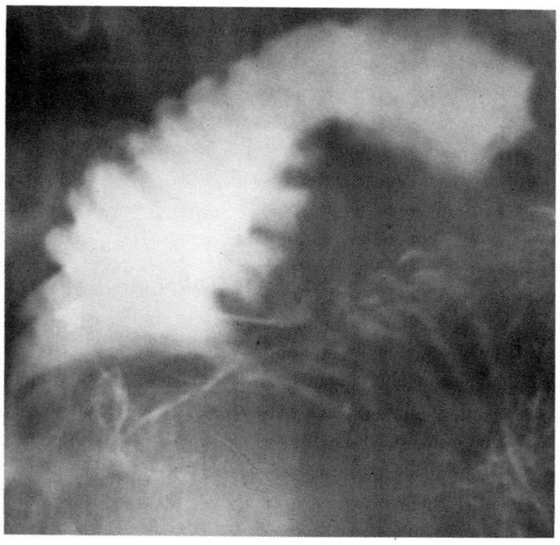

Figure 35 **Posttraumatic hematoma.** A large filling defect is seen at the junction between the second and third portion of the duodenum with almost complete obstruction and significant prestenotic dilatation.

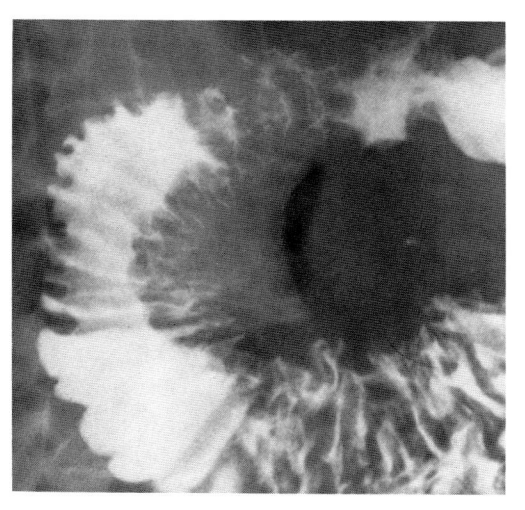

Figure 36 **Pancreatic carcinoma.** An extrinsic impression on the inner border of the second portion of the duodenum with mucosal destruction is seen.

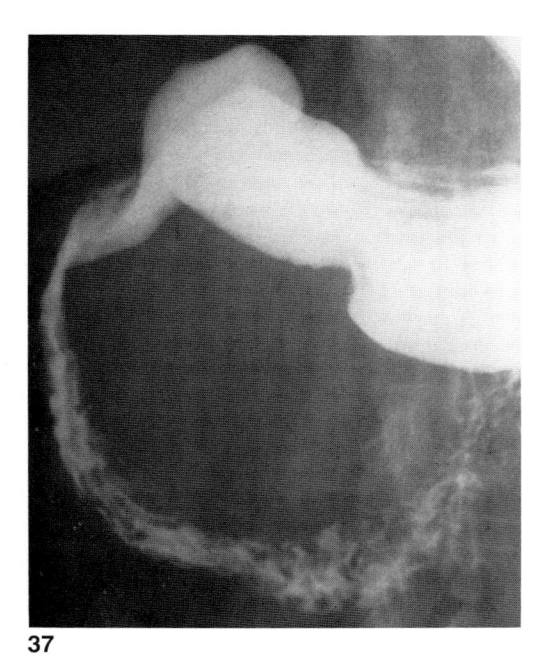

Figure 37 **Extrinsic defects caused by distended gallbladder and cystadenoma of the pancreas.** The extrinsic impression on the anterolateral aspect of the junction between the first and second portions of the duodenum is caused by a distended gallbladder, whereas the widening of the duodenal loop is caused by a large cystadenoma in the head of the pancreas.

Figure 38 **Non-Hodgkin's lymphoma** involving aortic lymph nodes. An extrinsic filling defect is seen in the inner aspect of the second and third portions of the duodenum. A markedly enlarged aortic lymph node is still faintly opacified from previous lymphography (arrow).

Figure 39 **Retroperitoneal hemangiosarcoma.** A marked widening of the duodenal loop by an extrinsic mass is seen. Mucosal destruction and nodular defects in the duodenum are caused by tumor invasion.

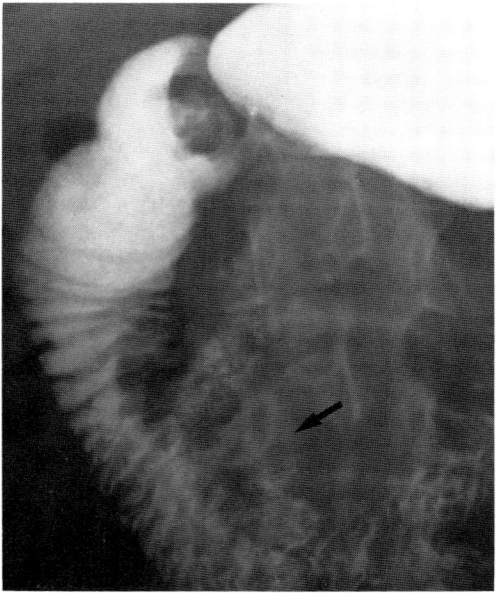

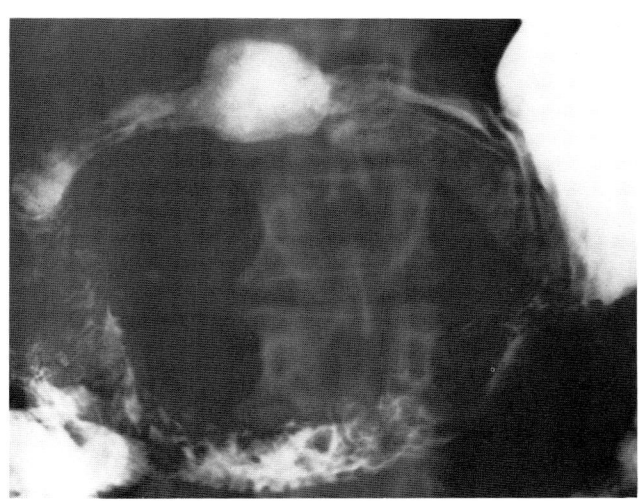

Table 4 Filling Defects in the Small Bowel (Jejunum and Ileum)

Disease	Radiographic Findings	Comments
Ectopic pancreas	Small submucosal nodule. Central umbilication is characteristic, but not always present.	Rare in small bowel (common in stomach and duodenum).
Duplication cyst	Intrinsic or extrinsic filling defect of varying size, usually in distal ileum.	Rare. May sometimes communicate with bowel lumen producing saclike structure.
Meckel's diverticulum (inverted) (Fig. 40)	Intraluminal filling defect in the middle or distal portion of ileum.	May progress to intussusception and cause small-bowel obstruction.
Endometrioma	Small, usually solitary extrinsic or intrinsic mass, preferentially located in the ileum.	Rare. Clinical symptoms related to menstrual cycle.
Nodular lymphoid hyperplasia (benign) (Fig. 41)	Multiple nodular filling defects with predilection for the terminal ileum, but may be found throughout small bowel and colon.	Usually in children and adolescents. May be associated with dysgammaglobulinemia.
Benign tumors and polyps (Fig. 42)	Single or multiple filling defects. May be pedunculated. Central ulceration secondary to necrosis occurs. *Leiomyoma:* extrinsic or intrinsic filling defect, almost always single, often ulcerated, and occasionally pedunculated. Preferentially located in the jejunum. *Polyps* (adenomatous and hamartomatous): Single or multiple, commonly pedunculated lesions, usually less than 5 cm in diameter. Preferentially located in the ileum. *Lipoma:* solitary relatively small filling defect that may be pedunculated. Characteristically changes shape when palpated. Preferentially located in the distal ileum and ileocecal valve area. *Hemangiomas:* commonly multiple and measuring less than 1 cm in diameter. Phleboliths are occasionally associated. *Neurofibromas:* single or multiple, sessile or pedunculated, with or without ulcerations.	Leiomyoma is the most common benign neoplasm of the small-bowel. 50% are smaller than 5 cm, 25% between 5 and 10 cm, and 25% larger than 10 cm in diameter. *Peutz–Jeghers* syndrome: multiple (hamartomatous) polyps in the small bowel often associated with colonic and gastric polyps and characteristic pigmentation of skin and mucous membranes. *Rendu–Osler–Weber* syndrome: familial disorder with multiple telangiectatic lesions. Spider telangiectasia or multiple nodular angiomas occur in the small bowel. Multiple polypoid lesions in the small-bowel are also found with *Cowden's* syndrome, *Canada–Cronkhite* syndrome, *Gardner's* syndrome, and *familial polyposis*. These conditions, however, are more common in the colon and therefore discussed in more detail in Table **5**, pages 182–184.
Carcinoid	One or, rarely, several small intraluminal masses, virtually always located in ileum (particularly the terminal portion) and characteristically associated with a fixed, kinked loop of bowel causing obstruction.	Most common neoplasm of the small-bowel. Besides the primary lesion, mesenteric lymph node metastases may also cause small-bowel obstruction. The carcinoid syndrome, characterized by skin flushing, diarrhea, and involvement of the right heart valves, is caused by extensive serotonin release into the blood. The syndrome is usually only found in the presence of extensive liver metastases.
Adenocarcinoma	A sharply demarcated nodular or annular filling defect with abnormal mucosal pattern is characteristic. Flat ulcerations are occasionally found. Most tumors are located in the jejunum. Presentation as a broad-based polyp occurs, but is relatively uncommon, whereas presentation as a pedunculated polyp is very unusual. Obstruction is a common complication.	Patients present commonly with small-bowel obstruction or, less frequently, with chronic gastrointestinal blood loss.
Leiomyosarcoma	Extrinsic or intrinsic (broad-based or rarely pedunculated) filling defect without site predilection. Deep central ulcerations occur in approximately half of the cases. Benign and malignant smooth muscle tumors cannot be reliably differentiated.	Approximately half of the smooth muscle tumors in small bowel are malignant, the other half benign (leiomyomas). Histologic differentiation between benign and malignant tumors is often very difficult, if not impossible. Other sarcomatous tumors are very rare.

Filling Defects in the Gastrointestinal Tract 179

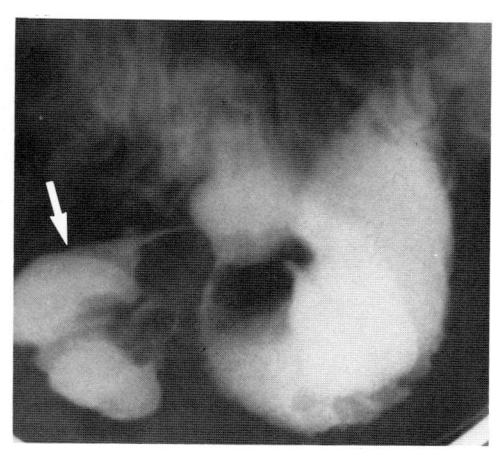

Figure 40 **Meckel's diverticulum.** A partially inverted Meckel's diverticulum (arrow) is seen causing an intraluminal filling defect and obstruction in the distal ileum.

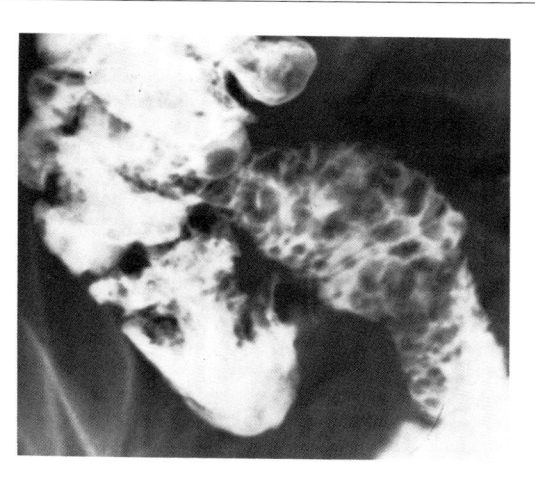

Figure 41 **Nodular lymphoid hyperplasia.** Multiple small nodular defects are seen in the terminal ileum and to a lesser degree in the cecum.

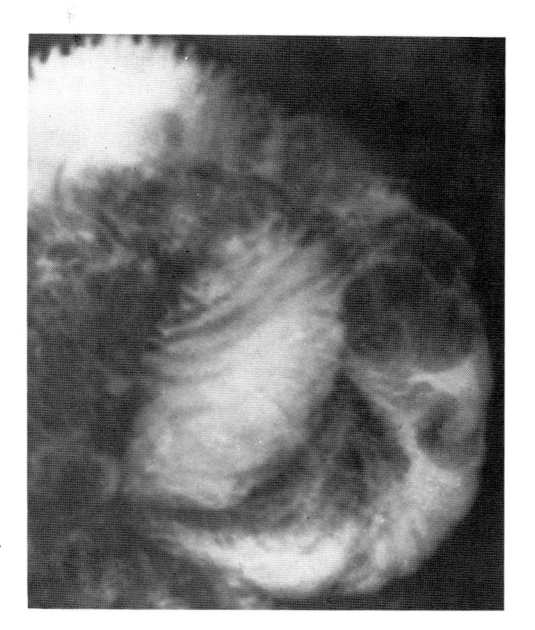

Figure 42 **Peutz–Jeghers syndrome.** Several polypoid ▶ lesions are seen in the jejunum with early obstruction caused by intussusception.

Table 4 (Cont.) Filling Defects in the Small Bowel (Jejunum and Ileum)

Disease	Radiographic Findings	Comments
Lymphoma (Fig. 43)	Single or multiple nodular extrinsic (secondary lymphoma) or intrinsic (polypoid to annular) masses without site predilection. Thickened folds, often with corrugated or tethered appearance, may be associated. Complete effacement of mucosal pattern and large ulcerations are commonly seen.	Primary and secondary small-bowel involvement occurs quite commonly with non-Hodgkin's lymphomas, whereas in Hodgkin's disease small bowel manifestations are rare and almost always secondary.
Metastases (hematogenous and mesenteric) (Fig. 44)	Single or multiple extrinsic or intrinsic masses without site predilection. Central ulcerations ("bull's eyes" or "target lesions") are particularly common in melanomas. A fixed loop of bowel associated with an extrinsic mass invading the bowel wall and causing an annular or eccentric defect is characteristic for mesenteric metastases. Mucosal tethering of the involved loop that is fixed by mesenteric metastases is a common finding.	Hematogenous metastases originate most commonly from melanoma, breast, and bronchogenic carcinomas. Mesenteric metastases (lymphatic spread or per continuitatem) are often found with carcinomas originating from the gastrointestinal or urogenital tract. Direct invasion of small bowel from a carcinoma in an adjacent organ (e.g., pancreas or colon) is also possible.
Kaposi's sarcoma	Multiple extrinsic or intrinsic nodules throughout the entire intestinal tract, often with central ulcerations.	Characteristic skin lesions (ulcerated hemorrhagic dermatitis).
Inflammatory pseudotumor	Localized submucosal filling defect or polypoid lesion.	May occasionally lead to an intussusception.
Intussusception (Fig. 45)	Intraluminal, often lobulated mass, characteristically with "coiled-spring" appearance.	Idiopathic only in infants and young children. In adults virtually always secondary to intraluminal mass (benign or malignant), an inverted Meckel's diverticulum or sprue.
Hematoma	Extrinsic mass may be caused by mesenteric hematoma. Often associated with intramural bleeding evident as "stacked-coin" appearance.	Usually with anticoagulation therapy or hemophilia. "Stacked-coin" appearance more striking in jejunum than ileum because of better developed jejunal folds.
Gallstone	Usually solitary intraluminal mass (radiolucent or opaque), most often seen in the distal ileum (narrowest portion) where the stone can become impacted and cause mechanical obstruction. Air or contrast reflux into the biliary system is diagnostic.	Elderly women are most often affected. In more than 50% of cases, gallstone perforation into the gut does not cause obstruction.
Food, foreign bodies, pills	Solitary or multiple freely mobile intraluminal filling defects of varying shapes and sizes.	Fruit pits trapped in a blind loop or area of narrowing can become calcified *(enterolith)*. *Air bubbles* may temporarily mimic round intraluminal masses.
Worm infestations (*Ascaris, Strongyloides,* hookworm or tapeworm) (Fig. 46)	Elongated radiolucent filling defects that can be coiled up and produce an intraluminal mass. Barium in the gastrointestinal tract of the worm is often seen presenting as a thin longitudinal line along the length of the worm.	No symptoms are found with mild infections, but large numbers of worms may produce abdominal pain and obstruction. A mass of coiled *Ascaris* contrasted by intestinal gas can occasionally be diagnosed without barium.
Pneumatosis intestinalis (primary or idiopathic) (Fig. 47)	Radiolucent cystic lesions along the contour of the bowel wall are diagnostic.	*Secondary pneumatosis intestinalis* is found with bowel necrosis (e.g., ischemic bowel disease and necrotizing enterocolitis in infants), peptic ulcer disease, inflammatory bowel disease, post gastrointestinal surgery, and in obstructive pulmonary disease. In these conditions, the air in the bowel wall tends to have a more streaky or crescent, linear appearance.

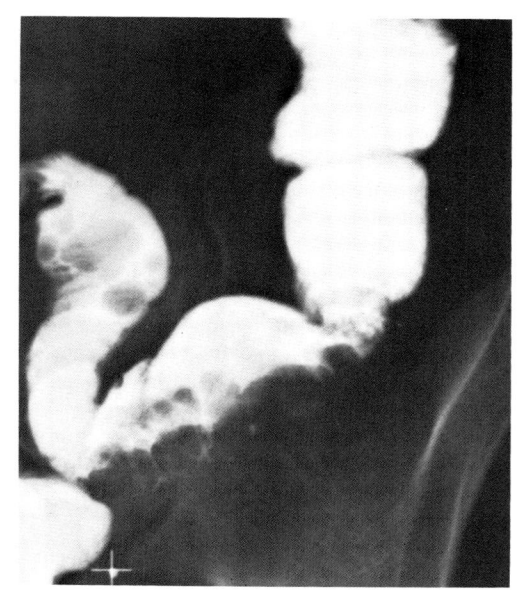

Figure 43 **Non-Hodgkin's lymphoma.** Extrinsic invasion of the ileum is seen producing nodular defects and mucosal tethering.

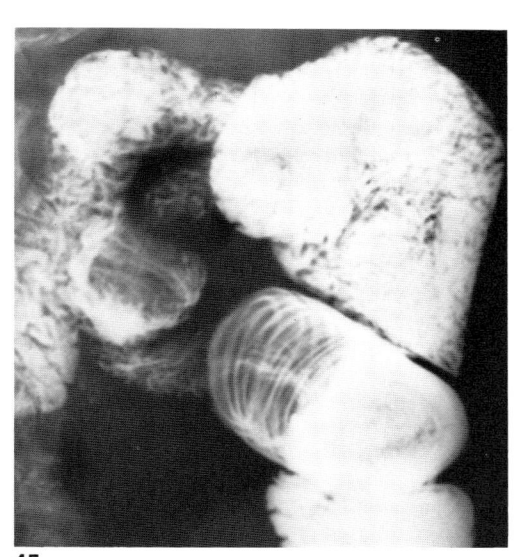

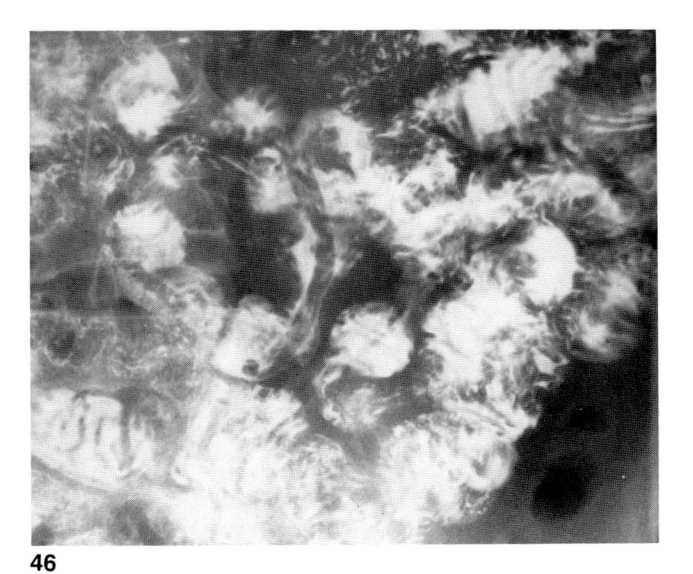

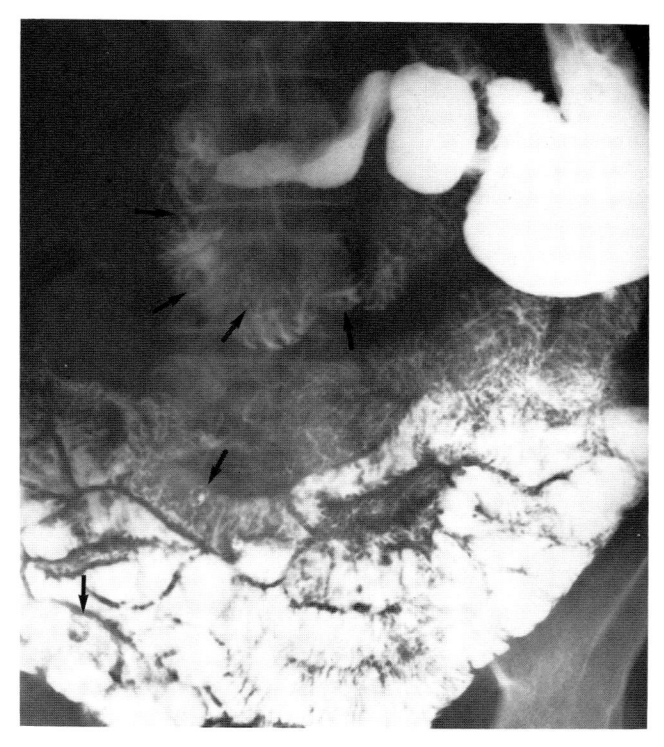

Figure 44 **Melanoma metastases.** Multiple small nodules with central ulcerations are seen throughout the small bowel (arrows).

Figure 45 **Intussusception in Hodgkin's lymphoma.** An intraluminal mass with characteristic "coiled-spring" appearance is seen in the jejunum.

Figure 46 ***Ascaris.*** Several tubular filling defects are seen in the small bowel.

Figure 47 **Pneumatosis intestinalis.** A radiolucent band consisting of numerous confluent radiolucent cystic lesions is seen.

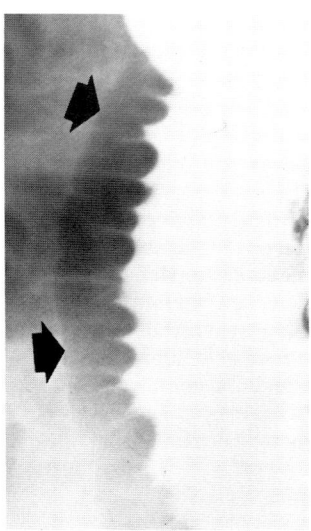

Table 5 Filling Defects in the Colon and Rectum

Disease	Radiographic Findings	Comments
Ileocecal valve (Fig. 48)	*Normal:* Intrinsic round to oval filling defect not exceeding 4 cm in diameter and arising from the medioposterior wall of the colon at the junction of the cecum and ascending colon. *Lipomatous infiltration or hypertrophy:* Enlarged, often slightly lobulated ileocecal valve with smooth surface and intact mucosa. *Ileal mucosal prolapse:* Radial folds in the form of a star are seen in a normal or slightly enlarged ileocecal valve viewed face-on.	Histologically, lipomatous infiltration is characterized by submucosal fatty infiltration and lack of a capsule. Enlargement of the ileocecal valve may also be caused by benign or malignant neoplastic and inflammatory diseases (e.g., *Crohn's disease, tuberculosis, amebiasis*). In these conditions, the mucosal surface may no longer be smooth. A *neoplasm* may furthermore cause an asymmetric or polypoid enlargement. Rarely, an *intramural hematoma* or *impacted gallstone* or foreign body may cause or simulate an enlarged ileocecal valve.
Appendix (inverted stump or intussusception)	Oval, round, or less commonly finger-like intrinsic filling defect arising from the medial wall of the cecum without visualization of the appendix. (DD: Extrinsic cecal filling defect caused by appendiceal abscess.)	Postoperative defects secondary to inversion of the appendiceal stump or incomplete resection of the appendix may measure up to 3 cm in diameter. Intussusception of the appendix usually occurs in the presence of an *appendiceal tumor* or *mucocele* (obstructed appendix filled with sterile mucus) that may present with peripheral calcifications.
Duplication cyst	Rare extrinsic spherical or tubular mass with intact mucosa anywhere in the colon, producing often partial to complete obstruction.	Occasionally, duplication may communicate with the colonic lumen, producing a double-barrel appearance.
Lipoma (Fig. 49)	Smooth, relatively sharply outlined, deformable, and somewhat radiolucent intrinsic filling defect, preferentially located in the right half of the colon. A pedicle that appears to be wider than the thin stalk of an adenomatous polyp may develop in larger lipomas.	*Leiomyomas* and other benign mesenchymal tumors are relatively rare in the colon.
Endometrioma	Usually solitary extrinsic or intrinsic, broad-based filling defect, preferentially located in the sigmoid. May cause tethering of the adjacent mucosa due to secondary fibrosis, or produce an annular constricting lesion that simulates a carcinoma.	Usually diagnosed between ages 20 and 40, rarely in postmenopausal females.
Polyp (adenomatous) (Fig. 50)	Solitary or multiple spherical filling defects with smooth surface, often measuring less than 1.5 cm in diameter. May be lobulated when larger. Pedicles are common and may occasionally measure several cm in length. A barium-coated, air-filled *diverticulum* must be differentiated (see Fig. 3, page 162).	Premalignant condition: Incidence of malignancy correlates with size of lesion. Sessile and broad-based polyps measuring more than 2 cm in diameter are malignant in almost half of the cases. *Hyperplastic polyps* are smooth sessile mucosal elevations of less than 5 mm in diameter without malignant potential. They are found at autopsy in up to 50% of colons of asymptomatic adults. Radiographically, they cannot be differentiated from tiny adenomatous polyps.
Polyposis (Figs. 51–53)	*Familial polyposis:* Innumerable, sessile polyps ranging from 1 to 2 mm to 1 to 2 cm in diameter. Small pedicles can occasionally be identified in some lesions. Usually the entire colon is involved, though left colon and rectum involvement is often more pronounced. Segmental colonic involvement is unusual. In less than 5% of cases, polyps are also found in the stomach and small bowel (Fig. 51).	Autosomal dominant inheritance. Sporadic cases without traceable family history occur rarely. Usually diagnosed in young adults. Carcinoma of the colon will develop in virtually all patients when untreated (approximately 15 years after the appearance of colonic polyps).

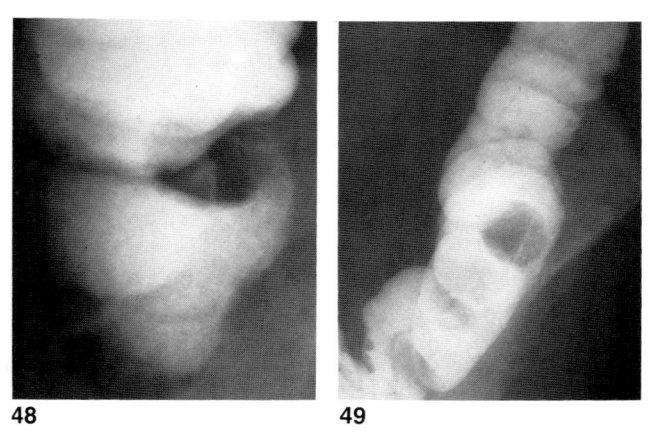

Filling Defects in the Gastrointestinal Tract   183

Figure 48 **Lipomatous infiltration of the ileocecal valve.** A slightly lobulated, smooth filling defect is seen originating from the medioposterior wall of the junction between the cecum and ascending colon.

Figure 49 **Lipoma.** A smooth and relatively sharply outlined filling defect is seen in the descending colon.

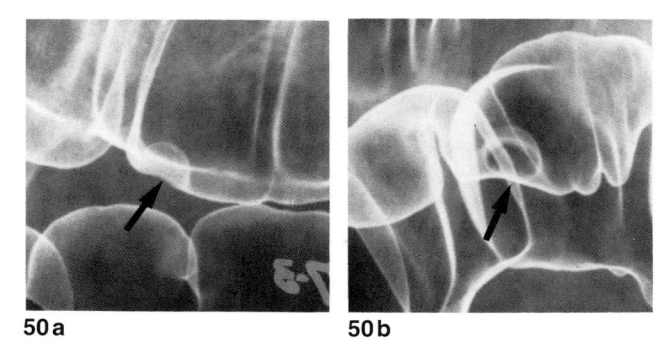

Figure 50a, b **Polyp a** in profile **a** and **b** in oblique projection. A small polyp (arrows) with the appearance of a bowler-hat is seen in **b**.

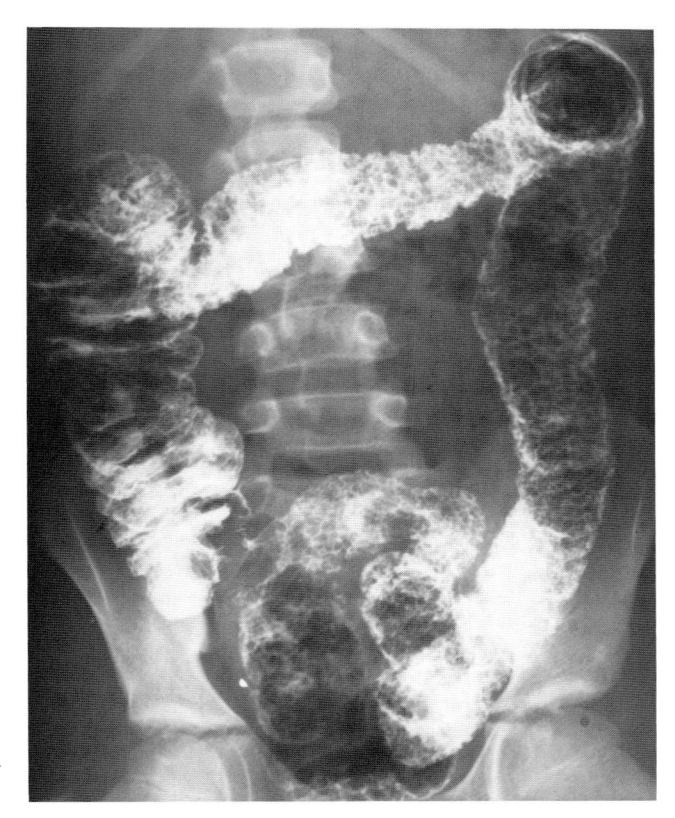

Figure 51 **Familial polyposis.** Innumerable small polyps ▶ throughout the colon and rectum are seen.

Table 5 (Cont.) Filling Defects in the Colon and Rectum

Disease	Radiographic Findings	Comments
	Gardner's syndrome: Colonic polyps (rarely stomach and small bowel) radiographically indistinguishable from familial polyposis. Osteomas and soft-tissue lesions (e.g., a desmoid of the mesentery presenting as a large extrinsic mass) may be seen.	Autosomal dominant syndrome consisting of colonic polyposis predisposing to carcinoma, osteomatosis, and cutaneous soft tissue lesions (mesenchymal tumors and cysts). Tendency for excessive scar formation (keloids).
	Turcot syndrome: Colonic polyposis with potential for malignancy associated with brain tumors (astrocytomas).	Autosomal recessive inherited.
	Canada–Cronkhite syndrome: Polyps in colon, small bowel, and stomach.	Gastrointestinal hamartomatous polyposis and ectodermal abnormalities (alopecia, hyperpigmentation, and nail atrophy). Develops in the elderly and has no familial or sexual predilection. Presents with malabsorption and severe diarrhea.
	Juvenile polyposis: Multiple hamartomatous colonic polyps, usually in children under 10 years of age, rarely in adults.	DD: *Multiple juvenile polyps:* One or a few polypoid lesions containing multiple mucin-filled cysts and abundant connective stroma are found in young children, presenting often with diarrhea and rectal bleeding. Polyps have a tendency to autoamputate or regress spontaneously.
	Cowden's syndrome (multiple hamartoma syndrome): Multiple polyps (rarely solitary lesions) may be found in the entire gastrointestinal tract.	Rare hereditary disorders associated with multiple tumors and malformations in different organs. Circumoral papillomatosis and nodular gingival hyperplasia are characteristic clinical features.
	Peutz–Jeghers syndrome: Only a few colonic polyps can be seen at best, since the disease primarily involves the small bowel.	See Table 4, page 178.
	Colonic neurofibromatosis: Multiple filling defects varying in diameter from one to several centimeters. Characteristic is the eccentric location of the lesions which are all located on the mesenteric side.	Associated with Recklinghausen's disease (cutaneous neurofibromas and "cafe-au-lait" pigmented skin lesions).
	Nodular lymphoid hyperplasia of the colon: Innumerable, tiny filling defects of uniform size, measuring only a few millimeters in diameter (Fig. 52).	Usually in children and rare in adults. DD: Polypoid lesions in lymphoma tend to be larger, vary in size, and are associated with thickened folds.
	Inflammatory pseudopolyps: Associated with radiographic evidence of inflammatory process (Fig. 53).	For example, ulcerative colitis, granulomatous colitis, amebiasis, and schistosomiasis.
	Pneumatosis cystoides coli: Round extrinsic and intrinsic filling defects with increased radiolucency (gas-containing cysts) that can already be seen on plain film radiographs).	May be idiopathic or caused by air spread from the mediastinum (e.g., in chronic obstructive pulmonary diseases) or associated with peptic ulcer disease or secondary to surgery.
Villous adenoma (Fig. 54)	Solitary, broad-based, often lobulated intrinsic filling defects that is commonly located in rectum or sigmoid. Tumor is often walnut-sized, but may range from 0.5 to 15 cm in diameter. Its appearance is characteristic when barium is trapped between villous strands, producing an irregular reticulated surface. Since the tumor is soft, it changes shape and may even be effaced by compression.	Usually diagnosed in the middle-aged and elderly, who may present with mucous diarrhea. Incidence of adenocarcinoma is high and increases with the size of the tumor.

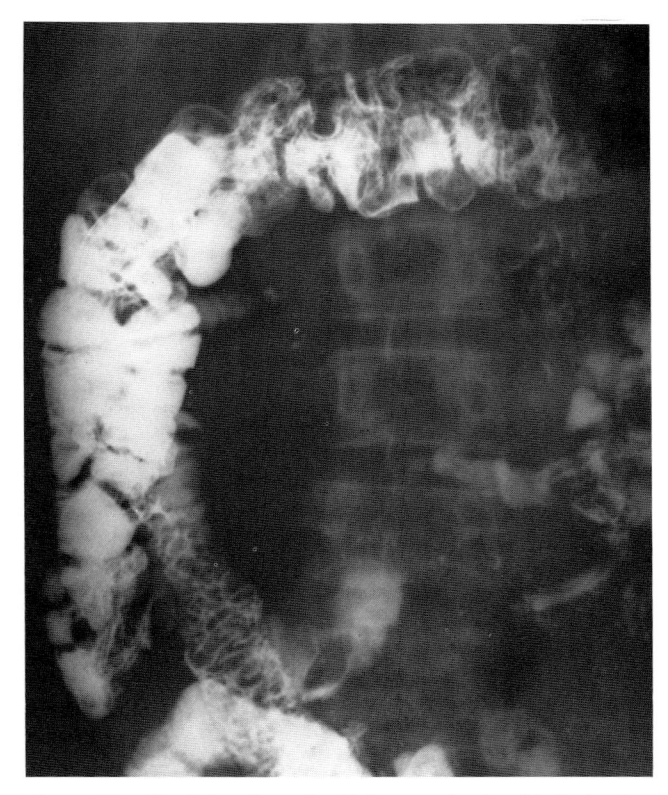

Filling Defects in the Gastrointestinal Tract 185

Figure 52 **Nodular lymphoid hyperplasia.** Multiple tiny polyps are seen in this small bowel follow-up examination in the colon. Note that the greatest number of lesions is characteristically seen in the terminal ileum.

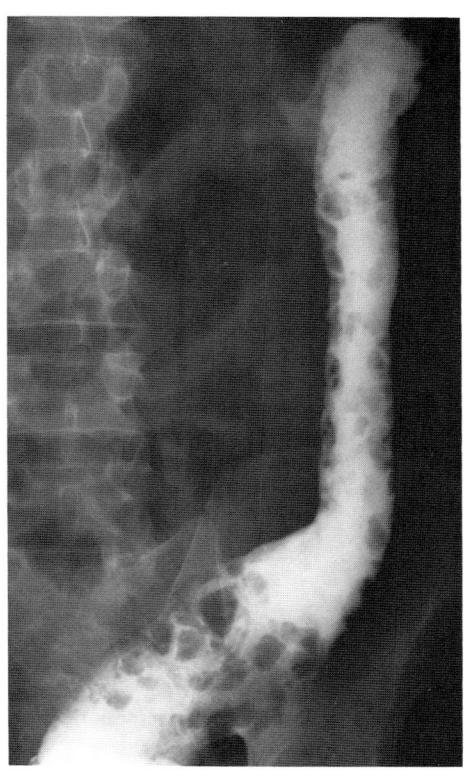

Figure 53 **Inflammatory pseudopolyposis** in ulcerative colitis. Numerous filling defects are seen in the descending and sigmoid colon.

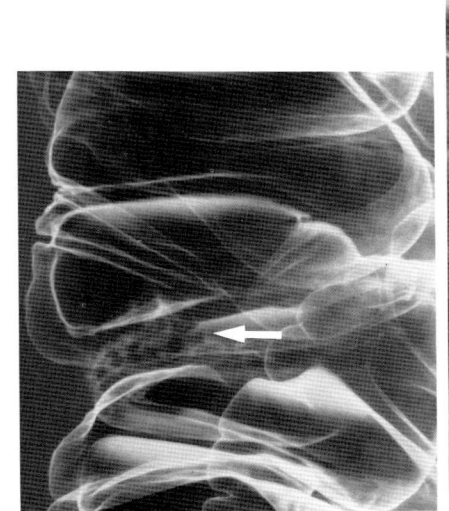

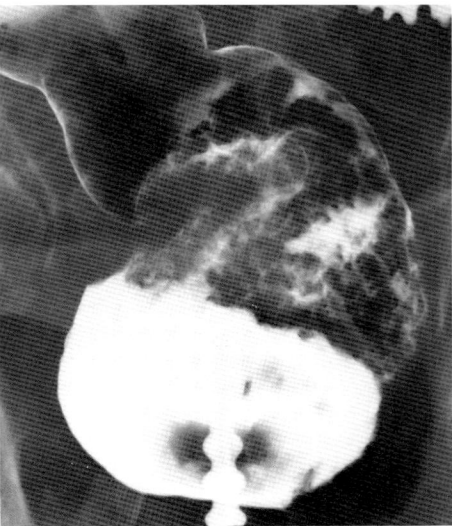

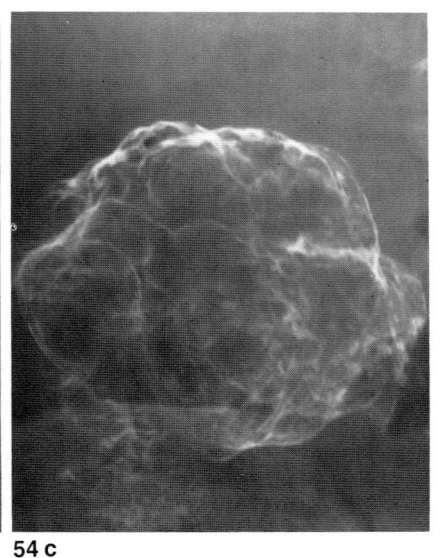

54 a 54 b 54 c

Figure 54 **Villous adenoma** (2 cases). **a** The small sponge-like lesion (arrow) in the ascending colon was histologically completely benign. **b** The bulky mass in the rectum, with an irregular reticulated surface, revealed a malignant transformation at its base histologically. **c** The postevacuation film often demonstrates the characteristic sponge-like pattern caused by barium trapped between villous strands best.

Table 5 (Cont.) Filling Defects in the Colon and Rectum

Disease	Radiographic Findings	Comments
Carcinoid	Two different clinicopathologic entities: 1 Benign, small sessile, polypoid lesion, measuring less than 2 cm in diameter and preferentially located in appendix or rectum. 2 Broad-based bulky intraluminal filling defect measuring several centimeters at the time of diagnosis and commonly associated with lymph node and liver metastases. Usually located in cecum or right colon.	The benign variety located in appendix and rectum occurs usually in the younger and middle-aged patient, and is much more common than the malignant colonic form, which is usually seen in the elderly patient.
Carcinoma (Fig. 55)	Usually, solitary polypoid or annular filling defects varying greatly in size. The surface may be smooth, ragged, or ulcerated. Fungating polypoid carcinomas are preferentially located in the cecum, ascending colon, or rectum, whereas annular ulcerating lesions, characteristically with "overhanging edges", are more commonly seen in the transverse, descending, and sigmoid colon. Abrupt transition from tumor to healthy mucosa is typical. Rarely curvilinear and/or mottled calcifications are seen in the primary and metastatic lesions (lymph nodes and liver).	Colon cancers present with occult blood in the stool, but are otherwise asymptomatic until late in their course, when complications develop. These include obstruction, perforation (peritonitis or, when sealed off, abscess formation), and invagination. Calcifications are seen in mucus-producing adenocarcinomas.
Lymphoma and sarcoma (Fig. 56)	Localized form may present as a polypoid or annular, often ulcerated mass, preferentially located in the cecum and less commonly in the rectum. Extrinsic filling defects can occur from lymphoma involving adjacent organs or lymph nodes.	Diffuse colonic involvement by lymphoma presenting with thickened folds, nodules and ulcerations is a more common presentation. Involvement of the colon by non-Hodgkin's lymphoma is much more common than involvement in Hodgkin's disease. Colonic sarcomas (e.g., *Kaposi's sarcoma* with diffuse involvement and *leiomyosarcoma* with localized involvement) are radiographically indistinguishable from lymphoma.
Metastases (Figs. 57, 58)	Present as solitary or multiple extrinsic filling defects with intact mucosa, or as an intrinsic mass lesion mimicking a primary colon carcinoma. In the pelvis, extrinsic metastases may simulate pelvic lipomatosis (vertical elongation, elevation, and narrowing of the rectum and urinary bladder).	Pathways of involvement: 1 Direct invasion from carcinomas in adjacent organs (e.g., gastrointestinal and urogenital systems). 2 Hematogenous (e.g., from breast carcinoma and rarely from bronchogenic carcinoma and melanoma). 3 Intraperitoneal seeding (transported by ascites).

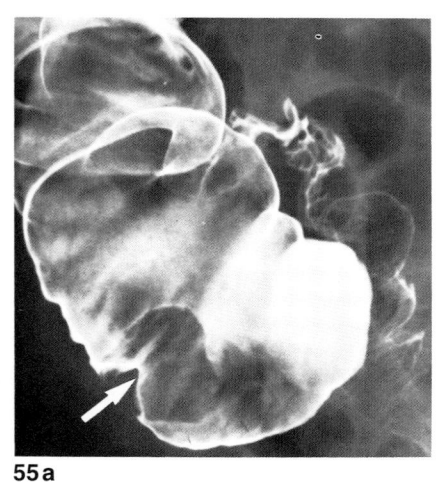

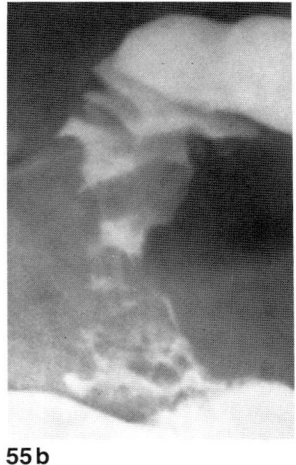

Filling Defects in the Gastrointestinal Tract   187

Figure **55a, b Colonic adenocarcinomas** in two different patients. **a** An irregularly outlined polypoid mass is seen in the cecum. Retraction of the colonic wall at the site of origin of the lesion strongly suggests malignant nature of the polypoid mass (arrow). **b** A circumferential, ulcerating mass lesion is seen in the sigmoid colon in the second case.

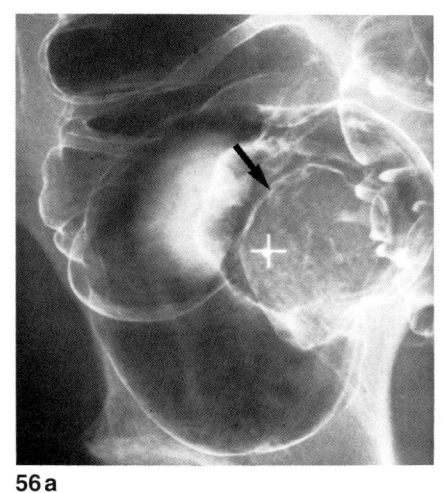

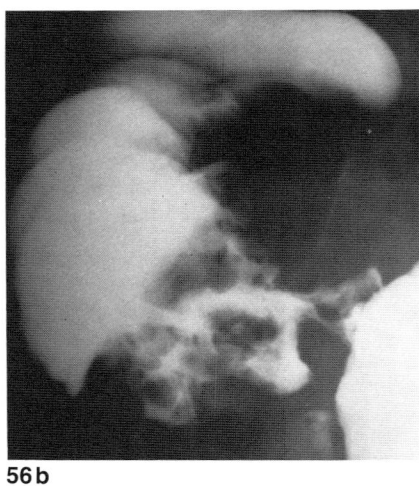

Figure **56a, b Non-Hodgkin's lymphoma** involving the cecum (2 cases). In **a** a round intraluminal mass (arrow) is seen, whereas in **b** an ulcerating and a destructive lesion is present. Radiographically, both cases are indistinguishable from adenocarcinomas at this location.

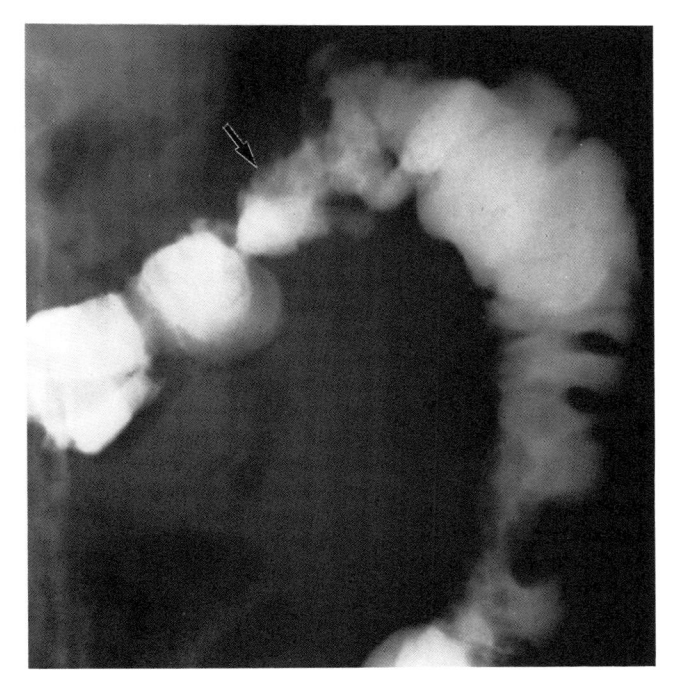

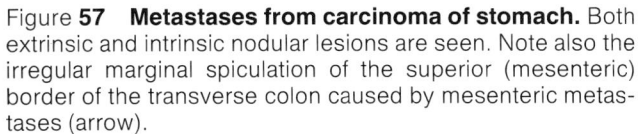

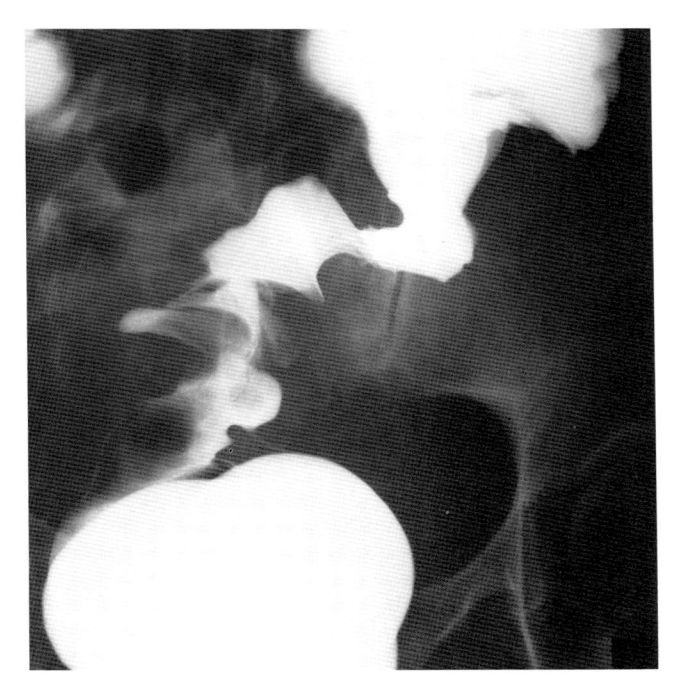

Figure **57 Metastases from carcinoma of stomach.** Both extrinsic and intrinsic nodular lesions are seen. Note also the irregular marginal spiculation of the superior (mesenteric) border of the transverse colon caused by mesenteric metastases (arrow).

Figure **58** Metastases from ovarian carcinoma. Circumferential narrowing of the shortened and fixed sigmoid with large filling defects is seen.

Table 5 (Cont.)　　**Filling Defects in the Colon and Rectum**

Disease	Radiographic Findings	Comments
Appendiceal abscess (Fig. 59)	Extrinsic filling defect, usually in the cecum and terminal ileum, but it may develop anywhere in the abdomen with an abnormally located or unusually long appendix. Extrinsic mass may have mottled appearance simulating fecal material or an air–fluid level on upright and decubitus films. An appendicolith (oval-shaped with laminated calcifications) within the lesion is diagnostic but is found only in a small minority of cases.	Perforated appendicitis is the most common cause of intra-abdominal abscess in a patient who has not previously undergone surgery.
Diverticulitis with abscess formation (Fig. 60)	Solitary or less commonly multiple, extrinsic filling defects, usually in the sigmoid colon. Barium may occasionally enter abscess cavity. In the acute stage, spasm of the involved colon segment is usually present and the adjacent diverticula may be draped over the abscess ("drape sign"). In the chronic stage, an intramural abscess is often associated with a markedly narrowed bowel lumen, simulating colonic carcinoma.	Predominant clinical symptoms are localized tenderness and fever.
Amebic colitis (Fig. 61)	Thumbprinting and multiple filling defects caused by pseudopolyposis and amebomas are seen besides ulcerations. The disease may involve any part of the colon, but the cecum is involved in up to 90% of cases. The ileum is not involved. Contrast reflux through a "gaping" ileocecal valve differentiates cecal amebiasis from a carcinoma.	An *ameboma* is a hyperplastic granuloma of the large bowel caused by secondary bacterial invasion of an amebic abscess. Radiographically, it usually presents as an annular, constricting mass lesion with apple-core appearance that is often indistinguishable from a carcinoma. Demonstration of small ulcers adjacent to the ameboma and the relatively young age of the patients are both helpful in differentiating it from carcinoma.
Tuberculosis	Localized tuberculosis of the colon is usually limited to the cecum, which appears shrunken and retracted. An intraluminal mass is rarely seen. A narrowed and ulcerated terminal ileum is commonly associated, but barium refluxes only infrequently into the terminal ileum because of spasm and thickening of the ileocecal valve.	With the exception of the cecum, localized tuberculous involvement of the colon or rectum is rare.
Actinomycosis	Cecal mass similar to tuberculosis, but greater tendency towards fistulization.	Develops secondary to appendicitis or appendiceal abscess.

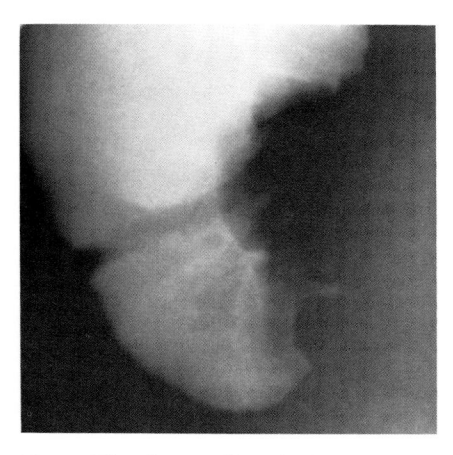

Filling Defects in the Gastrointestinal Tract

Figure **59 Appendiceal abscess.** An extrinsic defect is seen on the medial aspect of the cecum. Other inflammatory mass lesions (e.g., Crohn's disease) cannot, however, be differentiated in the absence of an appendicolith.

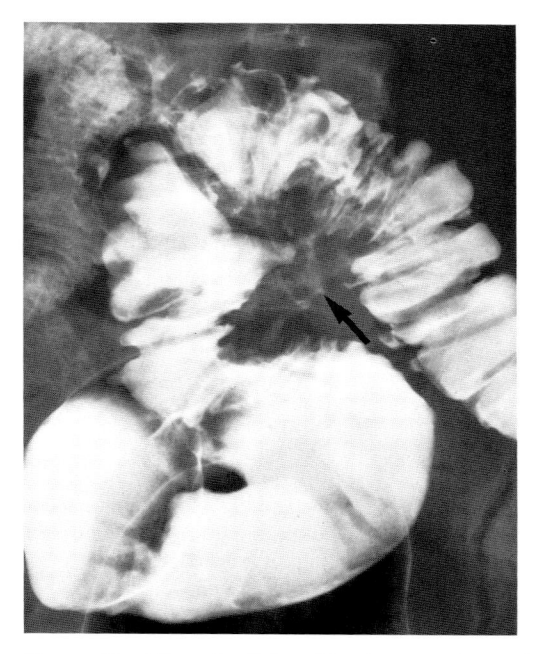

Figure **60 Diverticulitis with abscess formation.** A mass lesion with barium entering the abscess cavity (arrow) and the edematous sigmoid draped around it is seen.

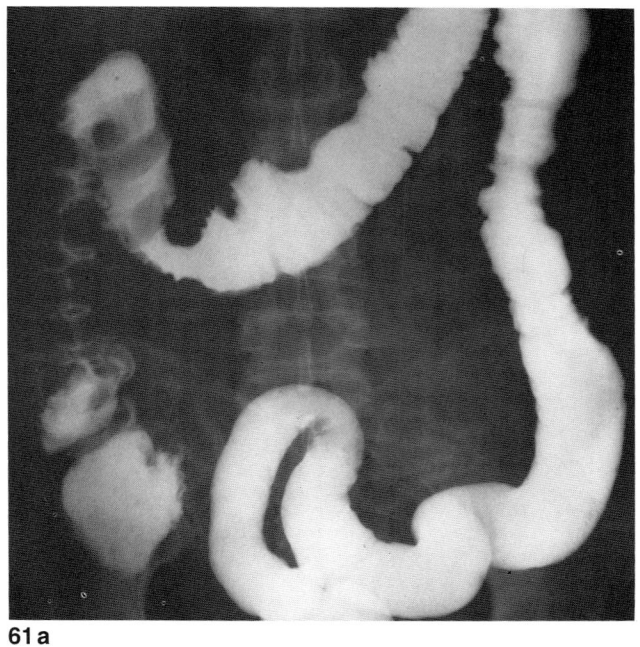

Figure **61 Amebic colitis. a** Thumbprinting and filling defects are limited to the right colon, whereas **b** tiny ulcerations, some of them with a "collar-button" appearance, are seen throughout the entire colon with the exception of the sigmoid.

61 a   61 b

Table 5 (Cont.) Filling Defects in the Colon and Rectum

Disease	Radiographic Findings	Comments
Ulcerative colitis (Fig. 62)	Pseudopolyps present usually as numerous small filling defects associated with other signs of the disease (ulceration, absence or irregularities of haustral folds, narrowing and foreshortening of the colon). Rarely, a pseudopolyp may present as large fungating mass. When localized, the rectosigmoid area is preferentially involved.	Can affect all ages, although two peaks occur, the first between 20 and 25 and the second between 50 and 60 years of age. Characteristic clinical presentation consists of intermittent episodes of diarrhea and rectal bleeding. Pseudopolyps can already be seen in the acute stage, where they represent edematous mucosal remnants, but they are usually more prominent in the subacute and chronic stages, when epithelial regeneration has occurred.
Crohn's colitis (Fig. 63)	Uniform filling defects ("cobblestone" appearance) may be created by swollen mucosa separated by deep, linear, longitudinal, and vertical ulcers. When localized, the right colon, including terminal ileum, is preferentially involved. Skip lesions and presence of fistulas are characteristic.	Occurs primarily in adolescence and young adults, presenting with diarrhea but without gross bleeding.
Inflammatory pseudotumor (Fig. 64)	A localized large intraluminal mass with irregular surface mimicking a carcinoma is occasionally found with ulcerative colitis and Crohn's disease.	The bulky mass is produced by a cluster of pseudopolyps.
Ischemic colitis (Fig. 65)	Pseudopolyps and "thumbprinting" are seen in addition to ulcerations in a more advanced stage that is often indistinguishable from ulcerative colitis. Preferential involvement of splenic flexure and left colon, but characteristically sparing the rectum.	Presents clinically in the elderly as acute episode of abdominal pain and bleeding.

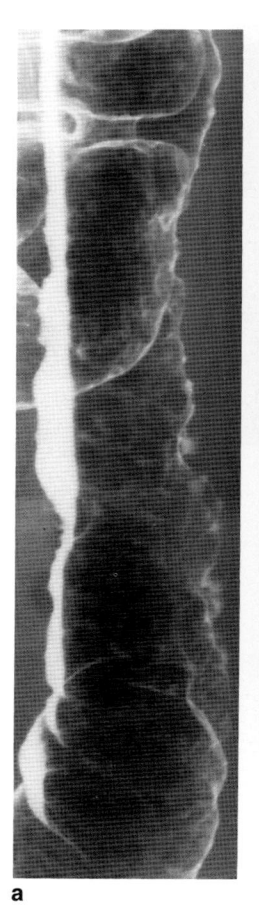

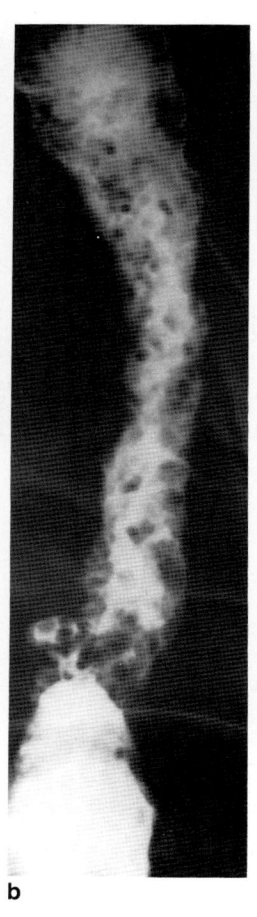

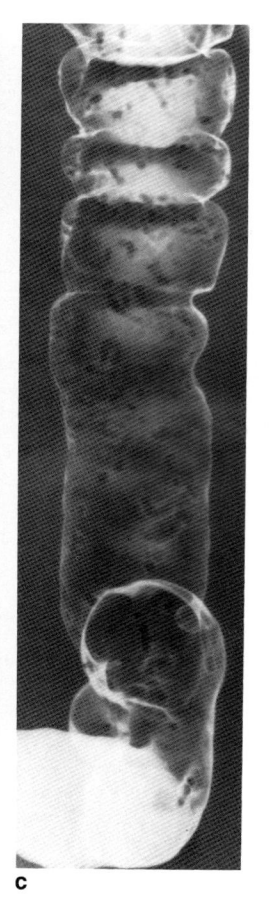

Figure 62 **Ulcerative colitis. a** Acute stage: marginal ulceration, including collar button ulcers, is evident. **b** (5 years after **a**): Multiple pseudopolyps, varying considerably in size, are now present, in addition to muccosal ulcerations and spasm. **c** (10 years after **a**). The pseudopolyps have decreased in size, the ulcers have healed, and a normal haustral pattern has returned.

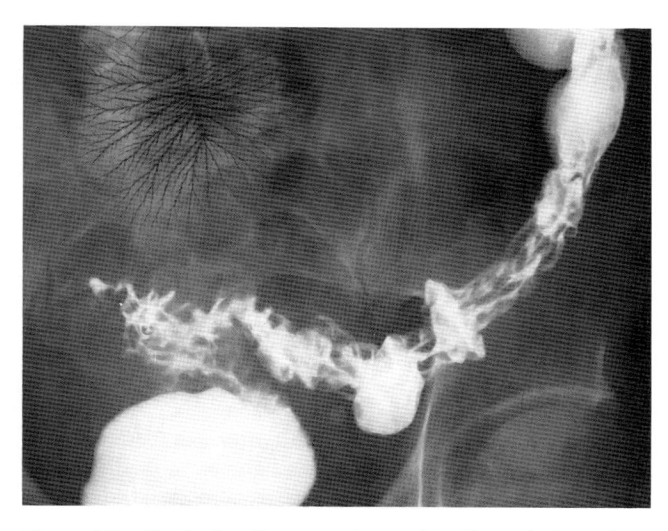

Figure **63 Crohn's disease.** A combination of ulceration, edematous mucosa and pseudopolyposis produces a cobblestone appearance in the foreshortened sigmoid. Note also that the rectum is not involved.

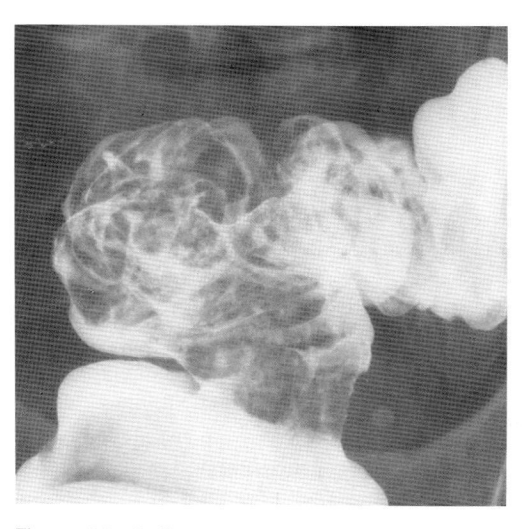

Figure **64 Inflammatory pseudotumor in Crohn's disease.** A localized fungating mass is produced in the foreshortened sigmoid by a cluster of pseudopolyps. (Same case as in Fig. **63**, 1 year later).

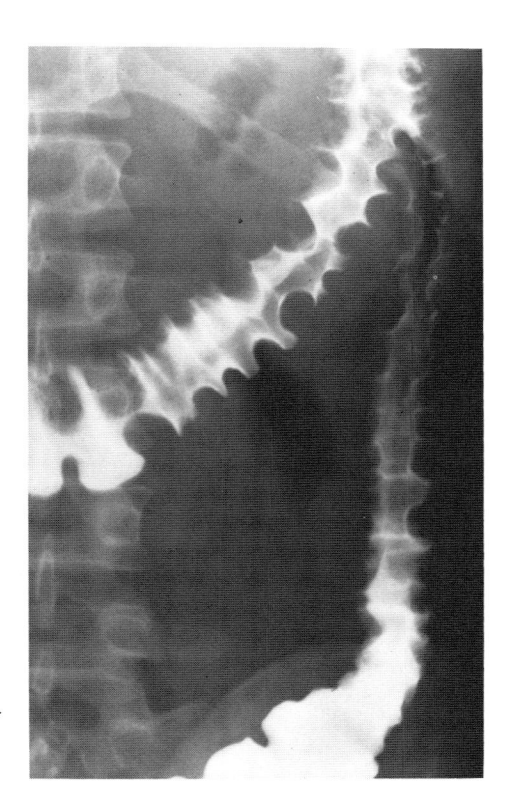

Figure **65 Ischemic colitis.** Large marginal filling defects ("thumbprinting") are seen in the distal transverse and descending colon.

Table 5 (Cont.) Filling Defects in the Colon and Rectum

Disease	Radiographic Findings	Comments
Pseudomembranous colitis (Fig. 66)	Large polypoid defects and "thumbprinting" to wide transverse bands of thickened colonic wall can be seen throughout the entire colon, but are usually most prominent in the transverse colon.	Usually develops after a course of antibiotic therapy. Severe diarrhea without significant rectal bleeding is the usual clinical presentation.
Schistosomiasis	Usually multiple polypoid filling defects measuring up to 2 cm, preferentially in the sigmoid and rectum. A single larger lesion is less common, and may cause obstruction and simulate carcinoma.	Filling defects are caused by granulomas, which are a late manifestation of the disease after heavy infestation and chronic exposure.
Colonic urticaria	Large, round or polygonal raised plaques in grossly dilated (usually right) colon, representing submucosal edema.	This condition is most often associated with an allergic reaction secondary to medication. Less common causes of submucosal edema presenting in this fashion include ischemia, chronic obstruction of various etiologies, and infections such as herpes zoster. "Thumbprinting" is, however, a far more common radiographic presentation of submucosal edema.
Worm infestations (Ascaris or Trichuris)	Solitary intraluminal filling defect by a bolus of ascaris or numerous irregular defects throughout the colon caused by excessive mucus production induced by *Trichuris trichiura* that are attached to the bowel wall.	*Trichuris trichiura* (whipworm) is a frequent inhabitant of the cecum and appendix of man. Infections (trichuriasis) are common in the subtropics and tropics.
Cystic fibrosis	Multiple poorly defined filling defects caused by viscous mucus adherent to the wall.	In children and young adults.
Colitis cystica profunda	Usually multiple filling defects measuring up to 2 cm in diameter and preferentially limited to the rectosigmoid area.	Filling defects are caused by submucosal cysts, lined with mucus-producing epithelium. Present clinically with bright rectal bleeding, mucus discharge, and diarrhea.
Pneumatosis cystoides coli (Fig. 67)	Multiple deformable round filling defects with increased radiolucency.	See under "polyposis" in this table, page 184.
Suture granuloma	Filling defect at anastomotic site that decreases in size characteristically with time.	Patient's history is important.
Intussusception (ileocolic or rarely colocolic) (Fig. 68)	Solitary filling defect, usually in the right colon. Obstruction and vascular compromise are often associated. "Coiled-spring" appearance is characteristic.	In adults, the leading points of intussusceptions are commonly Meckel's diverticula, lymphoma, mesenteric nodes, or polyps.
Hemorrhoids (internal)	Multiple polypoid filling defects in the rectum, usually associated with tubular filling defects caused by the veins from which the hemorrhoids arise.	May cause intermittent bleeding that is characteristically found on the outside of the stool.
Amyloidosis	Rare cause of single or multiple filling defects in the rectum and colon.	Since histologic involvement of rectal submucosa in both primary and secondary amyloidosis is common, rectal biopsies are often diagnostic even with a normal-appearing rectum.
Adhesions and fibrous bands	May produce extrinsic filling defects simulating a tumor.	Usually secondary to previous abdominal surgery. *Enlarged appendices epiploicae* may rarely produce similar filling defects.
Feces, artifacts, undigested food particles, air bubbles	Solitary ("fecaloma") or multiple intraluminal filling defects, which may be freely mobile or adherent to the wall and confused with polypoid lesions.	Undigested food particles caught in a diverticulum may calcify and produce *enteroliths*. Rarely, a *gallstone* trapped in the sigmoid may present as an intraluminal filling defect.

Filling Defects in the Gastrointestinal Tract 193

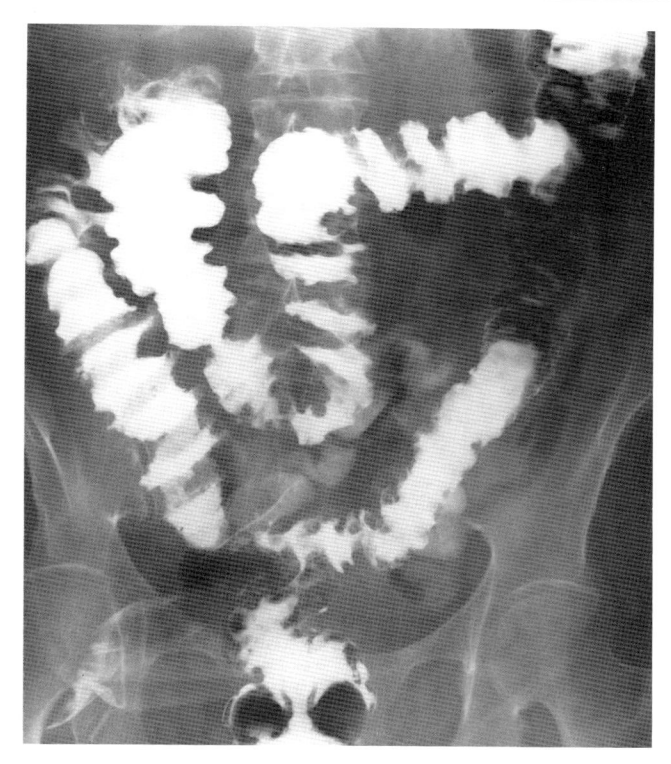

Figure 66 **Pseudomembranous colitis.** In addition to ulcerations, extensive submucosal edema is evident throughout the entire colon from the markedly thickened haustra and "thumbprinting."

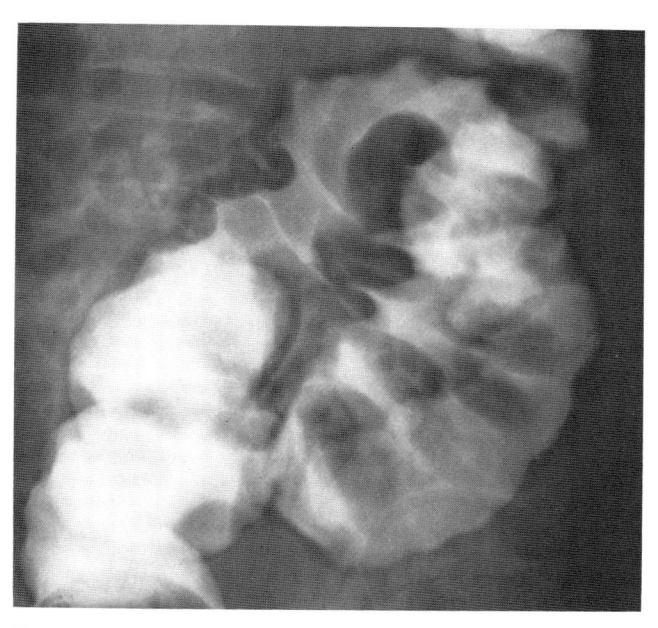

Figure 67 **Pneumatosis cystoides coli.** Multiple round filling defects with increased radiolucency are seen in the descending and sigmoid colon. In some areas, the cystic lesions have become confluent and form a broad radiolucent band along the barium column.

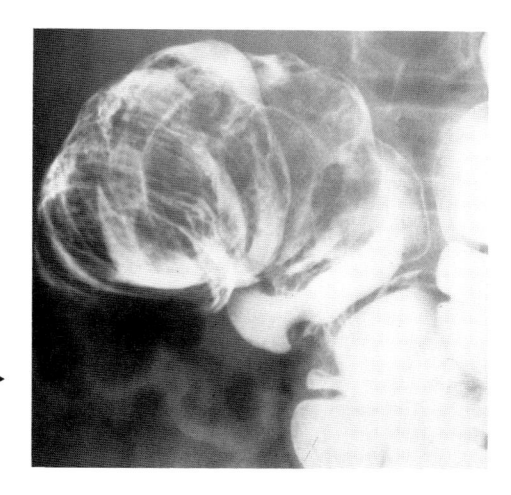

Figure 68 **Intussusception in non-Hodgkin's lymphoma.** Complete obstruction in the hepatic flexure by an intraluminal mass with "coiled-spring" appearance is seen in the hepatic flexure.

Chapter 8 Ulcers, Diverticula, and Fistulas in the Gastrointestinal Tract

Ulcers

An *ulcer* in the gastrointestinal tract is defined as a loss of mucous surface, causing gradual disintegration and necrosis of the tissues. Partial or complete loss of the mucosa only, without penetration into the submucosa, is generally called an *erosion*. In this chapter, solitary ulcerations, either single or multiple, will be discussed. Erosions and ulcers may be widespread and therefore create a generalized abnormality of the mucosal surface. Such conditions are discussed in Chapter 5, page 609. Single ulcers also cause abnormalities of the surrounding mucosa, either due to inflammatory changes or scarring.

Although deformity of the mucosal surface may be helpful in locating an ulcer, an ulcer crater should be demonstrated, preferably both in profile and en face, to make a definitive diagnosis. An ulcer crater on the dependent wall in the double-contrast examination and in the single-contrast examination may collect a pool of barium. An ulcer crater on the nondependent wall in a distended organ or elsewhere, if filled by a blood clot, will be seen as a ring shadow. Artifacts such as the stalactite phenomenon (a hanging drop of barium), patchy coating, precipitation, and flaking of barium or insufficient separation of the anterior and posterior walls (kissing artifact) may create shadows that simulate an ulcer or other mucosal abnormalities. Colonic or small-bowel diverticula may mimic the ring shadow of an ulcer.

Malignant versus Benign Ulcers

It is a common practice to obtain an endoscopic and histologic verification as soon as an ulcer in the gastrointestinal tract has been demonstrated radiographically. Certain features are helpful in the differential diagnosis of benign and malignant ulcers (Figs. **1** and **2**). This applies especially to the stomach, where both malignant and benign ulcerations occur frequently, whereas in the duodenum, the most common site of ulcers, the vast majority are benign. If a lesion is highly suggestive of malignancy on radiologic grounds, negative endoscopic or cytologic findings should not be taken as definitive evidence of its benign nature. Such lesions require follow-up studies.

Diverticula

A *diverticulum* is a circumscribed pouch created by herniation of the lining mucous membrane through a defect in the muscular coat of the wall. *True diverticula* are herniations of the mucous membrane and the submucous layers, whereas intestinal *false diverticula* are formed by protrusion of the mucous membrane alone through a tear in the muscular coat. Protrusion as a result of pressure from within are called *pulsion diverticula*. *Traction diverticula* are bulgings of the full thickness of the wall of the esophagus caused by adhesions resulting from some external lesion. If a diverticulum is shown by double contrast en face, the appear-

Figure 1 **Radiologic features of a benign gastric ulcer:** (1) Penetration beyond the normal contour of the stomach, (2) mucosal folds radiate into the orifice of the crater, (3) a smooth mound of edema surrounding a sharply defined crater, (4) signs of undermining of the mucosa (Hampton's line, ulcer collar).

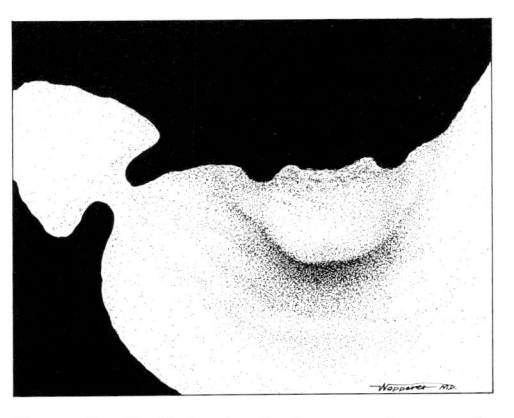

Figure 2 **Radiologic features of a malignant gastric ulcer:** (1) nodularity of the tissue surrounding the ulcer crater and in the orifice and floor of the crater, (2) tumor rim, (Carman's meniscus sign), (3) the crater fails to project beyond the normal gastric lumen, (4) radiating mucosal folds do not reach the orifice of the ulcer, (5) the crater is wider than it is deep.

ance may simulate the ring shadow around a polyp. The meniscus of barium in a diverticulum fades centrally, whereas around a polyp it fades peripherally. Criteria for differentiating are presented in Figure **3**, page 197. When seen in profile, they are easily differentiated. The mucosal lining and a narrow and long neck relative to the pouch itself help to differentiate a diverticulum from an ulcer.

Fistulas

A fistula refers to an abnormal communication from the gastrointestinal tract into another part of the bowel (enteric–enteric), to another organ (internal), or to the surface of the body (external). A fistula permitting the escape of pus is often called a *sinus tract*. The demonstration of fistulas in the barium examination of the gastrointestinal tract depends on the patency of the channel at the given moment. Fistulas may be better demonstrated by thin barium alone than in a double-contrast examination. Fistulas that open to the surface of the body may be cannulated and filled with contrast (fistulography). Fistulas may be congenital or secondary to an ulcer, chronic inflammation, malignancy, or trauma.

Table 1   Ulcers, Diverticula and Fistulas in the Esophagus

Disease	Radiographic Findings	Comments
Reflux esophagitis (Fig. 3)	Penetrating marginal ulcer in the region of the junction between the esophagus and stomach or hiatal hernia. The ulcer is a niche-like projection surrounded by ulcer collar and esophageal spasm.	Gastroesophageal reflux is often demonstrated. May be complicated by penetration into adjacent structures. Healing may result in stricture. For earlier signs of reflux esophagitis, see Chapter 5, page 108.
Barrett's esophagus (Fig. 4)	Esophageal ulceration usually at a distance from the cardia. Usually deep, penetrating, and identical to other peptic ulcerations. Often associated with a narrowed segment (spasm or stricture).	An ulcer in an islet of gastric mucosa in the esophagus complicating reflux esophagitis. A sliding hiatal hernia with gastroesophageal reflux is commonly demonstrated. In contrast to marginal ulceration of reflux esophagitis, Barrett's ulcer is separated by a variable length of normal-appearing esophagus from the hiatal hernia or cardia. Bears a high risk of malignant transformation.
Granulomatous esophagitis	Single or multiple ulcers, narrowing of the lumen, and numerous nodular filling defects. Fistulous tracts are common.	*Tuberculosis* of the esophagus is rare and usually associated with terminal disease in the lungs. *Crohn's disease, syphilis,* and *histoplasmosis* of the esophagus are likewise rare. Crohn's disease is suggested by concomitant Crohn's disease elsewhere. *Actinomycosis* of the adjacent tissues may also cause fistulization.
Carcinoma of the esophagus (Figs. 5–8)	The ulcer crater is surrounded by a bulging mass which projects into the esophageal lumen. The ulcerated surface is rigid. Purely ulcerating appearance with a flat meniscoid mass is rare. Bronchoesophageal or tracheoesophageal fistulas occur.	Esophageal carcinomas often present signs of ulceration but other radiographic features like narrowing or mass are more prominent. *Lymphomas or metastases* with "bull's eye" ulcerating lesions, (e.g., melanoma), are rare in the esophagus. 50% of acquired esophageal fistulas are due to malignancy in the mediastinum.

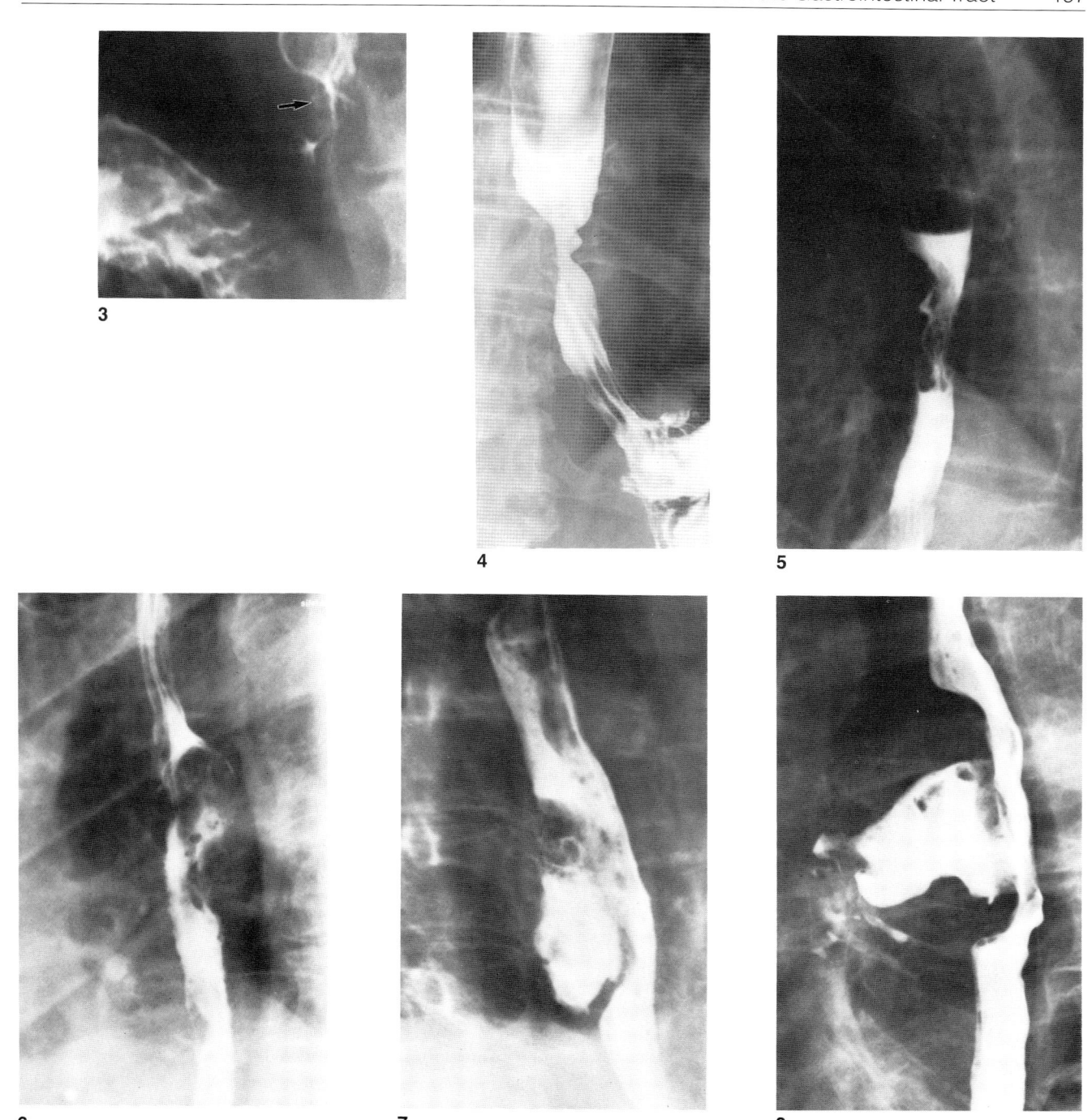

Figure 3 An **ulcer niche in the distal esophagus** (arrow) surrounded by an ulcer collar and spasm.

Figure 4 **Barrett's esophagus.** An ulcer and stricture is present about 10 cm above the esphagogastric junction. Esophageal folds below the ulcer are slightly thickened.

Figure 5 **Carcinoma of the esophagus.** A crater surrounded by a mass.

Figure 6 **Bull's eye ulcer of the esophagus.** Primary melanoma of the esophagus, a rare entity.

Figure 7 **Carcinoma of the esophagus.** A large ulceration with Carman's meniscus sign is seen.

Figure 8 **Adenocarcinoma of the esophagus.** A large ulceration and an esophagobronchial fistula are seen.

Table 1 (Cont.) Ulcers, Diverticula and Fistulas in the Esophagus

Disease	Radiographic Findings	Comments
Leiomyoma (Fig. 9)	A large mass with central ulceration, no concentric narrowing of the lumen.	Carcinoma may have an identical appearance.
Corrosive esophagitis	Ulceration associated with sloughing of destroyed mucosa, eventually associated with gradual narrowing of the esophagus. A fistula may follow esophageal perforation.	Ulceration always occurs following ingestion of corrosive materials. Alkali tends to produce more extensive changes in the esophagus than acid.
Drug-induced ulcer	Solitary esophageal ulceration complicating drug treatment. The ulcer itself has no distinctive features.	Associated with delayed esophageal transit time (supine position, hiatal hernia, reflux, abnormal peristalsis, stricture, left atrial enlargement). The most common cause is potassium chloride tablets.
Intramural esophageal pseudodiverticulosis	Innumerable pinhead-sized outpouchings project from the lumen and end at the same level. A proximal esophageal stricture is common.	Dilated esophageal glands probably secondary to an inflammatory process.
Zenker's diverticulum (Fig. 10, 11)	A saccular outpouching protrudes posteriorly in the upper esophagus (C5–6 level). It may extend downward and posteriorly, displace the cervical esophagus anteriorly, and cause narrowing of the lumen.	A pulsion diverticulum at a point of weakness between the oblique and circular fibers of the cricopharyngeal muscle. May be seen as a retroesophageal air–fluid level on plain films.
Diverticula of the thoracic esophagus (Fig. 12)	Most are seen in the middle third opposite the bifurcation of the trachea. May have a funnel, cone, tent, or fusiform shape and usually best visualized in the left anterior oblique projection. Perforation of a diverticulum may rarely cause mediastinitis and a fistulous tract.	Most are traction diverticula that develop in response to the pull of fibrous adhesions following infection of the mediastinal lymph nodes and often seen adjacent to a calcified lymph node. Pulsion diverticula of the midesophagus or traction diverticula of the cervical esophagus are rarely demonstrated.
Epiphrenic diverticula	A broad, short-necked outpouching in the distal 10 cm of the esophagus with normal mucosal appearance and an absence of spasm.	A pulsion-type diverticulum, usually associated with motor abnormalities of the esophagus, which may simulate an esophageal ulcer.
Congenital tracheoesophageal fistula (Fig. 13)	Type III: Most common (85 to 90%); the upper segment of esophagus ends in a blind pouch at the level of the bifurcation or slightly above. The lower segment is connected to trachea. Air in the stomach. Type I: The next most common type; both the upper and lower segments of the esophagus are blind pouches, no air below the diaphragm. Type II: The upper esophageal segment communicates with the trachea, no air below the diaphragm. Type IV: Either both segments of the esophagus are connected with the trachea or there is a single fistulous tract (H-fistula).	Results from failure of complete separation of the trachea and upper alimentary tract. An H-fistula may not be detected in infancy and may cause only occasional symptoms, whereas the others are symptomatic immediately after birth. Associated anomalies include: Vertebral or rib abnormalities Atrial or ventricular septal defects Tetralogy of Fallot Duodenal or anal atresia.
Traumatic laceration or perforation of the esophagus	Pneumomediastinum is a common initial finding in esophageal perforation, followed by development of mediastinitis and a fistulous tract. Laceration may be seen as a persistent linear collection of contrast material.	Perforation is usually a complication of esophagoscopy, dilatation of the esophagus, crush injury, or rarely due to severe vomiting (*Boerhaave's syndrome*). The mucosal–submucosal laceration and hemorrhage of the esophagus following severe vomiting, called *Mallory–Weiss syndrome*, is always located at the esophagogastric junction, and is rarely detected radiographically.

Ulcers, Diverticula and Fistulas in the Gastrointestinal Tract 199

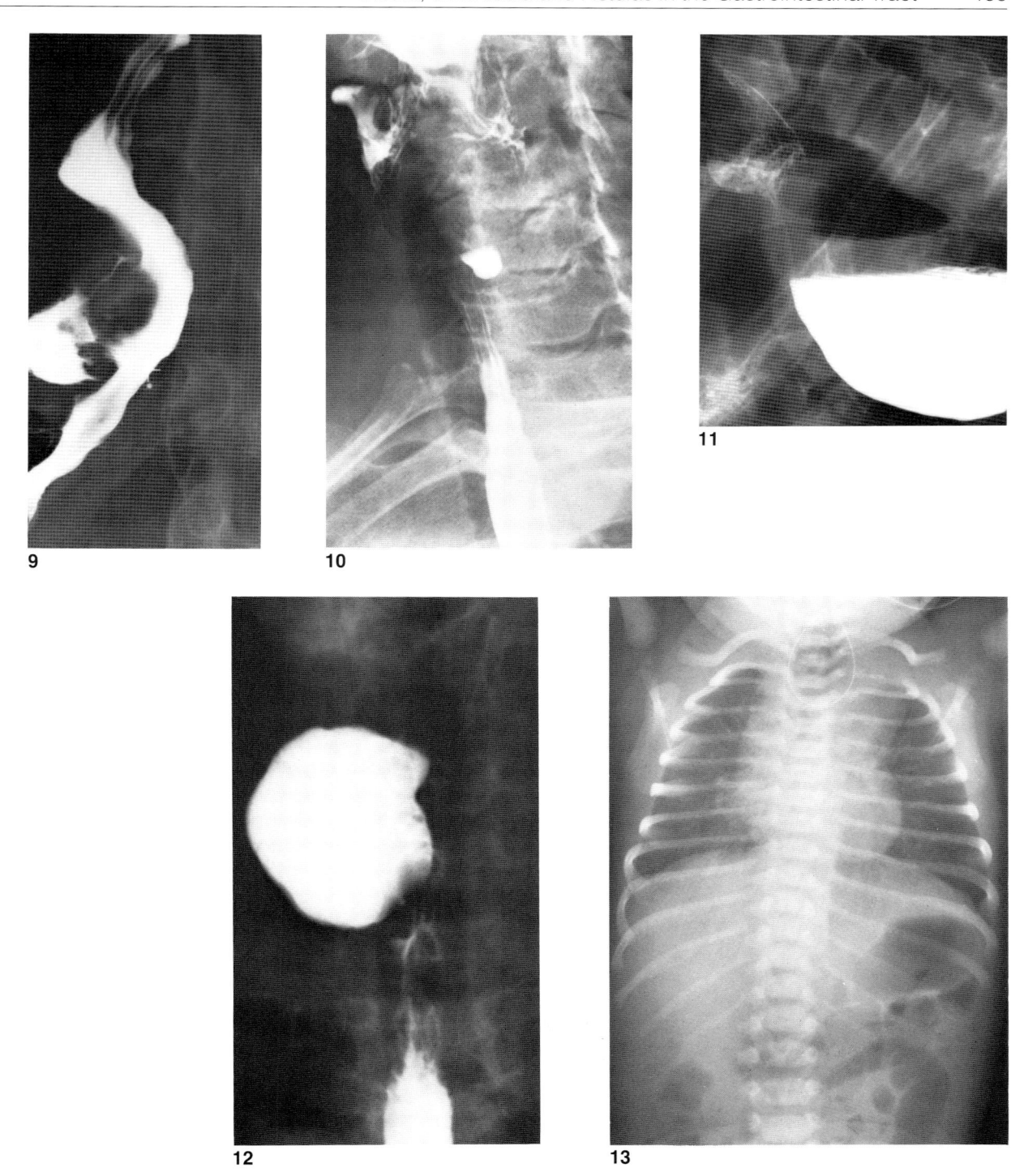

Figure 9 **Leiomyoma** of the esophagus. A large ulcerated mass mimics esophageal carcinoma, but luminal narrowing is not present.

Figure 10 **Zenker's diverticulum.** Barium remains in the posterior saccular outpouching at the pharyngoesophageal junction after swallowing.

Figure 11 A large **Zenker's diverticulum** presents as a retroesophageal air–fluid level and barium collection.

Figure 12 **Giant pulsion diverticulum** of the upper esophagus.

Figure 13 **Congenital tracheoesophageal fistula.** The nasopharyngeal tube makes a loop in the blind, air-containing pouch of the upper esophagus. Air in the bowel indicates a connection between the lower esophagus and the trachea.

Table 2 Gastric Ulcers, Diverticula, and Fistulas

Disease	Radiographic Findings	Comments
Peptic ulcer disease (Figs. 14–16)	Signs of benign gastric ulcer: Ulcer projects outside the normal gastric lumen. Undermining of mucosa with minimal edema, a lucent line (Hampton line) parallels the base of the crater. Edema may create an ulcer collar, an ulcer mound, or trapping of barium in the ulcer. Smooth, slender mucosal folds extend into the edge of the crater or, in the absence of folds, the surrounding tissue has a smooth contour. Diminishes to one half or less within 3 weeks and often disappears completely in 6 weeks, but residual deformity may remain.	A large ulcer mound can simulate a neoplasm by extending beyond the limits of the ulcer. The size or shape of the ulcer has no practical value as far as malignancy is concerned. Benign ulcers of the greater curvature may demonstrate features that suggest malignancy (intraluminal location, nodular surroundings). Practically all ulcers above the level of the cardia are malignant. A nonulcerating deformity tends to have an elliptic orientation perpendicular to the lumen, whereas true ulcerations, if elliptic, tend to be orientated along the long axis of the lumen.
Gastritis	A crater with signs of a benign ulcer may be seen in the absence of a peptic ulcer disease.	May not cause radiographic signs. Other radiographic features (e.g., thickening of mucosal folds, enlargement of areae gastricae or hypersecretion) are more characteristic.
Granulomatous infiltration of the stomach (Fig. 17)	Ulcer associated with mucosal abnormalities and usually disease elsewhere in the gastrointestinal tract (Crohn's disease) or lungs (tuberculosis).	Involvement of the terminal ileum suggests Crohn's disease.
Leiomyoma Leiomyosarcoma (Fig. 18)	Usually a large mass with central ulceration, often in the gastric fundus.	Leiomyoma and leiomyosarcoma are radiographically indistinguishable.
Radiation injury	Peptic ulcer like radiographic findings without a history of relationship to meals. A high incidence of perforation and hemorrhage.	A complication of a dose more than 45 Gy to the high para-aortic or upper abdominal area, which occurs from 1 month to 6 years (average 5 months) after treatment.
Pseudolymphoma	A large ulcer surrounded by a mass and associated with enlarged rugal folds.	A benign proliferation of lymphoid tissue that can simulate malignant lymphoma. May represent a reaction to chronic peptic ulcer disease. May not be distinguishable from malignant lymphoma in frozen sections or biopsy.

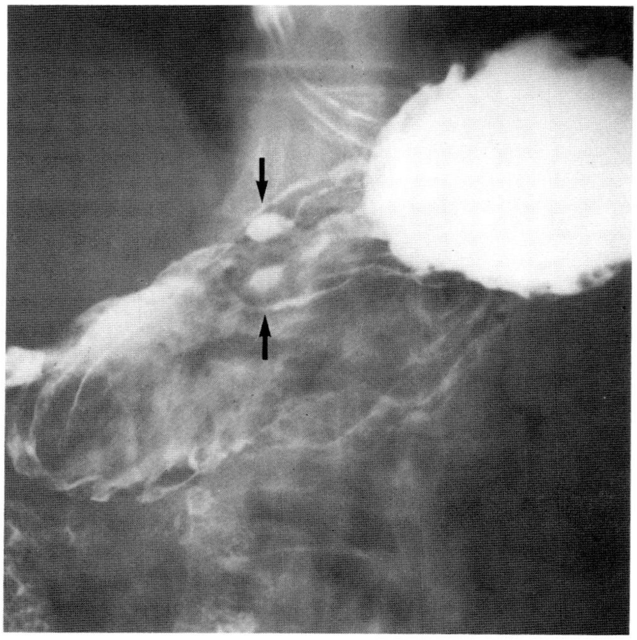

Figure 14 **Two superficial gastric ulcers** (arrows) seen as collections of barium surrounded by mucosal edema.

Ulcers, Diverticula and Fistulas in the Gastrointestinal Tract 201

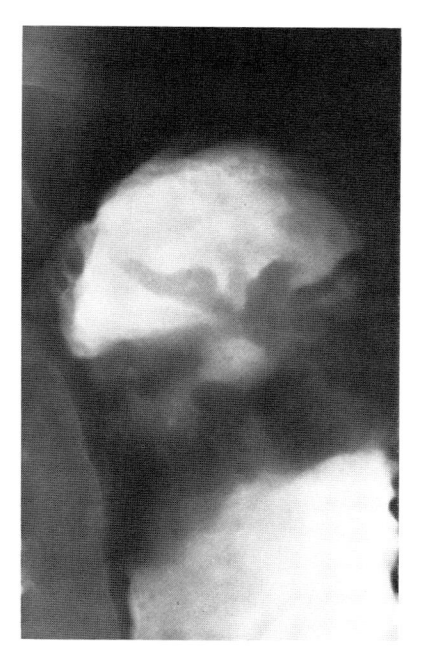

Figure 15 **Benign gastric ulcer** in the fundus – a rare location for a benign ulcer. Mucosal folds here tend to be thick. The folds extend into the edge of the crater.

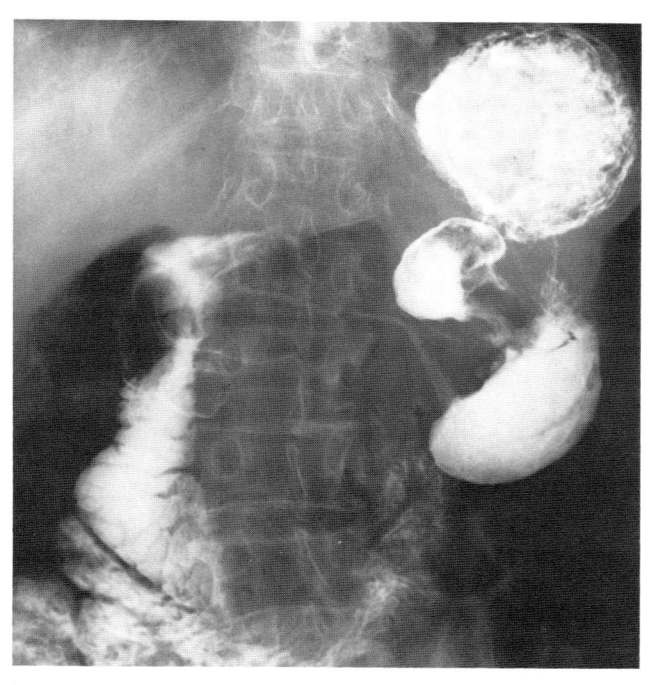

Figure 16 **Giant benign gastric ulcer** with the appearance of a diverticulum.

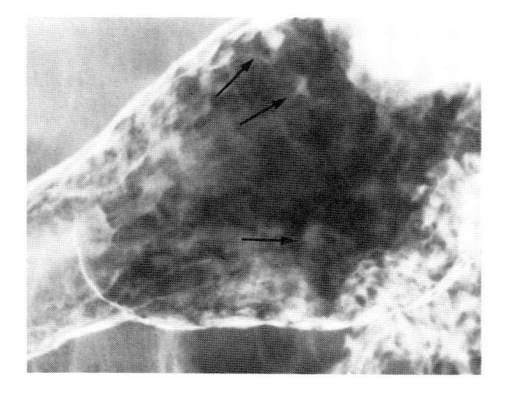

Figure 17 **Crohn's disease** involving the distal stomach. Tiny aphthoid ulcers and mucosal irregularity are seen in the antrum (arrows).

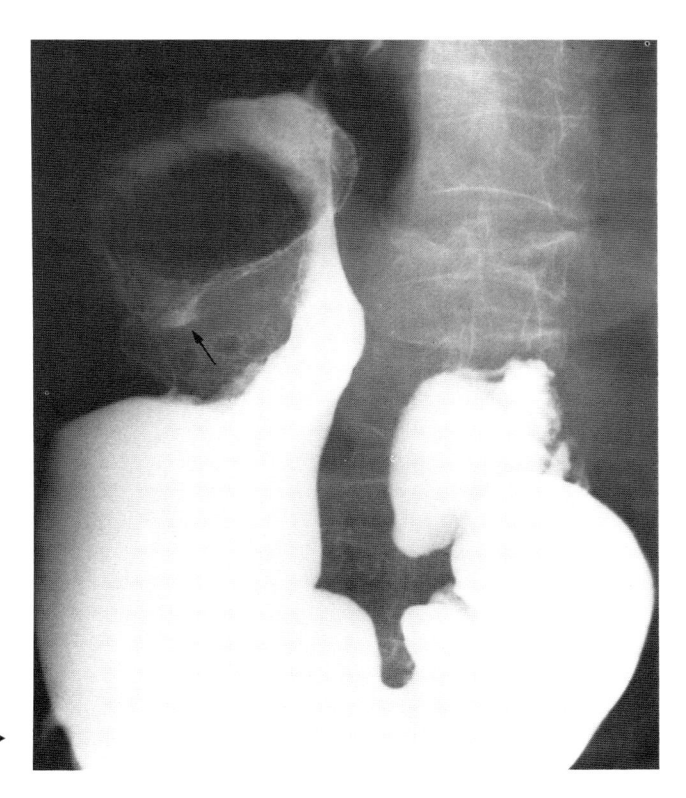

Figure 18 **Leiomyosarcoma.** A large intramural mass in ▶ the fundus with a central ulceration (arrow) is seen.

Table 2 (Cont.) Gastric Ulcers, Diverticula, and Fistulas

Disease	Radiographic Findings	Comments
Gastric carcinoma (Fig. 19, 20)	Signs of a malignant gastric ulcer: The ulcer projects inside the normal lumen. Radiating folds merge into a mound of polypoid tissue around the crater or may be clubbed. Gastric mucosa surrounding the ulcer is abnormal. A rim of tumor may be seen (Carman's meniscus sign). Practically all ulcers above the level of the cardia are malignant.	The radiographic appearance is extremely variable. Most gastric carcinomas can ulcerate.
Lymphoma (Fig. 21)	A large ulcerated mass, usually indistinguishable from other malignancies. A single huge ulcer or multiple ulcers suggest lymphoma.	About 2% of all gastric neoplasms are lymphomas, usually associated with diffuse disease. Enlargement of the spleen and retrogastric lymph nodes are often observed.
Metastatic lesion	Bull's eye lesion(s) with central, relatively large ulceration.	Most commonly seen in malignant melanoma but can occur in carcinoma of the breast and lung. Direct extension from neighboring organs can cause gastric ulceration.
Eosinophilic granuloma	A discrete polypoid mass (unlike eosinophilic gastroenteritis) that may demonstrate central ulceration.	Gastrointestinal eosinophilic granuloma is most frequent in the stomach, but may rarely occur elsewhere in the bowel. This entity is neither related to eosinophilic gastroenteritis nor to the histiocytosis X complex.
Marginal ulceration post partial gastrectomy (Fig. 22)	A benign ulcer is usually situated in the jejunal side, within first few centimeters of the anastomosis. It usually has a tent-shaped or conical configuration, but it may be superficial and undetectable. Secondary signs such as edema, flattening, or rigidity of the jejunum are helpful.	A postoperative complication of gastric surgery for the treatment of duodenal peptic ulcer disease, usually within 2–4 years of partial gastrectomy. May be difficult to detect radiographically due to postoperative distortion.
Gastric stump carcinoma	Gastric stump carcinoma may present as an ulcer on the gastric side.	Any ulcer on the gastric side of the anastomosis should be considered malignant unless proved otherwise, since carcinoma in gastric remnant occurs frequently (up to 20% in 20 years).
Erosive gastritis (superficial gastric erosions) (Fig. 25, page 205).	Tiny flecks of barium (erosion) surrounded by a radiolucent halo (edema). Defects in the epithelium do not penetrate beyond the muscularis mucosae and are rarely detected on conventional barium examination.	May be the cause of gastrointestinal bleeding. Usually an incidental finding, but may be associated with gastric irritation (alcohol, drugs), Crohn's disease, or candidiasis.
Ectopic pancreas (Fig. 23)	A smooth submucosal mass, usually 2 cm or less in diameter, that has a central dimple. This represents the orifice of the duct from pancreatic tissue and may mimic an ulcerated lesion.	Most common on the distal greater curvature of the gastric antrum within 3–6 cm of the pylorus.
Double pylorus	An accessory channel connects the lesser curvature of the prepyloric antrum with the duodenal bulb (gastroduodenal fistula). An ulcer is usually seen within or adjacent to the accessory channel.	Associated with peptic ulcer disease.

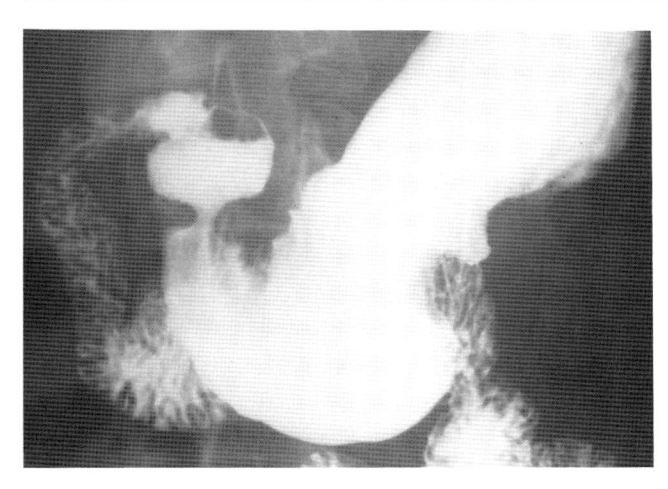

Figure 19 **Gastric carcinoma** with characteristic features of a malignant ulcer. The ulcer projects inside the lumen. Its margins are irregular.

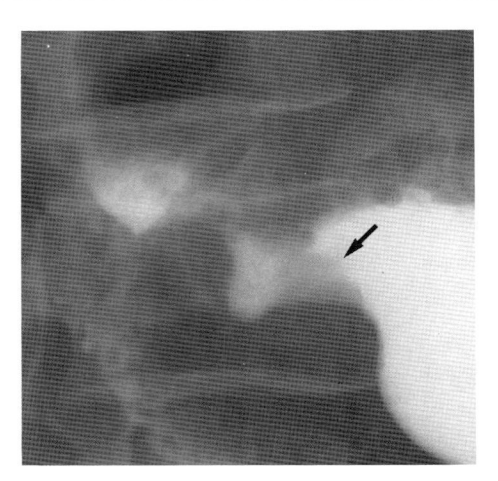

Figure 20 **Gastric carcinoma** with Carman's meniscus sign (arrow).

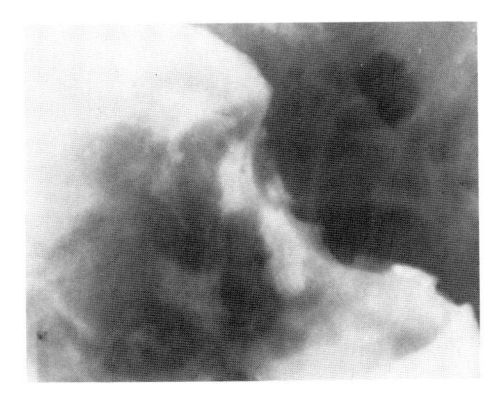

Figure 21 **Lymphoma.** A large mass with multiple ulcerations is typical of lymphoma.

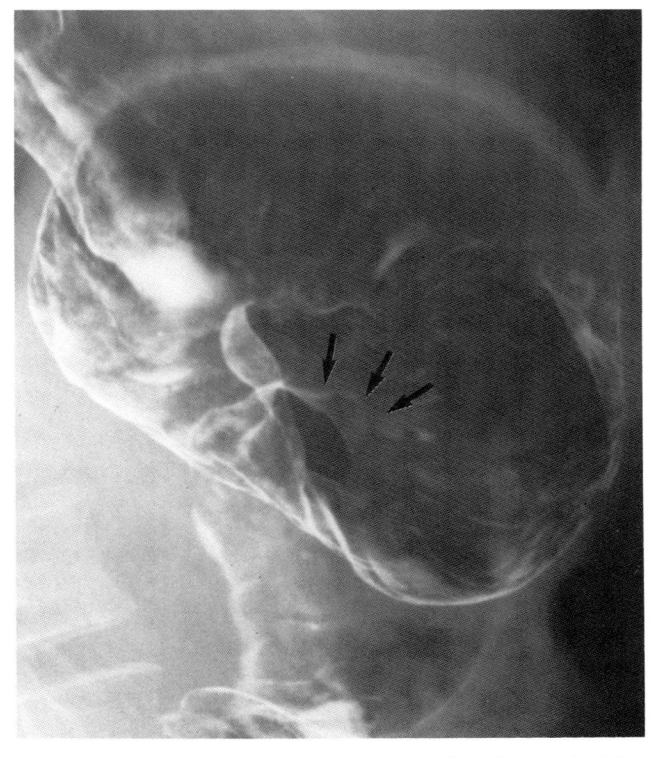

Figure 22 **Superficial marginal ulceration** (arrows) of the gastric stump. The marginal mucosal ulceration is difficult to detect radiographically.

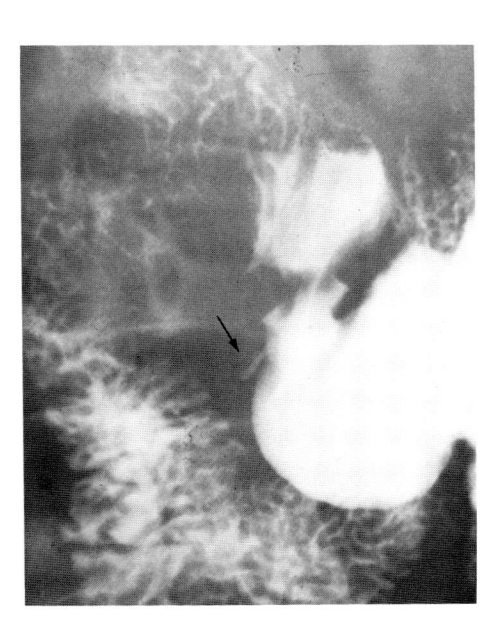

Figure 23 **Ectopic pancreas** in the distal greater curvature. The duct mimics a penetrating narrow ulcer crater. An indentation is seen in greater curvature (arrow).

Table 2 (Cont.) Gastric Ulcers, Diverticula, and Fistulas

Disease	Radiographic Findings	Comments
Hypertrophic pyloric stenosis (Fig. 24)	A small triangular outpouching from the greater curvature side of the long, narrowed pyloric canal is pathognomonic (Twining recess) and may mimic an ulcer.	Radiographically, adult and infantile forms are identical. Gastric ulcer is a common complication in adults but it does not involve the hypertrophied pyloric canal.
Gastric diverticulum (Fig. 25)	An outpouching of the gastric wall in the region of fundus or cardioesophageal junction. A narrow neck and gastric folds running into it allow it to be differentiated from a large ulcer.	Most gastric diverticula are congenital. A small congenital intramural gastric diverticulum may simulate dilated pancreatic duct of an ectopic pancreatic rest. Acquired diverticula may occur at the stoma after gastroenterostomy, or following healing of a perforated peptic ulcer. *Pseudodiverticulum* of the greater curvature may result from fibrosis and shortening of the lesser curvature (e.g., in severe peptic ulcer disease).
Gastrojejunal fistula (gastrojejunostomy) (Fig. 26)	Some or all of the contrast medium bypasses the duodenum.	Gastrojejunostomy is usually created surgically for the therapy of gastric retention.
Gastrocolic fistula	May not be detected on upper gastrointestinal series but frequently during barium enema.	Usually a complication of gastric or colonic carcinoma, more rarely pancreatic carcinoma. Benign ulcer of the greater curvature or posterior wall of the antrum in patients receiving steroids, chronic ulcerating bowel disease, or marginal ulceration following gastric surgery are rare causes.
Internal fistula involving the stomach	Passage of barium into an irregular cavity through a fistulous tract. Extraluminal gas (in pseudocyst, abscess, or biliary tree).	The most common cause is spontaneous (or surgical) communication into a pancreatic pseudocyst. Cholecystogastric fistulas are rare.
External fistula involving the stomach	May not be completely visualized on the upper abdominal series if not adequately drained and associated with abscesses.	Usually a complication of surgery on the pancreas, failing gastrointestinal anastomosis or postoperative abscess.

Ulcers, Diverticula and Fistulas in the Gastrointestinal Tract   205

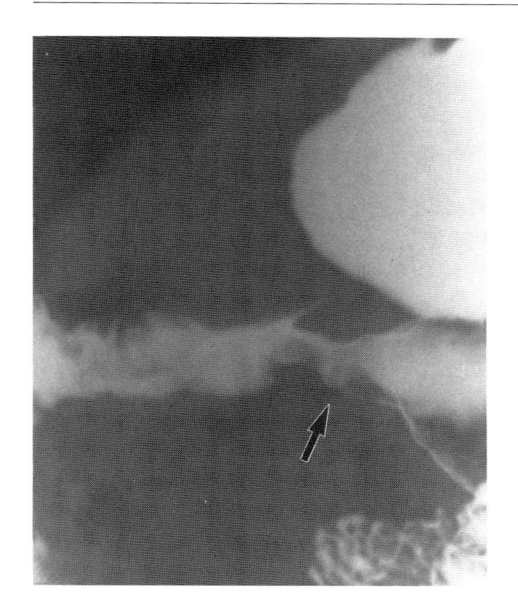

Figure 24 **Hypertrophic pyloric stenosis.** The pyloric canal is long. An outpouching on its greater curvature side (arrow) is pathognomonic and mimics an ulcer.

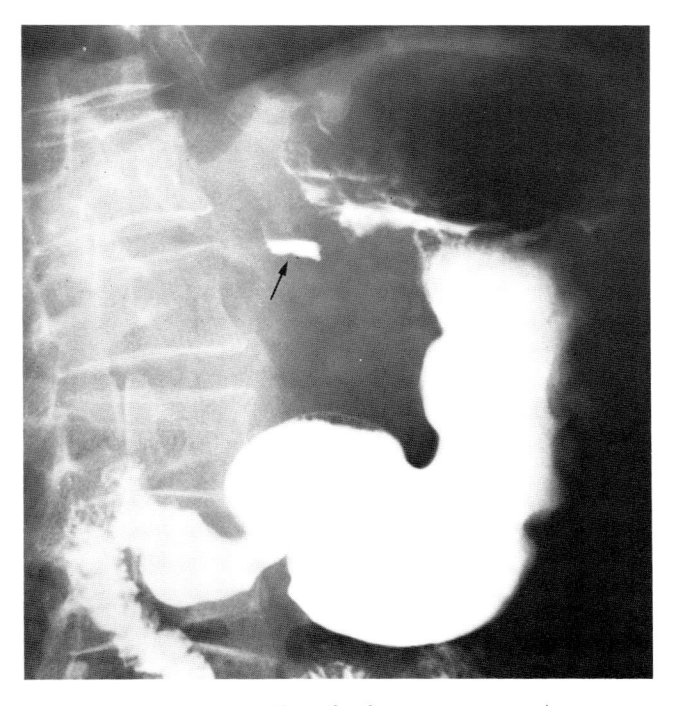

Figure 25 **Gastric diverticulum** near the cardioesophageal junction (arrow). The patient also has gastric carcinoma of the greater curvature.

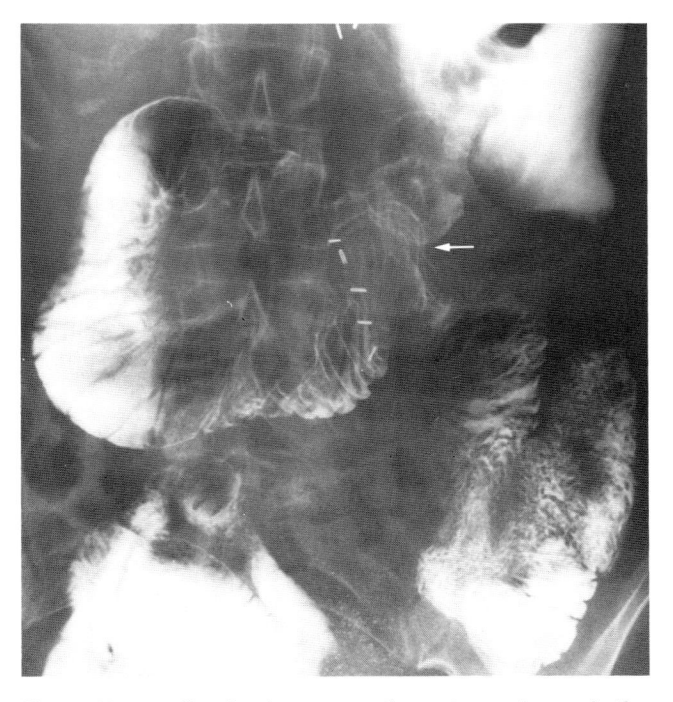

Figure 26 A **fistula between the stomach and the duodenojejunal junction** following radiotherapy of left renal carcinoma. Usually this kind of bypass is surgically performed (gastrojejunostomy).

Table 3 Ulcers, Diverticula, and Fistulas in the Duodenum

Disease	Radiographic Findings	Comments
Peptic ulcer of the duodenal bulb (Fig. 27)	Demonstration of the ulcer crater both in supine air contrast and compression radiographs is necessary. Thickened folds radiating toward the crater help in the localization. Only a minority of patients have deformity of the duodenal cap, spasm, or tenderness. Spasm, edema, or scarring may cause gastric outlet obstruction and nonvisualization of the bulb without hypotonization.	85% of ulcer craters are round, 15% are linear. Multiple ulcers occur in 10 to 15% of cases. Ulcers occur with equal frequency in anterior and posterior walls of the bulb. A *giant duodenal bulb ulcer* may appear like a normal bulb in shape but is fixed and rigid and has irregular margins (ulcer within an ulcer).
Postbulbar peptic ulcer (Fig. 28)	A shallow, flattened niche on the medial aspect of the upper second portion of the duodenum, associated with eccentric local spasm or later with ring stricture. Penetration into the pancreas may cause pancreatitis and widening of the duodenal sweep.	One fourth of duodenal ulcers in *Zollinger–Ellison syndrome* are postbulbar or even more distal. Postbulbar ulceration may occur also in the benign peptic ulcer disease, but multiple distal ulcers and thickened gastric folds suggest the presence of an islet cell tumor of the pancreas and Zollinger–Ellison syndrome.
Leiomyoma Leiomyosarcoma (Fig. 29)	An intramural ulcerated mass lesion. May mimic a mound of edema surrounding a peptic postbulbar ulcer.	Differentiation between leiomyoma and leiomyosarcoma is radiographically impossible.
Adenocarcinoma	Narrowing of the duodenum and ulceration may occur at any point along the sweep.	Gardner's syndrome and Peutz–Jeghers syndrome have an increased risk of developing an otherwise rare duodenal adenocarcinoma.
Spread of carcinoma from adjacent organs	Tumor may invade duodenum and cause ulceration and deformity at any point.	Pancreatic carcinoma tends to involve the inner wall of the sweep, others (colon, right kidney, gallbladder) the outer aspects of the sweep or bulb.
Metastases	Hematogenous metastases may ulcerate and create a target lesion appearance.	
Lymphoma	Solitary involvement of the duodenum is rare and has variable appearances, including ulcerations.	Lymphoma may mimic all common duodenal deformities (ulcer, pancreatitis, Crohn's disease, hyperplasia of Brunner's glands).
Crohn's disease Tuberculosis	Granulomatous disease is characterized by duodenal nodularity and postbulbar ulceration.	Crohn's disease is almost invariably associated with the same process elsewhere in the gastrointestinal tract. Duodenum is involved in approximately 1%.
Ectopic pancreas	May simulate a postbulbar small ulceration surrounded by edema, but characteristic spastic incisure is absent.	
Duodenal diverticulum (Fig. 30, 31)	Most common in the medial side of the sweep and in the periampullary region. Diverticula have a smooth, rounded shape. They are often multiple. They may contain inspissated food particles. A large gas-filled diverticulum may mimic an abscess, dilated cecum, or a pancreatic pseudocyst on plain films.	An incidental finding in up to 5% of barium examinations and usually asymptomatic. Duodenal diverticulitis may mimic cholecystitis, peptic ulcer disease, or pancreatitis, and may be complicated by hemorrhage, retroperitoneal perforation, abscess, or fistulas. Opening of bile and pancreatic ducts into a diverticulum (3%) may predispose to obstructive biliary or pancreatic disease.
Duodenal pseudodiverticula	Exaggerated outpouchings of the inferior and superior recess of the duodenal bulb secondary to a peptic ulcer ("clover leaf deformity").	
Duodenocolic fistula	A communication between abnormal duodenum and colon is better demonstrated on barium enema than on upper gastrointestinal series.	May be associated with Crohn's disease involving the duodenum or carcinoma of the colon infiltrating into the duodenum. Other enteroenteric fistulas, e.g., *duodenojejunal*, may be present in Crohn's disease.

Ulcers, Diverticula and Fistulas in the Gastrointestinal Tract 207

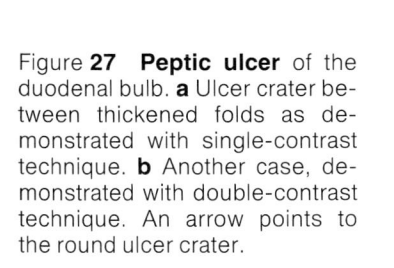

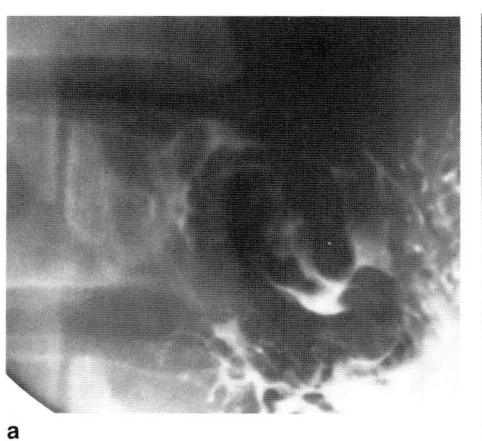

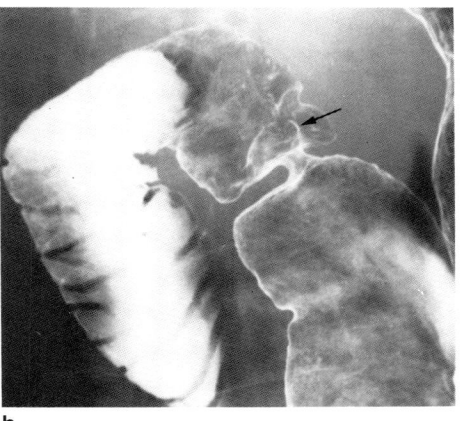

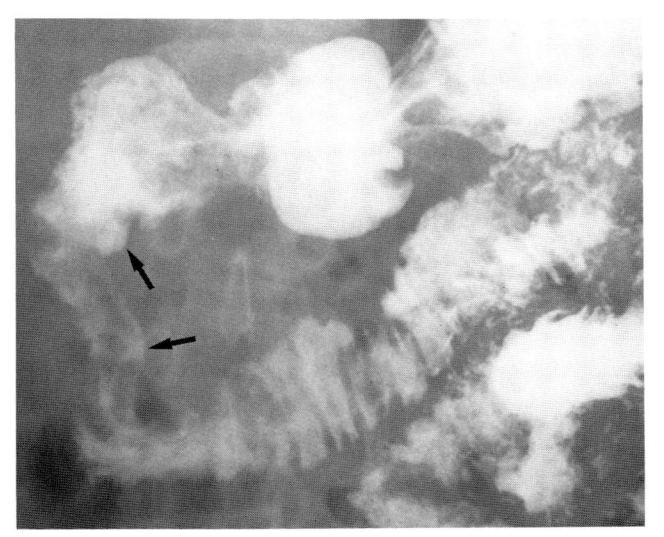

Figure 27 **Peptic ulcer** of the duodenal bulb. **a** Ulcer crater between thickened folds as demonstrated with single-contrast technique. **b** Another case, demonstrated with double-contrast technique. An arrow points to the round ulcer crater.

Figure 28 **Zollinger–Ellison syndrome.** Postbulbar ulcers (arrows) on the medial side of the descending duodenum. Irregular duodenal folds and increased secretions.

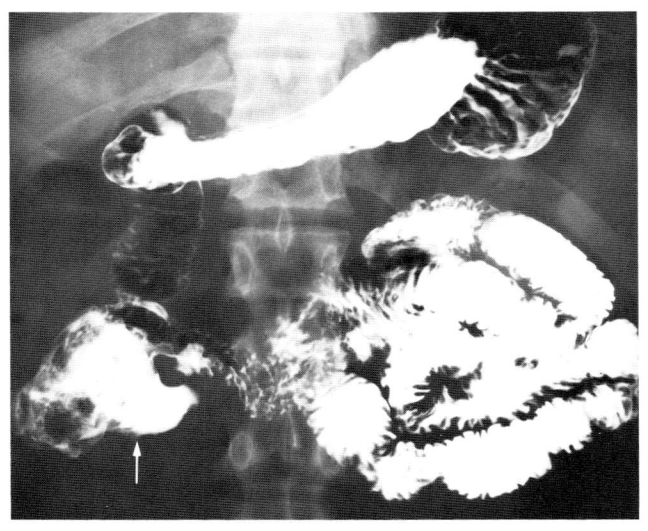

Figure 29 **Leiomyoma of the duodenum.** A large ulcerated mass lesion (arrow) is seen at the junction between the second and third portions of the duodenum.

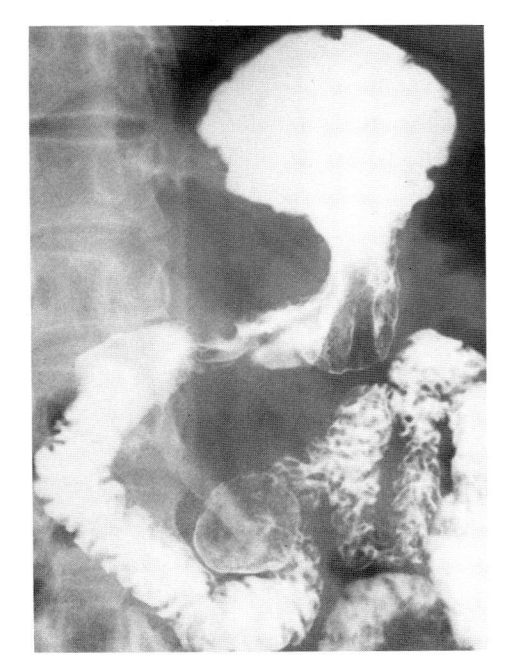

Figure 30 **Duodenal diverticulum** in the distal duodenum, filled with food.

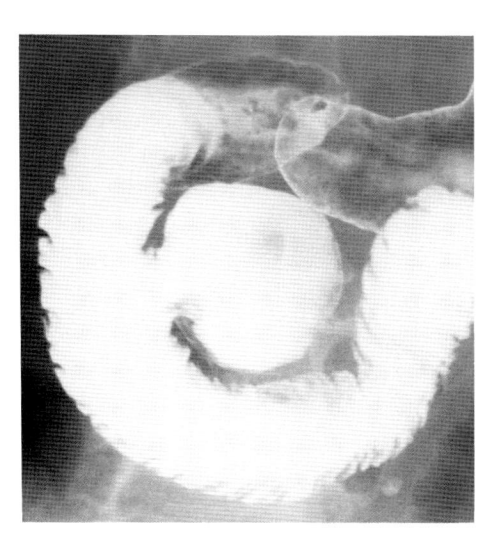

Figure 31 A large **duodenal diverticulum** on the medial side of the descending duodenum. A food particle causes a filling defect.

Table 3 (Cont.) Ulcers, Diverticula, and Fistulas in the Duodenum

Disease	Radiographic Findings	Comments
Cholecystoduodenal fistula (Fig. 32)	Plain films demonstrate gas in the gallbladder or biliary tree, and on upper gastrointestinal series barium usually refluxes into the fistula. (The fistula may occasionally extend to the stomach, hepatic flexure, or jejunum, but most commonly into the duodenum.)	Most (90%) are secondary to acute cholecystitis, usually complicating a gallstone disease. Penetrating duodenal or gastric ulcer, trauma, or tumor are rare causes. The fistula may be surgical (cholecystoduodenostomy, choledochoduodenostomy).
Duodenorenal fistula (Fig. 33)	A communication to the right perirenal space may be demonstrated on upper gastrointestinal series. A communication to the renal pelvis is best demonstrated on retrograde pyelography.	Secondary to a rupture of a right perirenal abscess into the duodenum (often in renal tuberculosis) or rarely due to a penetrating duodenal ulcer.

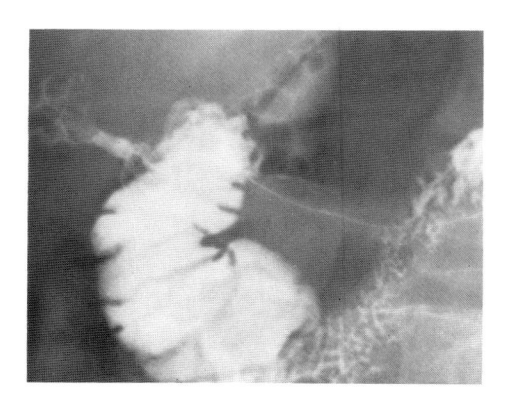

Figure 32 **Cholecystoduodenal fistula** in a patient with gallstone ileus.

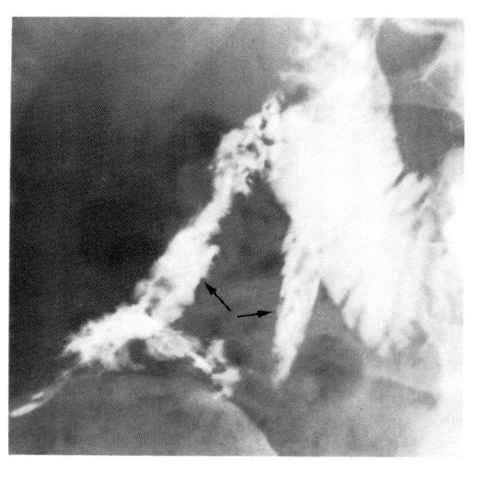

Figure 33 **Duodenorenal fistula** secondary to rupture of a perirenal abscess into the duodenum. The abscess contains mottled gaseous lucencies. Two fistulous tracts (arrows) are demonstrated with water-soluble contrast medium.

Table 4 Ulcers, Diverticula, and Fistulas in the Small Bowel

Disease	Radiographic Findings	Comments
Zollinger–Ellison syndrome (peptic ulcer disease)	Peptic ulcer of the proximal jejunum may occur. Association with multiple duodenal ulcers and enlarged gastric rugae is characteristic.	See also page 206.
Partial gastrectomy (peptic ulcer disease)	Benign ulcer in the jejunum may occur near the gastrojejunostomy stoma.	An ulcer on the gastric side of the soma has to be considered malignant unless proved otherwise.
Carcinoid tumor	Most small-bowel carcinoids present as one or more filling defects or as small-bowel obstruction. An intramural or intraluminal mass with gross ulceration (bull's eye lesion) is a less common manifestation.	The most common tumor in the small intestine. Most are located in the distal ileum. *Carcinoid syndrome* refers to systemic effects of circulating serotonin. Most symptomatic patients have extensive metastases. Urinary excretion of 5-hydroxyindoleacetic acid is elevated.
Leiomyoma Leiomyosarcoma	A pedunculated or intramural mass with a deep, pit-like ulcer crater is characteristic. May cause small-bowel obstruction.	Leiomyoma is the most common benign tumor of the small intestine (most frequent in the duodenum). About one-sixth of them are malignant leiomyosarcomas, but these tumors are radiographically indistinguishable.
Adenocarcinoma	A plaque-like ulcerated mass is an infrequent presentation. An annular short constrictive process and/or bowel obstruction is a typical presentation.	Most occur in the duodenum or jejunum. May rarely present as a bull's-eye lesion.
Lymphoma	A relatively long lesion involving the entire circumference of the bowel wall with extensive ulceration is a typical presentation of a solitary small-bowel lymphoma.	Primary lymphoma of the small intestine occurs usually in the jejunum or ileum, very rarely in the duodenum. Separation of bowel loops due to a mesenteric mass is common.
Metastatic melanoma	Round or oval nodules with sharply demarcated borders and a relatively large ulcer (bull's-eye lesion).	Gastrointestinal metastases can be the first clinical presentation of metastatic melanoma. Ulcerated metastases to the jejunum or ileum from other, more common carcinomas are rare.
Kaposi's sarcoma	Metastases to the small bowel are relatively common and they characteristically appear as multiple bull's-eye lesions.	A systemic disease with multiple soft bluish nodules of the skin with hemorrhages, similar to infectious granulomas but has a neoplastic character. Common in AIDS and in elderly men in parts of Africa, eastern Europe, and northern Italy.
Jejunal diverticula	Thin-walled, atonic outpouchings with narrow necks on the mesenteric side of the small bowel. Leakage of gas through diverticula may cause pneumoperitoneum without peritonitis.	Jejunal diverticulosis may cause malabsorption secondary to overgrowth of bacteria. Jejunal diverticulitis is a rare complication, which may cause a mesenteric abscess or mass displacement of the jejunal loops.
Pseudodiverticula	Large sacs with squared, broad bases involving the antimesenteric side of the small bowel.	Pseudodiverticula result from smooth-muscle atrophy and fibrosis. They are characteristic of *scleroderma*. In *Crohn's disease* they are associated with strictures. They may also occur in *lymphoma*.
Meckel's diverticulum	Rarely demonstrated radiographically as a wide-necked outpouching that arises from the antimesenteric side of the distal ileum.	Rudimentary omphalomesenteric duct, usually within 100 cm from the ileocecal valve. It has an incidence of 1% to 4% in autopsies. Usually asymptomatic, but may cause bleeding, intestinal obstruction, or inflammation (simulates appendicitis clinically).
Ileal diverticula	Small outpouchings near the ileocecal valve, which resemble those commonly seen in the sigmoid colon.	Usually asymptomatic and rarely cause complications. If infected, they simulate late appendicitis clinically.

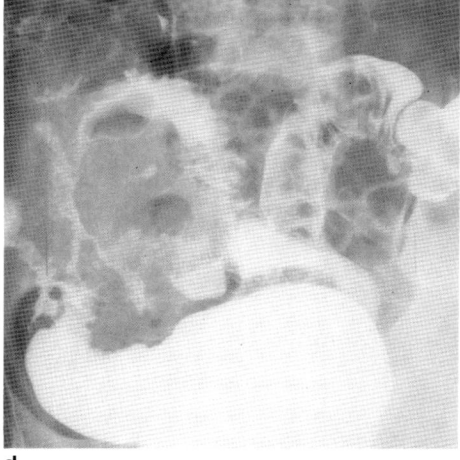

Table 4 (Cont.) Ulcers, Diverticula, and Fistulas in the Small Bowel

Disease	Radiographic Findings	Comments
Enteric-enteric fistulas (Fig. 34)	Fistula formation associated with abnormal bowel mucosa, stricturation, and mesenteric thickening of the involved segments. The distal ileum is almost invariably affected.	Fistulas are a hallmark of chronic *Crohn's disease* (seen in 50%), whereas they are rare in *ulcerative colitis* (0.5%). Enteric–enteric fistulas are most common, but fistulas extending to bladder, vagina, an abscesses, or perianal skin also occur. Enteric–enteric fistulas involving the small bowel may occur also secondary to *primary* or *metastatic malignancy, radiation therapy,* ulcerative colitis, and infections (*tuberculosis, pelvic inflammation, actinomycosis, amebiasis, shigellosis*).
Diverticulitis	Single or multiple fistulous communications between the colon and small bowel occur in 10% of patients with diverticulitis.	
Postoperative gastrojejunocolic fistula	In barium enema examination, contrast extends directly from the transverse colon into the stomach.	A grave complication of marginal ulceration after gastric surgery. Associated with diarrhea, weight loss, or bleeding.

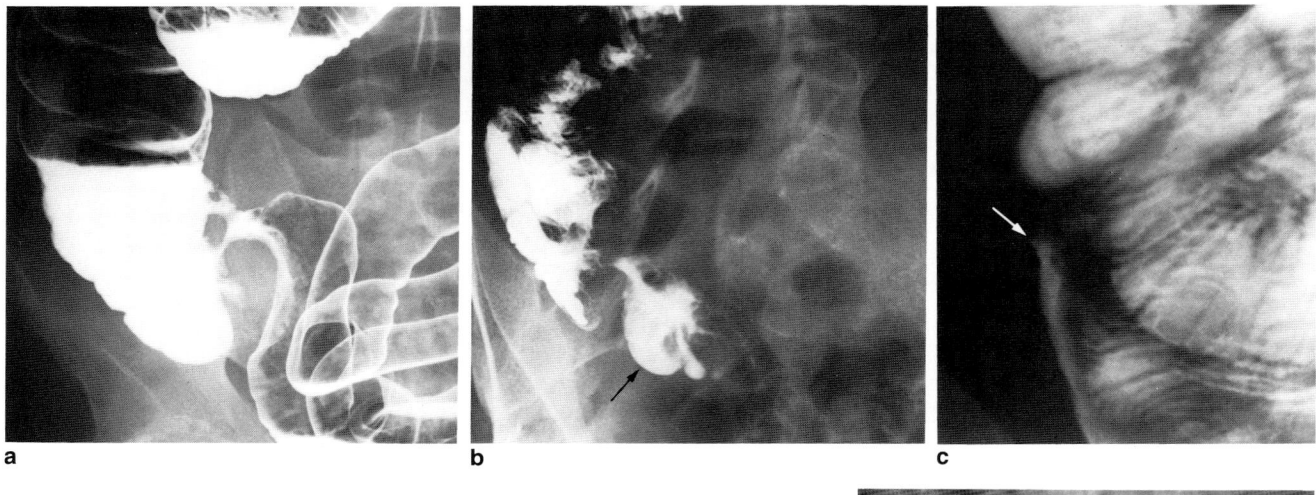

Figure 34a–d **Crohn's disease. a** Ileocolic fistulas through a mass between the distal ileum and cecum. **b** Pseudodiverticulum (arrow) of the distal ileum, narrowing of the ileal lumen. **c** External fistula (arrow) originating from the jejunum and descending towards pelvis. **d** Numerous fistulous tracts through a mass in the right iliac fossa.

Table 5 Ulcers, Diverticula, and Fistulas in the Colon and Rectum

Disease	Radiographic Findings	Comments
Ulcerative colitis (Fig. 35)	Discrete and widely separated marginal ulcers are unusual. Monotonous symmetric ulceration of the mucosa is more characteristic. Enteric–enteric fistulas are rare (about 0.5%).	See Chapter 5, page 126, for the patterns of mucosal changes. Generalized ulceration occurs also in *Shigella, Salmonella,* and *Staphylococcus* infections, in *pseudomembranous colitis,* and in severe *strongyloidiasis.*
Crohn's disease	Aphthoid ulcers surrounded by normal mucosa. Deeper irregular ulcers may penetrate beyond the contour of the bowel and coalesce to form long (over 10 cm) tracts parallel to the longitudinal axis of the colon. Fistulous tracts to adjacent bowel, bladder, vagina, perineum, or abdominal wall are common.	Similar deep ulcers and fistulas involving primarily cecum may occur in *tuberculosis* and *amebiasis.* Cecal ulceration may be also a manifestation of *cytomegalovirus* infection. Aphthoid ulcers may occur in amebiasis, tuberculosis, and *Yersinia* infections and in *Behçet's syndrome.*
Ischemic colitis	Single or multiple ulcers surrounded by pseudopolyposis and "thumbprinting" mucosal edema.	Most common in the splenic flexure and sigmoid. The disease may resolve rapidly or progress to stricture formation.
Radiation-induced colitis	Spasm, fine serrations of the bowel wall and superficial to penetrating ulcerations can be found in the field of irradiation. Fistulas and strictures develop often.	The most common site of localized injury is the anterior rectal wall, since it often receives the highest radiation dose during the treatment of gynecologic, prostatic and bladder carcinomas.
Lymphogranuloma venereum	Multiple shaggy ulcers of the rectum associated with fistulas and sinus tracts of varying length, sometimes progressing to tubular rectal stricture.	Sinus tracts can be short and blind or connected to a perianal abscess. Involvement of the whole rectum (rarely distal colon) and barium spicules projecting from the lumen distinguish this condition from other causes of rectal ulceration.
Solitary rectal ulcer syndrome	Preulcerative nodulation is followed by ulcer formation within 15 cm of the anal verge and near the valve of Houston. Longstanding ulceration leads to fibrosis and rectal stricture.	A rare condition that may be difficult to differentiate from inflammatory bowel disease or malignancy. Manifests mainly in young patients as rectal bleeding. Probably associated with pelvic muscle discoordination during defecation.

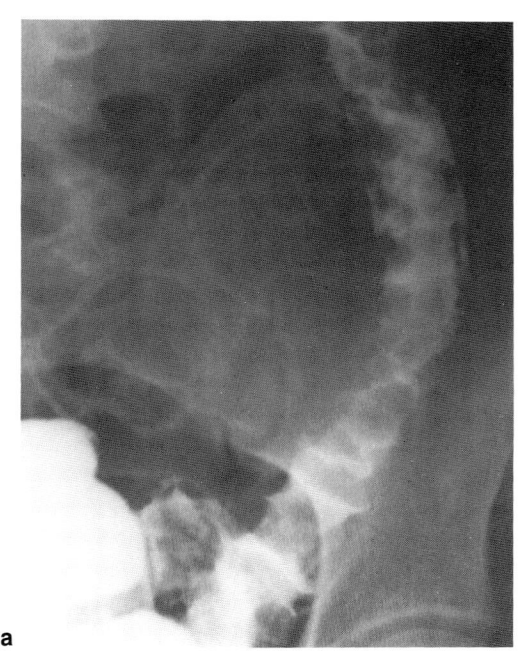

Figure 35a, b **Ulcerative colitis. a** Pseudopolyps originating from the ulcerated mucosa create the appearance of double tracking in the descending colon. **b** Discrete ulcerations (arrow) are seen at the hepatic flexure.

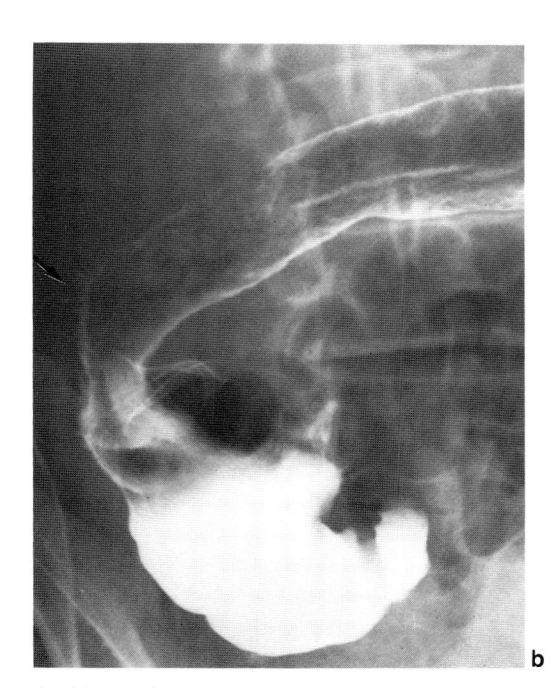

Table 5 (Cont.) Ulcers, Diverticula, and Fistulas in the Colon and Rectum

Disease	Radiographic Findings	Comments
Nonspecific benign ulceration of the colon	Usually single (in 20% multiple) colonic ulcer arising usually from the antimesenteric wall. Radiographically, a carcinoma of the colon is usually suspected due to the mass-like effect of the inflammatory reaction.	A diagnosis of exclusion only. Most frequent in the cecum and ascending colon where it can clinically mimic appendicitis. May perforate.
Carcinoma of the colon	Early saddle cancer may be seen as a flat, plaque-like lesion, which shows central ulceration. Double tracking of the sigmoid colon, representing pericolic sinus tracts or fistulas, may occur.	A more common pattern in left colon is an annular "apple-core" tumor with eventual mucosal destruction or a large fungating mass in the right colon. *Rectal carcinoids* may also ulcerate.
Metastatic carcinoma	May rarely present as bull's-eye lesions or enteric–enteric fistulas.	*Lymphomas* and *leucemias* may also rarely present as mucosal ulcerations or ulcerating mass lesions in the colon.
Diverticulosis (Figs. 36, 37)	Round outpouchings beyond the confines of the lumen, usually less than 2 cm in diameter. They commonly occur in the sigmoid colon, but may also involve other segments of the colon. They are very rare in the rectum.	A huge sigmoid diverticulum probably represents a slowly progressing diverticular abscess. Diverticula appear around the mesenteric tenia. The distensibility of the colon is retained in the absence of inflammation.
Diverticulitis (Fig. 38)	A complication of diverticulosis in which perforation of a diverticulum leads to the development of a peridiverticular abscess. Extravasation of barium beyond the diverticulum, either as a tiny projection of contrast from the tip of the diverticulum or as obvious filling of a pericolic abscess, is diagnostic. A more common but less specific sign is the demonstration of a pericolic soft-tissue mass (abscess). Colonic obstruction, short (3 to 6 cm) parasigmoid tracts (double tracking) and fistulas may be associated.	Clinically, the most common presentation is "left-sided appendicitis." Colonic cancer associated with diverticular disease can be difficult to differentiate from diverticulitis, although the latter usually involves a longer segment. Fistulas into the small bowel (10%) and adjacent organs may occur, mimicking Crohn's disease. Colocutaneous fistulas may complicate surgical treatment.
Pseudodiverticula (Fig. 39)	Sacculations with squared, broad basis on the antimesenteric border at the colon. Characteristic of *scleroderma* and *healing ischemic colitis*.	Pseudodiverticula are produced by fibrosis involving primarily the mesenteric border of the colon.

Ulcers, Diverticula and Fistulas in the Gastrointestinal Tract 213

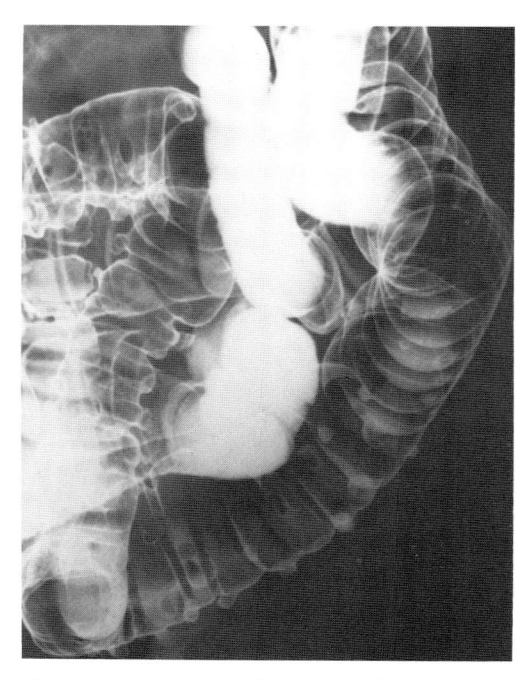

Figure 36 **Sigmoid diverticulosis.** Several diverticula are seen in profile and end-on.

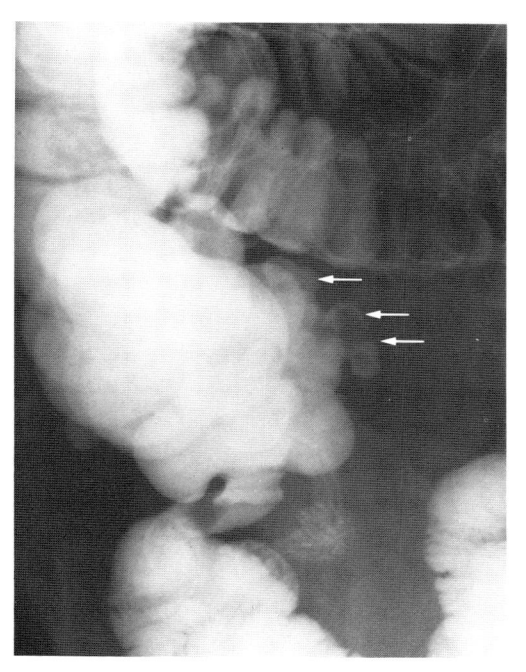

Figure 37 **Cecal diverticulosis.** Several diverticula contain fecal material or gas (arrows).

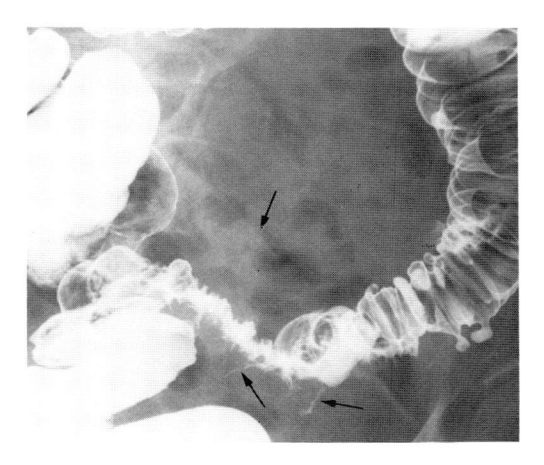

Figure 38 **Sigmoid diverticulitis.** Narrowing of a segment with short fistulous tracts (lower arrows) and perisigmoid soft tissue mass (long arrow) is seen.

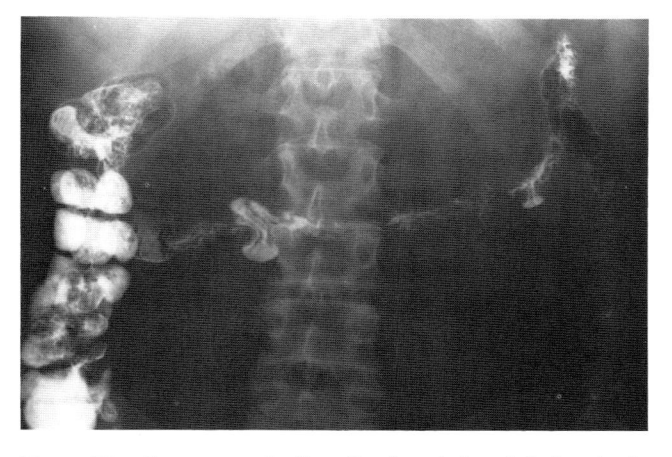

Figure 39 **Two pseudodiverticula** of the inferior (antimesenteric) margin of the transverse colon in scleroderma are seen.

Table 5 (Cont.) Ulcers, Diverticula, and Fistulas in the Colon and Rectum

Disease	Radiographic Findings	Comments
Fistulas involving the colon or rectum (Figs. 40–42)	Fistulous tracts are not always demonstrated by barium enema despite passage of feces or gas through the fistula. Urinary fistulas are best demonstrated by voiding cystourethrography.	*Acquired fistulas* are usually associated with Crohn's disease or radiation necrosis, less commonly with other inflammatory disease or malignancy. *Congenital fistulas* (rectovesical, rectovaginal, rectourethral, rectoperineal and rectofourchette fistulas) may be associated with an imperforate anus.

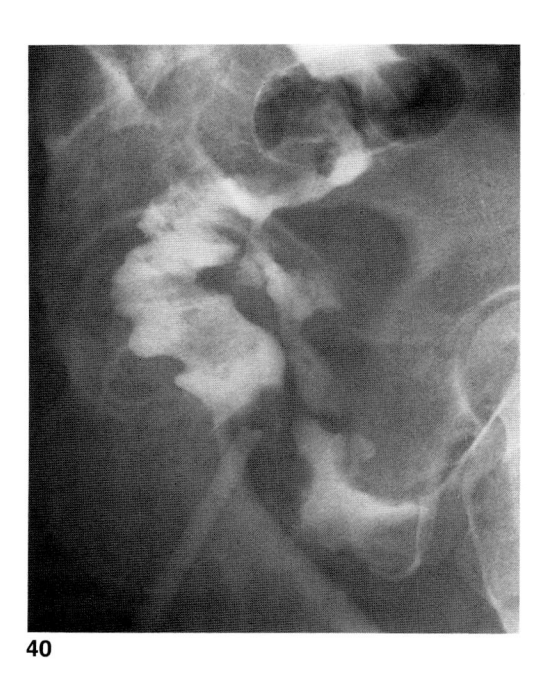

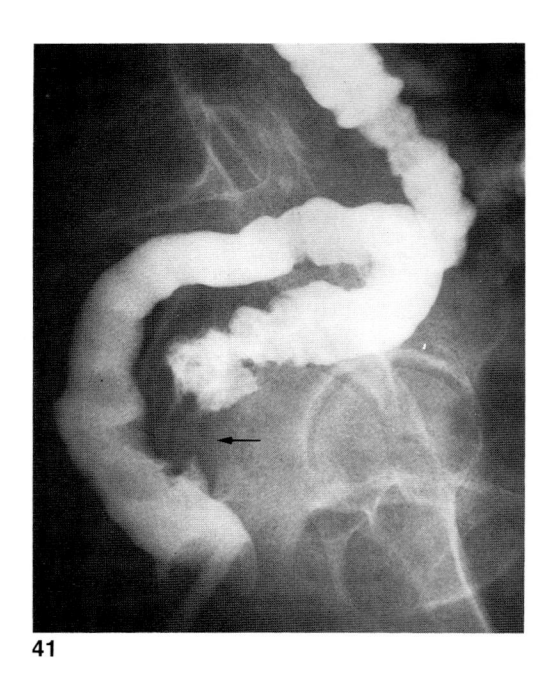

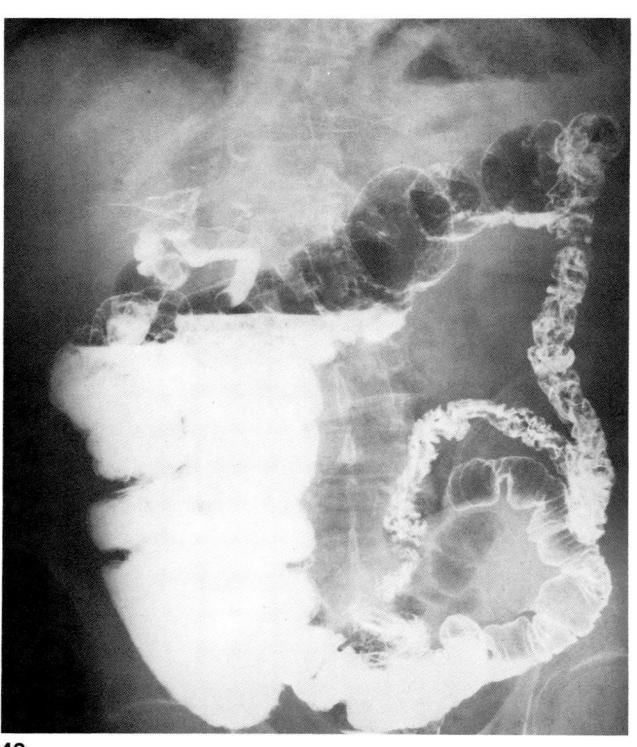

Figure **40 Rectouterine fistula** as a complication of radiotherapy of carcinoma of the cervix. Contrast medium leaks from the anterior wall of the rectum into the uterine cavity and further into the vagina.

Figure **41 Rectosigmoid fistula** (arrow), a complication of radiotherapy of carcinoma of the cervix.

Figure **42 Choledochocolic fistula.** Filling of the biliary tree during barium enema is seen. A complication of carcinoma of the right kidney.

Chapter 9 Gallbladder and Bile Duct Abnormalities

Plain Radiography

The normal gallbladder and the biliary ducts are not seen on plain radiography with the possible exception of thin patients, in whom a very faint density caused by the gallbladder is occasionally recognizable. Therefore, the presence of gas or calcification is required in the biliary system before it becomes visible on plain radiography.

Gas in the biliary system is virtually limited to two conditions: (1) an abnormal communication between the gastrointestinal and biliary tracts allowing the reflux of air (and also barium) from the bowel into the biliary system and (2) the presence of gas-producing organisms within the biliary system (Fig. 1). Biliary gas has to be differentiated from other gas collections in the right upper quadrant. Both the duodenal bulb and a large duodenal diverticulum can be confused with an air-filled gallbladder, but an upper gastrointestinal barium examination will clearly identify these structures. Hepatic and subhepatic abscesses may be more difficult to differentiate because of their anatomic proximity to the gallbladder and a symptomatology similar to that of emphysematous cholecystitis. In these cases, ultrasonography appears most useful to locate the abnormal gas collection. Other pathologic gas collections (e.g., retroperitoneal and abdominal wall abscesses) are easily differentiated from air in the gallbladder with conventional radiography in two projections, since they will project outside the expected gallbladder area in at least one view.

Differentiation between *gas in the biliary ducts* and *gas in the portal system* can at times be difficult. As a general rule, gas in the biliary tree tends to be located in the larger ducts near the hilum of the liver, whereas portal vein gas is preferentially seen in the liver periphery. The most common cause of gas in the portal system is bowel infarction, that may also be evident radiographically (adynamic ileus with thickened folds and/or haustra, "thumb prints," and streaky or linear crescent gas in the bowel wall), thus supporting the diagnosis of intraportal gas (Fig. 2). Small mottled gas collections within the liver parenchyma can also be seen with *liver abscesses,* which are often multiple, but with only a small minority containing gas.

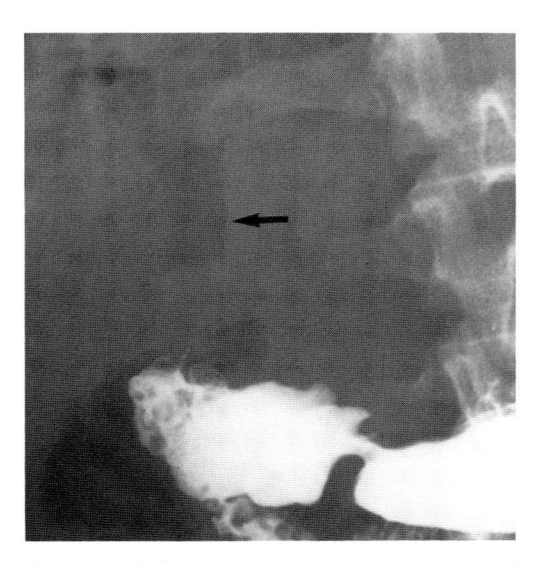

Figure 1 **Biliary gas secondary to choledochoduodenostomy.** The dilated extrahepatic bile ducts (arrow) are contrasted by gas, whereas the barium has not yet refluxed into the biliary system.

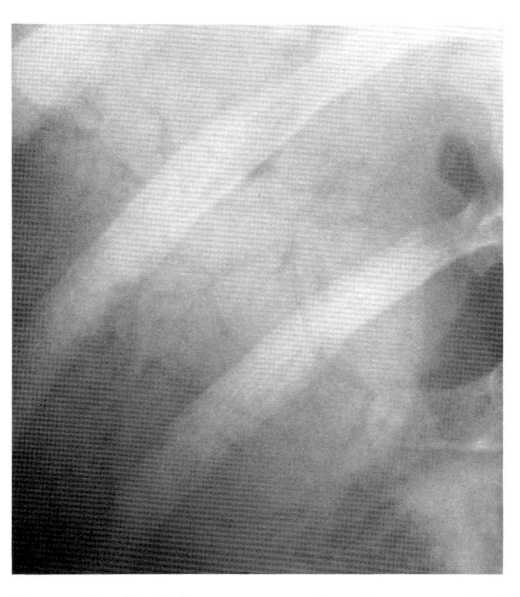

Figure 2 **Portal gas secondary to mesenteric infarction.** Irregular tubular radiolucencies are seen in the liver periphery. The supine abdominal film of this patient is shown in Fig. **23**, page 602.

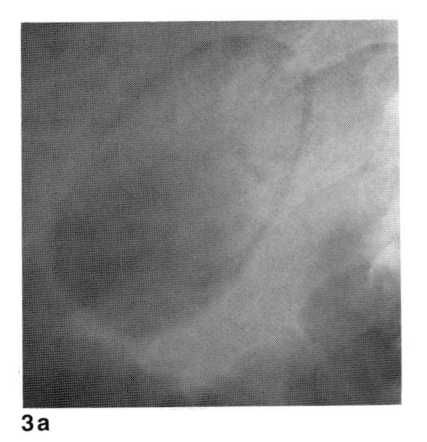

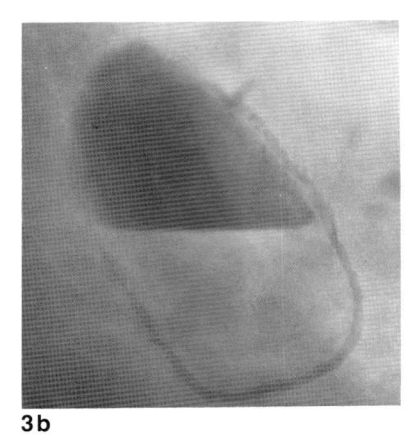

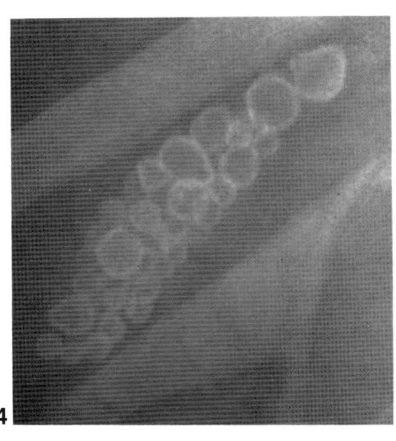

Figure **3a, b** **Emphysematous cholecystitis** in a diabetic patient **a** in supine and **b** in right lateral decubitus projections. Both intramural and intraluminal gas are seen in the gallbladder. On the lateral decubitus film, an air–bile level is seen.

Figure **4** **Gallstones.** Multiple Gallstones are evident as ring-like densities with a radiolucent center.

In *emphysematous cholecystitis,* gas is seen in either the lumen or the wall of the gallbladder, or in both (Fig. **3**). The gallbladder usually has a generous size. Although cystic duct obstruction is almost always associated, cholelithiasis may not be present. Upright or decubitus films may disclose an air–bile level.

The incidence of emphysematous cholecystitis is approximately 5 times greater in males than females, and is associated with diabetes in a majority of cases. Gallbladder perforation is an extremely serious but not unusual complication. Gas-forming organisms of the *clostridium* group are the most common germs, but *Escherichia coli, anaerobic Streptococci,* and others have also been implicated. Ascending cholangitis caused by these organisms generally does not produce enough gas in the bile ducts to be detectable by conventional radiography.

Spontaneous or postoperative *cholecystoenteric fistulas* are the most common cause of gallbladder air. However, in these cases the gallbladder is small to normal in size and air is never seen in the gallbladder wall, but commonly in the lumen of bile ducts. *Gallstone perforation* into the duodenum or less commonly into the colon is the most common cause of a spontaneous cholecystoenteric fistula. Rarely, a *carcinoma* of the gastrointestinal tract, pancreas, or biliary system may produce an enterocholic fistula that is radiographically evident by intraluminal air in the bile ducts and/or gallbladder. Perforation of a peptic ulcer into the biliary system is even more unusual. By far the most common cause of intrabiliary air results from *surgical procedures* such as choledochoduodenostomy, cholecystoenterostomy, and sphincterotomy. On upper gastrointestinal examination, barium refluxes freely into the biliary system in these cases. Small amounts of gas in the common bile duct are occasionally seen with an *incompetent Oddi's sphincter.* This may be drug-induced (cholecystokinin, anticholinergica), caused by local inflammation and scarring (e.g., postbulbar ulcer disease), or a carcinoma originating in the region of the ampulla of Vater. The sphincter incompetence is rarely idiopathic. Similarly, gas or contrast material reflux into the pancreatic duct can occasionally also be seen in these conditions.

Gallstones are by far the most common cause of calcification in the biliary system, despite the fact that only approximately 20% contain sufficient calcium to be radiopaque. Ultrasonography is, therefore, the procedure of choice to diagnose cholelithiasis, since both calcified and noncalcified gallstones are readily demonstrated by this technique. There is a great variation in the radiographic appearance and size of gallstones. They are present as homogeneous or ring-like densities, which is unfortunately also the radiographic manifestation of many other calcified right upper quadrant lesions (Fig. **4**). Calcifications in the right kidney, retroperitoneum, and costal cartilage may all project into the gallbladder area on an anteroposterior film, but can easily be differentiated from gallstones in an oblique or lateral view. Ultrasonography or oral cholecystography may, however, be required to differentiate gallstones from vascular, hepatic, and lymph node calcifications located in the proximity of the biliary system. Faceted gallstones or the demonstration of stellate radiolucencies representing gas within the gallstones ("Mercedes-Benz" sign) are relatively rare but diagnostic findings for cholelithiasis (Fig. **5**).

Opacification of the gallbladder on plain radiography (without the administration of any contrast medium) is caused by innumerable sand-like calcified particles dispersed in a thick, paste-like bile. It is termed *milk of calcium* or *limy bile syndrome* (Fig. **6**). In this condition, the gallbladder is chronically inflamed and the cystic duct obstructed by a stone that is often calcified. The visualization of a cystic duct stone and the often slightly granular appearance of the milk of calcium bile may help to differentiate this condition from a gallbladder opacified by contrast medium. One has to be aware that the gallbladder may occasionally remain opacified for up to two weeks after intravenous or oral cholecystography and that vicarious biliary excretion of a urographic

Gallbladder and Bile Duct Abnormalities 217

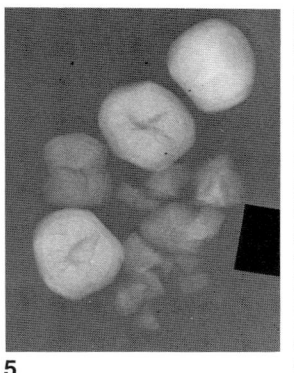

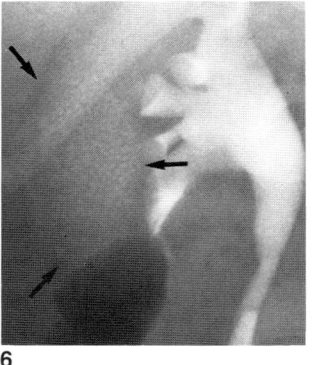

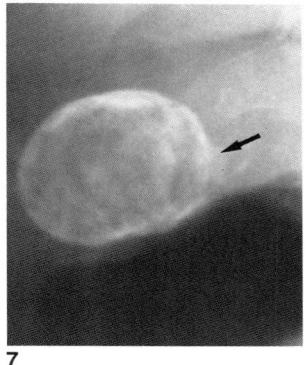

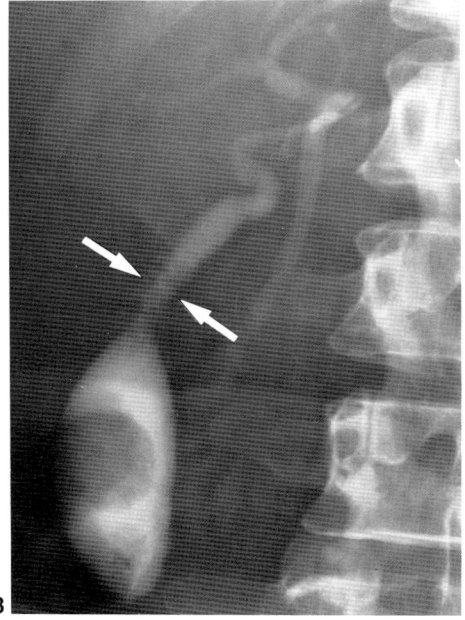

Figure 5 **Gallstones** with "Mercedes-Benz" sign. Gas within the gallstones is evident as stellate radiolucencies.

Figure 6 **Milk of calcium bile** or **limy bile syndrome.** The gallbladder contains innumerable sand-like calcific densities (arrows) that were coincidentally seen during intravenous urography.

Figure 7 **Porcelain gallbladder.** Calcification of the gallbladder wall is seen. Note the additional density next to the gallbladder neck representing the obstructing cystic duct stone (arrow).

Figure 8 **Rokitansky–Aschoff sinuses.** Multiple punctate collections of contrast medium along both sides of the markedly contracted gallbladder neck after a fatty meal are seen (arrows). Note also the unusually good visualization of the normal bile ducts in oral cholecystography. The apparent filling defects in the gallbladder fundus are caused by superimposed gas in the colon.

contrast agent resulting in gallbladder opacification occurs with poor renal function, with an acute unilateral ureteral obstruction and a normally functioning contralateral kidney, or when large urographic contrast material dosages are used.

Porcelain gallbladder refers to calcifications in the gallbladder wall that can occur in chronic cholecystitis (Fig. 7). Gallstones are almost always present with one usually obstructing the cystic duct. Malignant degeneration of the porcelain gallbladder develops with a high enough frequency to warrant prophylactic cholecystectomy even in asymptomatic patients. Rarely, a *mucinous adenocarcinoma* of the gallbladder can disclose fine punctate calcifications.

Contrast Examination

Visualization of the gallbladder and/or bile ducts can be achieved by oral or intravenous administration of biliary contrast agents or by direct injection of contrast into the biliary system. The latter is attained by transhepatic or endoscopic retrograde cholangiography and postoperative T-tube cholangiography.

Diagnostic visualization of the biliary system by oral and intravenous cholecystangiography is virtually limited to nonjaundiced patients. In the presence of normal liver function, failure to visualize gallbladder after two 3 g doses of an oral cholecystographic agent administered on two consecutive days is highly suggestive of gallbladder disease (e.g., *cholecystitis*). Rare causes of *nonvisualization* that are related neither to the liver nor to the biliary system include diseases and abnormalities of the gastrointestinal tract, malabsorption syndromes, and interference by a variety of drugs with the cholecystographic agents in the resorption from the gut or the biliary excretion. In the noncholecystectomized patient, opacification of the bile ducts during intravenous cholangiography without gallbladder opacification is virtually diagnostic of cystic duct obstruction. The diameter of the common bile duct on intravenous cholangiography ranges from 1 to 15 mm (average 5 mm) in healthy individuals, although a diameter larger than 10 mm is quite unusual in noncholecystectomized patients. After cholecystectomy, the average bile duct diameter tends to be larger than in the noncholecystectomized patient. A diameter in excess of 15 mm strongly suggests bile duct obstruction in any patient.

The differential diagnosis of filling defects in the opacified gallbladder and bile ducts is discussed in Tables 1–3. *Mucosal outpouchings* (diverticula) from the gallbladder are usually multiple and present radiographically as small oval collections of contrast material adjacent to the gallbladder wall. They are referred to as *Rokitansky–Aschoff sinuses* (Fig. 8), are best seen after gallbladder contraction (e.g., after a fatty meal), and represent one of several manifestations of gallbladder adenomyomatosis (see also Tables 1 and 2). The differential diagnosis of saccular lesions originating from bile ducts is the subject of Table 4. It has to be remembered that in a jaundiced patient, gallbladder and bile duct lesions are only visualized with direct (e.g., transhepatic or endoscopic retrograde) cholangiography, whereas oral and intravenous cholangiography normally result in nonvisualization of the biliary system in these cases.

Table 1 Linear or Band-Like Filling Defects in the Opacified Gallbladder

Disease	Radiographic Findings	Comments
Septate gallbladder	Septa of variable length and number in a normal-sized gallbladder.	Rare. Stasis in different gallbladder compartment predisposes to infection and gallstone formation.
Phrygian cap (Fig. 9)	A radiolucent line, caused by an incomplete circumferential septum of varying thickness, partially separates the fundus from the body.	Developmental anomaly without clinical significance.
Gallstones (Fig. 10)	A layer of innumerable tiny calculi may form a thin to thick radiolucent band on upright or lateral decubitus films, but cannot be seen on supine examination.	
Cystic fibrosis	Multiple web-like trabeculations in a small gallbladder with marginal irregularities.	Opacification of the gallbladder with oral cholecystography is usually poor.
Adenomyomatosis (Fig. 11)	Localized adenomyomatosis of the "circumferential" type may cause compartmentalization of the gallbladder ("hourglass gallbladder"). Gallstones are often present in distal compartment.	Adenomatosis consists of mucosal proliferation, increased thickness of the muscularis, and mucosal outpouchings. Disease may be localized or diffuse. In the latter case, mucosal outpouchings may present as multiple oval contrast collections of varying size and may be seen adjacent to the gallbladder wall.

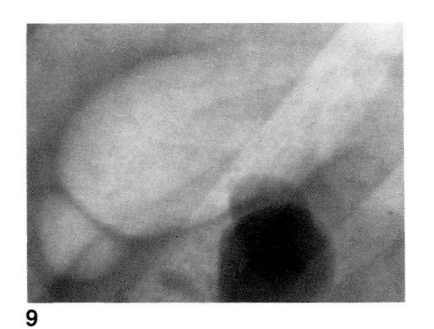

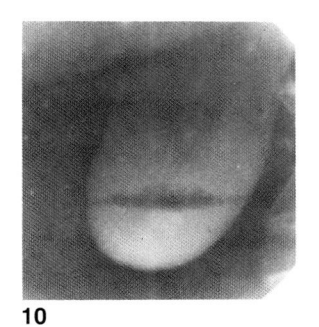

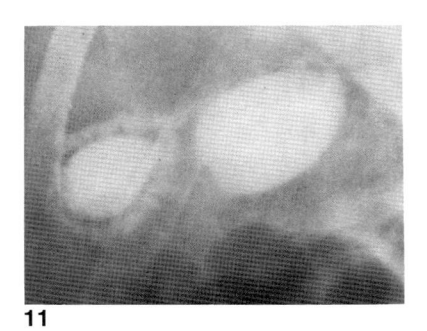

Figure 9 **Phrygian cap.** The radiolucent line between the fundus and the body of gallbladder is caused by an incomplete circumferential septum.

Figure 10 **Gallstones.** A layer of numerous small cholesterol stones forms a radiolucent band on this film taken with horizontal beam in upright position.

Figure 11 **Adenomyomastosis.** Compartmentalization of the gallbladder producing an "hourglass" deformity is seen. Note also the multiple Rokitansky–Aschoff sinuses presenting as a string of beads around the circumference of the distal compartment.

Table 2 Round or Mass-Like Filling Defects in the Opacified Gallbladder

Disease	Radiographic Findings	Comments
Gallstones (Fig. 12)	Single or multiple filling defects, varying greatly in shape and size, ranging from 1 mm to 5 cm. Characteristically, gallstones are freely movable, thus changing the location within the gallbladder in different positions. Rarely, a stone may become adherent to the wall and simulate a mural lesion.	80% are composed predominantly of nonradiopaque cholesterol. A higher incidence of gallstones is found with cirrhosis, diabetes, pancreatitis, Crohn's disease, and hyperparathyroidism. Bilirubin stones are associated with excessive red blood cell destruction (hemolytic anemias).
Cholesterolosis Cholesterol polyp (Fig. 13)	Single, or more commonly several, round to oval filling defects of varying size, but usually measuring less than 1 cm. They can be differentiated from gallstones by their fixed location in the gallbladder.	Abnormal deposits of cholesterol esters in fat-laden macrophages in the lamina propria ("strawberry gallbladder").
Adenomyoma (Fig. 14)	Solitary filling defect characteristically located in the fundus of the gallbladder. An "ulcer niche" is occasionally seen in the center of the lesion representing a solitary Rokitansky–Aschoff sinus.	Localized manifestation of adenomyomatosis caused by focal hyperplasia of the gallbladder wall.
Adenomyomatosis (Fig. 15)	Multiple small filling defects often associated with other manifestations of the disorder such as compartmentalization or narrowing of the fundus and Rokitansky–Aschoff sinuses.	May be associated with symptoms of chronic gallbladder disease.
Benign tumors, intramural cyst, or ectopic tissue	Extremely rare causes of one or more small mural filling defects in the gallbladder.	Benign tumors include adenomas, papillomas, carcinoids, and different mesenchymal tumors. Intramural cysts include epithelial and mucus retention cysts. Ectopic tissue implanted into the gallbladder wall may originate from the pancreas or stomach.
Carcinoma (Fig. 16)	Nonvisualization of gallbladder is the common presentation in oral or intravenous cholecystangiography. Irregular filling defect may be found in an opacified gallbladder.	May originate in gallbladder or represent a local extension of a biliary or hepatic carcinoma. Other less common malignancies include hematogenous *metastases* (e.g., from melanoma) and *sarcomas* (e.g., leiomyosarcoma).
Inflammatory pseudotumors	Solitary or multiple filling defects developing during the course of chronic cholecystitis.	*Xanthogranulomatous cholecystitis* is a rare form of chronic cholecystitis that presents with nodular lesions and is usually associated with cholelithiasis. *Parasitic granulomas* can occasionally be found with ascariasis and paragonimiasis.
Extrinsic mass	Extrinsic filling defects measure usually several centimeters and tend to be semicircular or may cause an hourglass deformity. Normal anatomical structures (e.g., dilated duodenum or colon) and mass lesions originating from liver, porta hepatis, and pancreas may produce extrinsic filling defects.	*Postoperative defects* may present in similar fashion. Small extrinsic defects may occasionally be caused by *vascular structures*.
Air in bowel	Superimposed bowel air may simulate one or more true filling defects. Projection of the air outside the opacified gallbladder on one film allows correct diagnosis.	

Gallbladder and Bile Duct Abnormalities 221

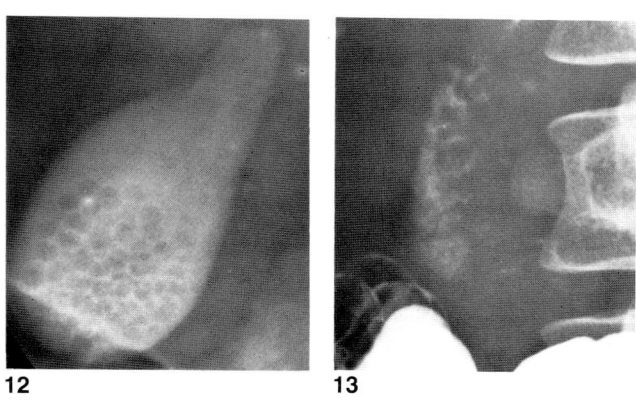

Figure 12 **Gallstones.** Multiple small filling defects caused by nonradiopaque cholesterol stones are seen.

Figure 13 **Cholesterolosis** ("strawberry gallbladder"). Multiple small polypoid filling defects are seen in the contracted gallbladder. As in this case, these small polypoid lesions are best appreciated in the contracted gallbladder after a fatty meal.

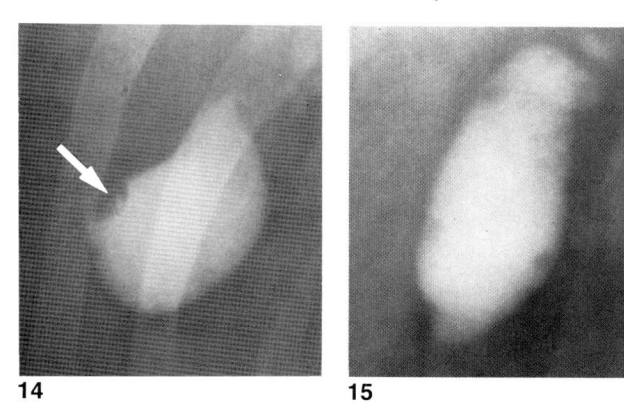

Figure 14 **Adenomyoma.** A solitary small defect is seen in the contracted gallbladder with a Rokitansky–Aschoff sinus presenting as central contrast collection (arrow).

Figure 15 **Adenomyomatosis.** Several small filling defects and a constricting narrowing of the gallbladder fundus are seen.

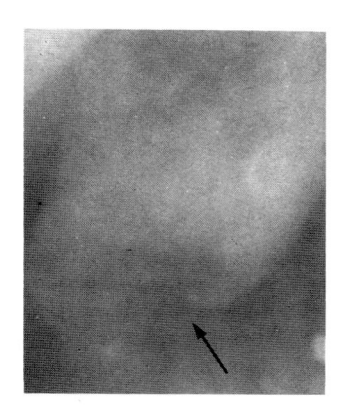

Figure 16 **Gallbladder carcinoma.** A relatively large, irregular filling defect in a poorly opacified gallbladder is seen.

Table 3 Filling Defects and/or Localized Stenosis of Opacified Bile Ducts

Disease	Radiographic Findings	Comments
Congenital membrane	Rare cause of partial obstruction of common hepatic duct by membranous diaphragm.	Usually diagnosed in young adults. Recurrent jaundice for many years characteristic. DD: *Biliary atresia* of the neonate is the result of a progressive inflammatory obliterative process during fetal life.
Calculi (Fig. 17)	Bile ducts usually dilated by partial or complete obstruction. Stones may be freely mobile. Impacted stones characteristically produce a convex filling defect with smooth border.	Visualization of bile ducts with intravenous cholangiography is only possible with partial but not with complete obstruction. *Mirizzi syndrome:* gallstone impacted in the cystic duct, causing partial common hepatic duct obstruction.
Cholangiocarcinoma and metastatic extrinsic or intrinsic carcinoma (Figs. 18–21)	Configuration of duct at point of obstruction is similar for extrinsic and intrinsic tumors. It may be blunt, rounded, jagged, tapered or show a "rat tail" deformity. *Pancreatic carcinoma* (Fig. 18): Obstruction usually associated with large mass and located at superior margin of pancreas (the level at which the common bile duct changes from a medial and slightly caudal course to a lateral and steeper caudal direction) or more distally. *Metastases* (Fig. 19): Obstruction of common hepatic duct often in porta hepatis. *Gallbladder carcinoma* (Fig. 19): Mass in gallbladder area associated with cystic duct obstruction, often combined with common hepatic duct obstruction when the latter is invaded. *Bile duct carcinoma* (Fig. 20): Originate in 95% anywhere in extrahepatic biliary ducts. May produce intraluminal masses of varying sizes or more commonly infiltrating stenotic lesions of varying length. *Ampullary carcinoma* (Fig. 21): Obstruction of the distal common bile duct, usually without traceable tumor. Occasionally an irregular or polypoid mass measuring less than 2 cm is found.	Middle-aged and elderly patients with unremittant progressive jaundice and pruritus. Opacification only with direct cholangiography possible, since intravenous cholangiography results in nonvisualization of the biliary system. *Klatskin tumors* are cholangiocarcinomas that originate from the junction between the right and left hepatic duct. They tend to grow slower and metastasize later than the usual cholangiocarcinomas. *Lymphoma* involving the nodes in the porta hepatis presents like metastasis.

Figure **17 Biliary calculi** with partial bile duct obstruction (intravenous cholangiography). An impacted stone, evident as smooth round filling defect with convex border (short arrow) causes partial biliary obstruction with pronounced dilatation of the extrahepatic bile ducts. A second larger and freely mobile stone is also seen in the dilated common bile duct (long arrow).

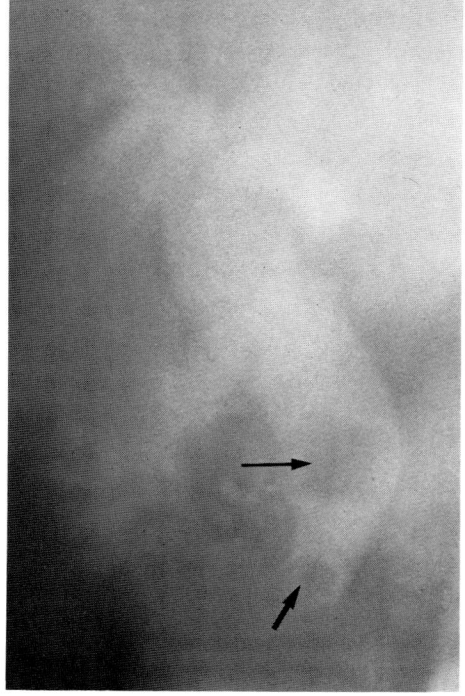

Gallbladder and Bile Duct Abnormalities 223

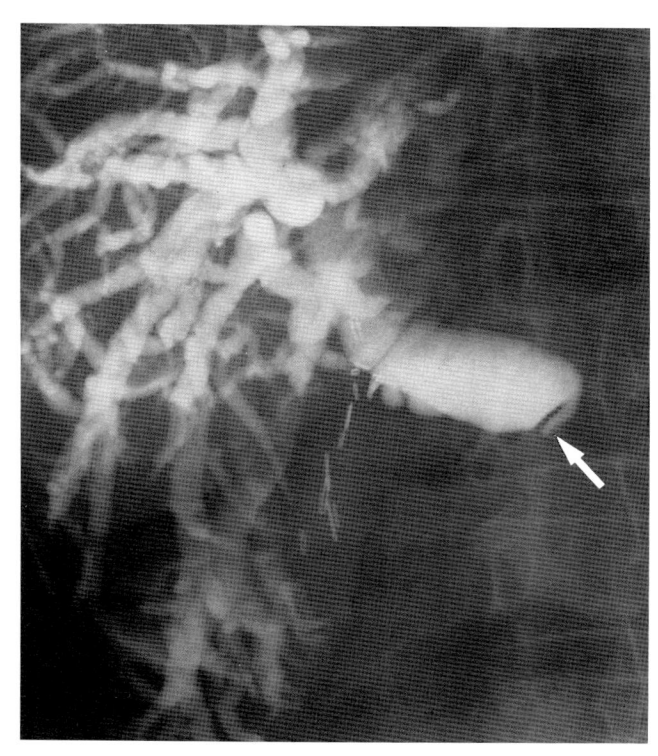

Figure 18 **Pancreatic carcinoma.** Obstruction of the common bile duct in characteristic location (level at which it changes from a medial and slightly caudal course to a lateral and steeper caudal direction) is present. The beak-like termination of the occluded duct is often seen in this condition (arrow). Cholecystectomy was performed in the past.

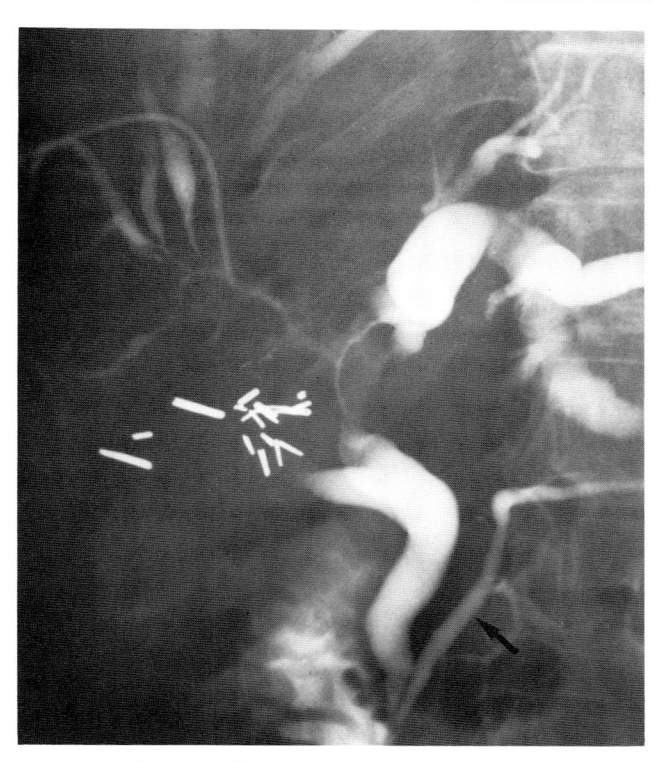

Figure 19 **Metastatic gallbladder carcinoma.** A large metastasis in the porta hepatis causes obstruction of the relatively smoothly tapered right hepatic ducts and a marked prestenotic dilatation of the left hepatic duct. Note also the contrast reflux into the pancreatic duct (arrow).

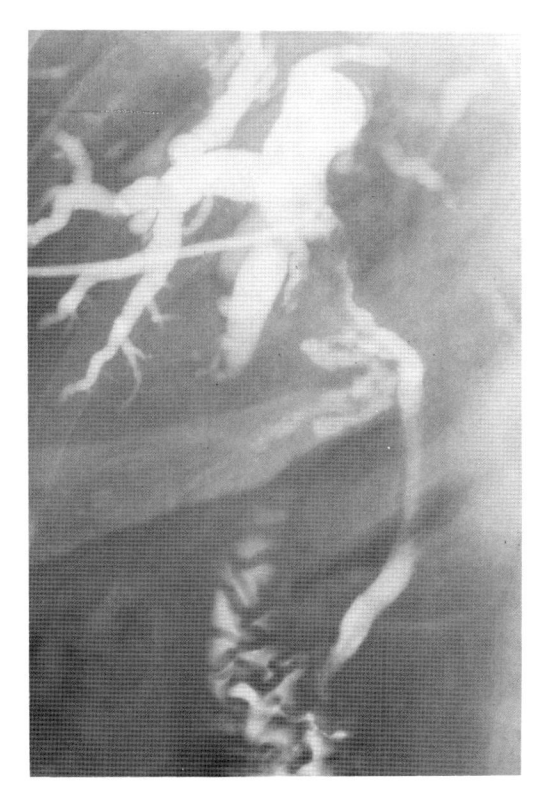

Figure 20 **Bile duct carcinoma.** Irregular stenosis of the common hepatic duct and, to a lesser extent, of the bile duct is seen.

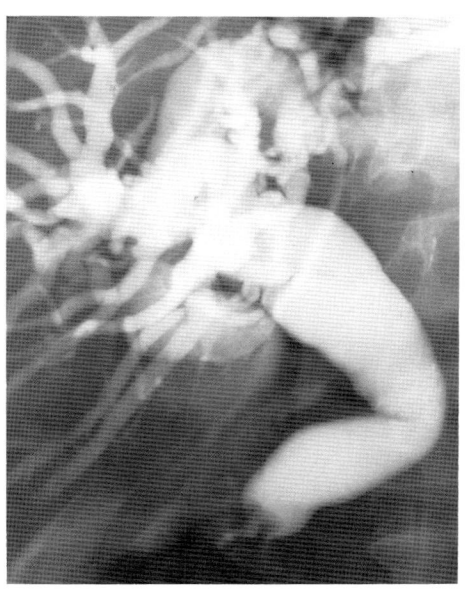

Figure 21 **Ampullary carcinoma.** An irregular stenosis of the ampullary portion of the bile duct combined with a polypoid lesion, producing an irregular filling defect in the obstructed common bile duct, is virtually diagnostic.

Table 3 (Cont.) Filling Defects and/or Localized Stenosis of Opacified Bile Ducts

Disease	Radiographic Findings	Comments
Benign tumors and inflammatory pseudotumors	Rare cause of a sessile polypoid filling defect that may or may not cause obstruction.	*Adenomas* and a wide variety of other benign neoplasms are encountered. *Papillomas* may be multiple, and the combination of intraluminal nodules and thick mucous production may cause biliary obstruction. *Tuberculosis, sarcoidosis,* and other granulomatous diseases involving the lymph nodes in the porta hepatis rarely cause extrinsic compression and obstruction of the biliary system.
Pancreatitis, chronic (Fig. 22)	Smooth stricture of distal common bile duct characteristic. Complete obstruction is rare. Pancreatic pseudocyst may cause displacement of bile ducts. Pancreatic calcifications are occasionally seen.	May present with recurrent cholangitis and obstructive jaundice. *Acute pancreatitis:* A reversible smooth narrowing of the distal common bile duct by the enlarged and edematous pancreas head is occasionally seen.
Inflammation/fibrosis of papilla of Vater	Incomplete distal common bile duct obstruction with or without contracted (spastic) Oddi's sphincter may simulate a polypoid lesion (DD: calculus or ampullary carcinoma).	Causes: Acute or chronic inflammatory disease (e.g., bile ducts, pancreas). Postoperative or postinstrumentation. Idiopathic (hypertrophy of Oddi's sphincter).
Cholangitis 1. recurrent or chronic 2. primary sclerosing (Fig. 23)	Diffuse or localized narrowing of the extrahepatic and intrahepatic ducts. Occasionally moderately dilated prestenotic segments alternate with strictured areas.	Usually secondary to longstanding partial biliary obstruction. Primary sclerosing cholangitis is often associated with ulcerative colitis and less commonly with Crohn's disease and retroperitoneal fibrosis.
Worm infestation (ascaris, liver flukes, echinococcus) (Fig. 24)	Characteristic filling defects by an ascaris (up to 20 cm in length) that may extend into the duodenum or be coiled in the bile duct, causing partial obstruction.	Ascaris and liver flukes ascend from the duodenum into bile ducts. Liver flukes (*Clonorchis sinensis* and *Fasciola hepatica*) are nematodes, measuring 1 to 2 cm in length. They inhabit the smaller bile ducts and produce oval to linear filling defects. Echinococcus: Round or irregular filling defects caused by cyst membranes, daughter cysts or scoleces discharged from a communicating hepatic cyst.
Postoperative and posttraumatic (e.g., hematomas and strictures)	Filling defects or smooth localized narrowing.	Following bile duct surgery or interventional radiologic procedures.
Blood clots	Mobile filling defects of varying shape, simulating radiolucent calculi or worms.	Usually postoperative, rarely with bleeding disorders.
Air bubble (Fig. 25)	Round, mobile, nonobstructive filling defects.	Only found with direct cholangiography.

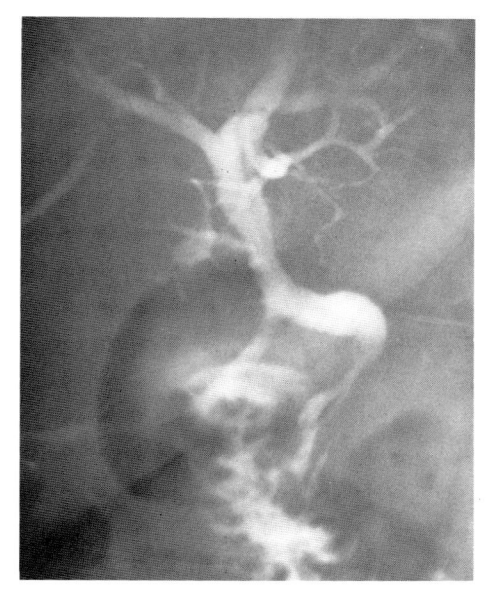

Figure 22 **Chronic pancreatitis.** A relatively smooth stricture of the distal common bile duct is seen that begins at the superior margin of the pancreas (the level at which the common bile duct changes from a medial course to a lateral and steep caudal direction).

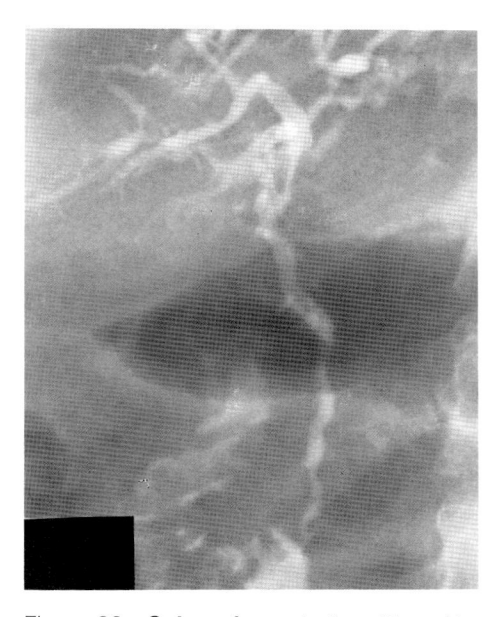

Figure 23 **Sclerosing cholangitis.** Alternating stenotic and nonstenotic segments in the common hepatic duct and bile duct, combined with small saccular outpouchings, are characteristic.

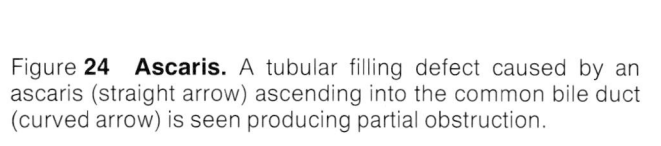

Figure 24 **Ascaris.** A tubular filling defect caused by an ascaris (straight arrow) ascending into the common bile duct (curved arrow) is seen producing partial obstruction.

Figure 25 **Air bubbles simulating biliary calculi.** Multiple small round radiolucencies are seen in a normal sized and nonobstructed common bile duct in this postoperative T-tube cholangiogram.

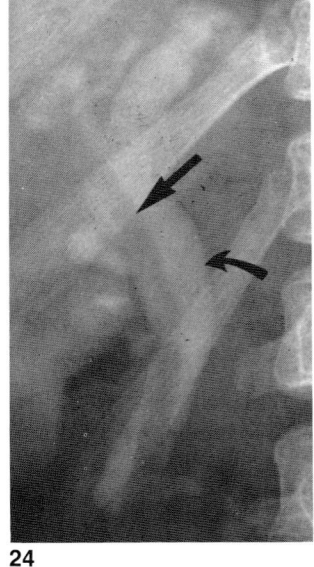

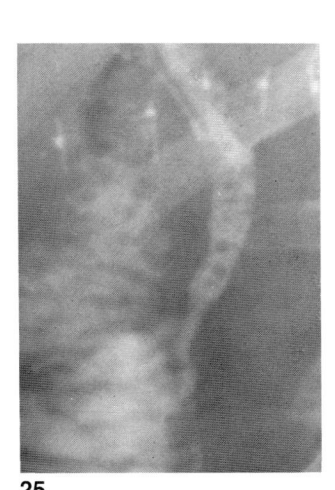

Table 4 Saccular and Diverticular Lesions of the Bile Ducts

Disease	Radiographic Findings	Comments
Congenital hepatic fibrosis	Irregular cystic spaces of varying sizes communicating with intrahepatic bile ducts (lollipop-tree appearance).	Rare disorder that radiographically simulates Caroli's disease. Associated with periportal fibrosis and portal hypertension.
Caroli's disease (Fig. 26)	Segmental saccular dilatation of intrahepatic bile ducts.	Congenital malformation, but usually first diagnosed in adulthood, when the following complications occur: intrahepatic stone formation, cholangitis, liver abscess, and septicemia. There is a high incidence of associated medullary sponge kidneys.
Choledochal cyst (Fig. 27)	Segmental dilatation of the common bile duct and adjacent portions of common hepatic duct and cystic duct. Separate segmental dilatation of intrahepatic and extrahepatic ducts represents a rare variant of the disease. Diverticulum-like extrahepatic and intrahepatic lesions ("congenital hepatic diverticulum") are also included in this entity and comprise about 1%.	Most common congenital bile duct lesion, with male : female ratio of 1 : 4. Present classically with jaundice, right upper quadrant mass, and/or abdominal pain in children or adults.
Choledochocele (Fig. 28)	Cystic dilatation of intramural portion of the common bile duct in duodenal wall with pancreatic duct entering it.	Insertion of the common bile duct into a duodenal diverticulum must be differentiated.
Hepatic abscesses (Fig. 29)	Multiple small intrahepatic contrast collections are characteristically found with direct cholangiography in severe suppurative cholangitis and are diagnostic for complicating abscesses.	Hematogenous hepatic abscesses rarely communicate with the biliary system.
Sclerosing cholangitis (Fig. 30)	Prestenotic dilatation with small saccular outpouchings can be seen in addition to localized areas of narrowing and may be the dominating radiographic feature. Involvement occurs in extrahepatic and major intrahepatic ducts.	Usually secondary to longstanding partial biliary obstruction. A rare primary form tends to occur with inflammatory bowel disease, especially ulcerative colitis.
Echinococcal cyst	Irregular intrahepatic cavity with or without marginal calcification and often sharply defined round filling defects (daughter cysts). Detached daughter cysts may produce filling defects in the extrahepatic ducts and lead to total obstruction.	Communication with the biliary tree is the most common complication of hepatic echinococcal disease. Intermittent pain and jaundice may be caused by periodic discharge of fragments of the cyst membrane or its contents.
Fistula	Irregular cavity communicating with the extrahepatic biliary system.	Usually postoperative.
Cystic duct remnant	Tubular structure in characteristic location in patients who have undergone cholecystectomy.	No clinical significance unless associated with stones or inflammation.

Gallbladder and Bile Duct Abnormalities 227

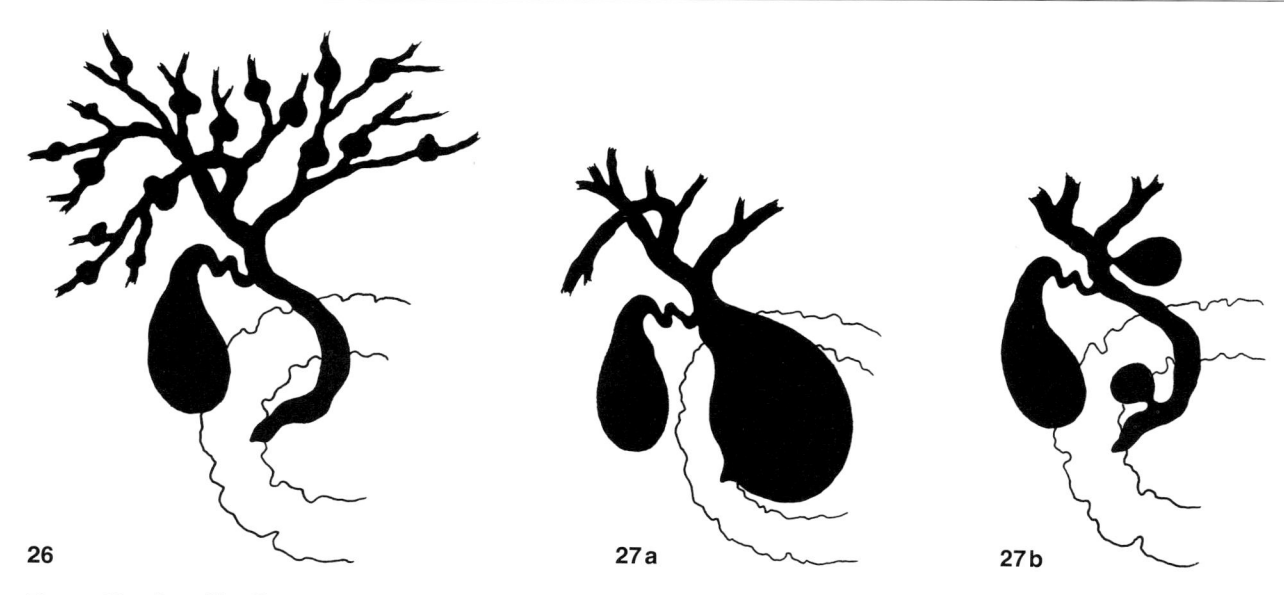

Figure 26 **Caroli's disease.** Multiple saccular dilatations of the intrahepatic ducts are characteristic.

Figure 27a, b **Choledochal cysts. a** A segmental dilatation of the common bile duct, which may reach such proportions that widening and extrinsic compression of the duodenal sweep occur, is the most common presentation. **b** Diverticulum-like outpouchings from the extrahepatic bile ducts and rarely the intrahepatic ducts are an unusual manifestation of the choledochal cyst entity.

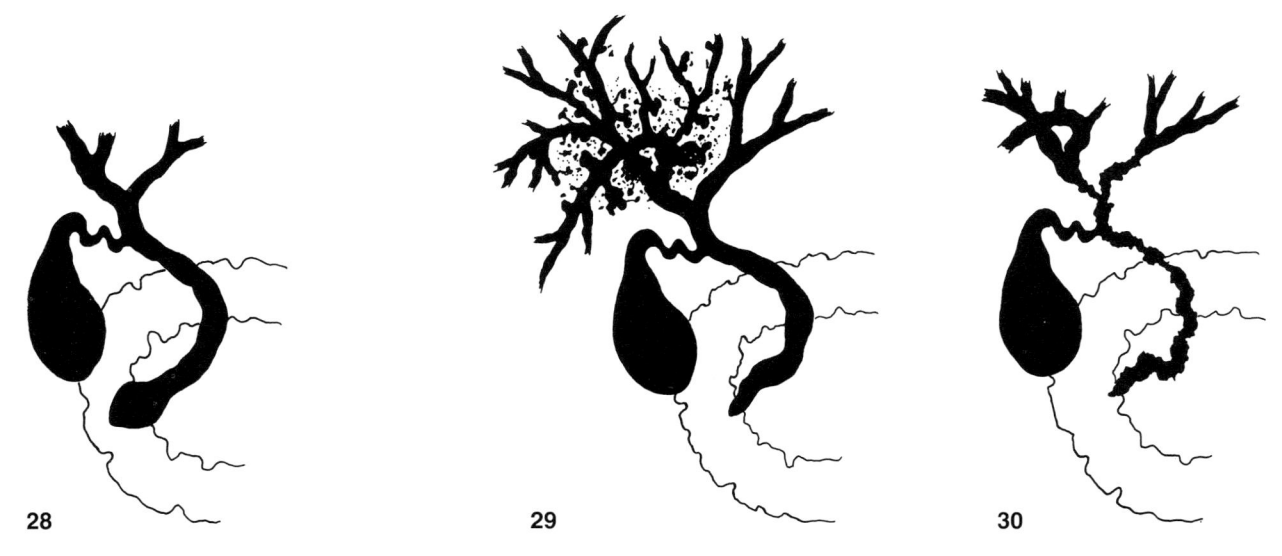

Figure 28 **Choledochocele.** Cystic dilatation of the intramural portion of the common bile duct. Produces a smooth filling defect in the second portion of the duodenum on an upper gastrointestinal examination.

Figure 29 **Hepatic abscesses.** Multiple intrahepatic contrast collections can be found in severe suppurative cholangitis.

Figure 30 **Sclerosing cholangitis.** Prestenotic duct ectasia with small saccular outpouchings may be interspersed with areas of localized narrowing.

References

Berk RN, Ferrucci JT, Leopold GR. Radiology of the gallbladder and bile ducts. Philadelphia: Saunders, 1983.

Cremin BJ, Cywes S, Louw JH. Radiological diagnosis of digestive tract disorders in the newborn. London: Butterworths, 1973.

Cummack DH. Gastrointestinal X-ray diagnosis. Edinburgh: Livingstone, 1969.

Davidson AJ. Radiologic diagnosis of renal parenchymal disease. 2nd ed. Philadelphia: Saunders, 1985

Elkin M. Radiology of the urinary system. Boston: Little, Brown, 1980.

Federle MP, Megibow AJ, Naidich DP. Radiology of AIDS. New York: Raven Press, 1988.

Freeman, BA. Textbook of microbiology. 22nd ed. Philadelphia: Saunders, 1985.

Friedland GW, Filly R, Goris ML, et al. Uroradiology: an integrated approach. Edinburgh: Churchill Livingstone, 1983.

Frimann-Dahl J. Roentgen examinations in acute abdominal diseases. 3rd ed. Springfield, IL: Thomas, 1974.

Kissane JM, ed. Anderson's pathology. 8th ed. St Louis: Mosby, 1985.

Kreel L. Outline of radiology. London: Heinemann Medical, 1971.

Laufer, I. Double-contrast gastrointestinal radiology with endoscopic correlation. Philadelphia: Saunders, 1979.

Lusted LB, Keats TE. Atlas of roentgenographic measurement. 5th ed. Chicago: Year Book Medical 1985.

Margulis AR, Burhenne HJ. Alimentary tract radiology. 4th ed. St Louis: Mosby, 1989.

Marshak RH, Lindner AE. Radiology of the small intestine. 2nd ed. Philadelphia: Saunders, 1976.

Marshak RH, Lindner AE, Maklansky D. Radiology of the colon. Philadelphia: Saunders, 1980.

Marshak RH, Lindner AE, Maklansky D. Radiology of the stomach. Philadelphia: Saunders, 1983.

McCort JJ, Mindelzun RE, Filpi RG, Rennell C. Abdominal radiology. Baltimore: Williams and Wilkins, 1981.

Meschan I. Analysis of roentgen signs in general radiology. Philadelphia: Saunders, 1984.

Meyers MA. Dynamic radiology of the abdomen: normal and pathologic anatomy. 3rd ed. Heidelberg: Springer, 1988.

Ney C, Friedenberg RM. Radiographic atlas of the genitourinary system. 2nd ed. Philadelphia: Lippincott, 1981.

Pollack HM ed. Clinical urography. Philadelphia: Saunders, 1990.

Radiological Clinics of North America, 1976;14(3). Philadelphia: Saunders.

Reeder MM, Felson B. Gamuts in radiology. 2nd ed. Cincinnati: Audiovisual Radiology of Cincinnati, 1987.

Robbins SL. Pathologic basis of disease. 4th ed. Philadelphia: Saunders, 1989.

Sabiston DC, Jr. Textbook of surgery: the biological basis of modern surgical practice. 13th ed. Philadelphia: Saunders, 1986.

Schinz HR. Lehrbuch der Röntgendiagnostik. Stuttgart: Thieme, 1989.

Seminars in Roentgenology 1973;13(3–4); 1982;17(2). New York: Grune and Stratton.

Silverman F, ed. Caffey's pediatric X-ray diagnosis: a textbook for students and practitioners of pediatrics, surgery and radiology. 8th ed. Chicago: Year Book Medical, 1985.

Singleton EB, Wagner ML, Dutton RV. Radiology of the alimentary tract in infants and children. Philadelphia: Saunders, 1977.

Sutton D. A textbook of radiology and imaging. 4th ed. Edinburgh: Churchill Livingstone, 1987.

Swischuk LE. Imaging of the newborn, infant and young child. 3rd. ed. Baltimore: Williams and Wilkins, 1989.

Taveras JM, Ferrucci JT. Radiology: diagnosis, imaging, intervention. Philadelphia: Lippincott, 1989.

Taybi H. Radiology of syndromes and metabolic disorders. 3rd ed. Chicago: Year Book Medical, 1990.

Teplick JG, Haskin ME. Surgical radiology. Philadelphia: Saunders, 1981.

Teschendorf W, Anacker H, Thurn P. Röntgenologische Differentialdiagnostik. 2 vols. 5th ed. Stuttgart: Thieme, 1975–78.

Williams PL, Warwick R, Dyson M, Bannister LH, eds. Gray's anatomy. 37th ed. Edinburgh: Churchill Livingstone. 1989.

Wyngaarden JB, Smith LH Jr, eds. Cecil's textbook of medicine. 18th ed. Philadelphia: Saunders, 1988.

Index

Entries under major organs are extensive but not exhaustive. Users are advised to look up specific conditions should they not be found as subentries of main headings.

A

abdomen
    abnormal gas patterns 1–29
        extraluminal gas collections 21–9
        large bowel distension 10–15
        in the neonate 16–20
        small bowel distension 4–9
    compartments of abdominal cavity 2–3
    organs
        abnormal position 57–81
        normal position 55–6
abetalipoproteinemia 118
abscess 2, 26–9
    air—fluid level 2
    appendix 188
    colonic involvement 99
    diagnosis 2
    gas collections 26–9
    intraperitoneal 28
    liver 26, 176, 215, 226
    Morrison's pouch 76
    pelvic 26
    subhepatic abscess 176
    subphrenic abscess 26, 57
acanthosis nigricans, esophagus 110
actinomycosis 130, 154, 188
acute abdomen
    abnormal gas patterns 1–29
        films required 1
        gasless 2
        infant 1–2
adenomyomatosis 220
adrenal neoplasms, displacing kidney 60, 62
adrenal and retroperitoneal calcifications 44–7
    neonatal adrenal hemorrhage 44
aerophagia, radiography 4
aganglionosis (Hirschsprung's disease) 13, 18, 104, 152
alpha chain disease, small bowel 120
amebiasis, large bowel 128, 129, 154, 188
amyloidosis
    esophagus 87
    large bowel 104, 130, 158, 192
    small bowel 117, 118, 119
    stomach 112, 142, 170
anus, imperforate 16
aortic aneurysm
    duodenal displacement 68
    longitudinal tubular calcification 46
aortic arch, double 163
appendicitis 14, 99
    'left-sided' 212
appendicoliths 37, 14, 99
appendix
    abscess 188
    inverted, intussusception 182
ascites, signs 70, 97

B

Behçet's syndrome 130
biliary tract 215–27
    air bubbles 224
    ascarids 224
    atresia 222
    benign tumors 224
    calcifications 36
    calculi 222
    cholangitis 224
    cholecystitis 115
        emphysematous 22, 216
    cholecystoduodenal fistula 208
    cholecystoenteric fistula 22, 215, 22, 215
    choledochal cyst, choledochocele 144, 172, 174, 226
    congenital membrane 222
    cystic duct remnant 226
    extraluminal gas 22–3
    filling defects and/or localized stenoses 222–5
        cholangiocarcinoma 222
        papilla of Vater 224
        posttraumatic 224
    intraluminal gas 215–16
    limy bile syndrome 216
    Oddi's sphicter, incompetence 216
    saccular and diverticular lesions 226
    worm infestation 224
    see also gallbladder; gallstones
bladder *see* urinary bladder
blastomycosis 154

C

calcifications 31–53
    adrenal and retroperitoneal
        cystic (curvilinear) 44
        longitudinal tubular 46
        mottled mass 46
        triangular 44
    alimentary tract
        calculus 37
        cystic 37
        parenchymal 38
    biliary tract
        calculous 36
        homogeneous 36
        punctate 36
    diffuse, widespread 52
    injection sites 31
    kidney 38–44
        nephrolithiasis 38
    liver
        capsular 33
        cystic 32
        disseminated 32
        general increase in density 33
        solitary 32–3
        vascular 33
    pancreas
        cystic 36
        disseminated 34
        solitary 36
    pelvic 48–53
        bladder wall 48
        female tract 50
        male tract 50
        tubular 48
    spleen 34
        capsular 34
        cystic 34
        disseminated 34
        general increase in density 34
        vascular 34
    ureters 44
calculi
    biliary 36
    bladder 48
    renal 38
Campylobacter colitis 128
Canada—Cronkhite syndrome 122, 167, 178, 184
candidiasis 130
cardiac disease, left atrial enlargement 163
Carman's meniscus sign 195
Caroli's disease 226
cecal volvulus 10, 100
cecum
    carcinoma 4
    displacement 74
    mobile 74
    see also large bowel
celiac disease 115, 124
Chagas' disease 86, 104, 124
Chilaiditi syndrome 13, 57, 76, 100
cholangitis *see* biliary tract
cholecystitis *see* gallbladder
cholelithiasis *see* gallstones
cholesterolosis 220
coffee bean sign 100, 101
colitis *see* large bowel, colitis
colon cut-off sign, pancreatitis and strictures 100
colon *see* large bowel
compartments of abdominal cavity 2
constipation, idiopathic 104
Cowden's disease 132, 167, 178, 184
cricopharyngeal achalasia 83–4
cricopharyngeal muscle, delayed opening 87, 163
Crohn's disease 108, 115, 117, 118
    esophageal stricture 136
    filling defects 190
    fistulas 210
    and granulomatous infiltration 200
    inflammatory pseudotumor 190
    mucosal changes, sequence
        large bowel 126
        small bowel 120
    narrowing
        duodenum 144
        small bowel 148
        stomach 142

cystic fibrosis 96, 116, 131, 192
cysts, duplication
　duodenum 144, 172
　large bowel 182
　stomach 167
　terminal ileum 178
　　neonate 18
cytomegalovirus colitis 130, 155

D

diaphragm
　Bochdalek's hernia 8, 57, 58, 64, 76
　eventration 57
　traumatic hernia 8
diarrhea, air—fluid levels 84, 92
diverticulitis
　abscess formation 188
　fistulas 210, 212
　and obstruction 99
diverticulosis
　mucosal patterns 130
　narrowing 154
　pseudodiverticula 104, 110, 138, 212
diverticulum
　defined 195
　differention from polyp 162
　types 195–6
　see also specific organs
duodenojejunal junction, abnormal position 68
duodenum
　abnormal position 68
　adenocarcinoma 206
　antral polyp prolapse 174
　atresia 16
　benign lymphoid hyperplasia 115
　Brunner's gland hyperplasia 115, 172
　carcinoma 144, 172
　choledochal cyst, choledochocele 144, 172, 174, 226
　cystic fibrosis 96, 116, 131, 192
　dilatation 90–1
　diverticula 206–8
　　pseudodiverticula 206
　double bubble, neonate 144
　duplication cyst 144, 172
　erosive duodenitis 116
　filling defects 172–7
　　halo sign 172
　fistulas 206–8
　　cholecystoduodenal fistula 208
　giardiasis 115
　hematoma 146, 176
　hemorrhage 116
　heterotopic gastric mucosa 172
　intraluminal diverticulum 172
　metastases 144, 174
　mucosae, abnormal patterns 105, 115–16
　　prolapse of gastric mucosa 174
　narrowing 144–7
　　iatrogenic strictures 146
　　Ladd's bands 144
　　midgut volvulus 144
　normal variant position 68, 69
　pancreatitis 68, 115
　papillary enlargement 174
　polyposis 116, 172
　postbulbar ulcers 144
　postoperative defect 176
　retroperitoneal mass 176
　ulcers 206–8
　　postbulbar 144, 206
　valvulae conniventes, deformation 107

varices 116, 174
vascular impressions 116
web 172
Whipple's disease 116
dysentery, bacillary 128, 154

E

echinococcal cyst 224, 226
emphysematous cholecystitis 22, 216
endometrioma 178, 182
endometriosis, narrowing of large bowel 152
enteroliths 180, 192
eosinophilic gastroenteritis
　duodenum 112
　esophagus 136
　small bowel 117, 118, 122
　stomach 112, 142
eosinophilic granuloma 202
esophagitis 86, 108–10, 136
　corrosive 198
　granulomatous 196
　infectious 136, 166
　reflux 138, 196
esophagus
　acanthosis nigricans 110
　achalasia 86
　AIDS, moniliasis 109
　amyloidosis 87
　atresia 16
　Barrett's 138, 196
　carcinoma 110, 136, 196
　corkscrew 85
　dilatation 85–7
　diverticula 196–9
　　pseudodiverticulosis 198
　　Zenker's diverticulum 198
　filling defects 162–6
　　benign tumors 164
　　carcinoma 164
　　cysts 164
　　food/foreign bodies 166
　　leiomyoma, leiomyosarcoma 164
　　normal/pathological 162, 163
　　spondylosis and spondylitis 166
　　varices 166
　　vascular structures 163
　fistulas 196–9
　　congenital tracheoesophageal 198
　hematoma 138
　intramural pseudodiverticulosis 110, 138
　leiomyoma, leiomyosarcoma 164, 206
　lymphoma 136, 163
　mediastinitis 138
　metastases 136
　motility disorders 86–7
　　abnormal contractions 85
　mucosae, abnormal patterns 105, 108–10
　narrowing 136–139
　　cartilagenous ring 136
　　iatrogenic strictures 138
　　motility disorders 138
　　Schatzki's ring 136
　presbyesophagus 85, 86
　trauma 198
　ulcers 196–9
　varices 110
　webs 136, 144

F

familial polyposis 122, 133, 167, 178, 182
fecal impaction 12, 99
fecaloma 192
female genital tract, calcifications 50–2
filling defects
　alimentary tract 161–93
　　duodenum 172–7
　　esophagus 162–6
　　large bowel 182–93
　　small bowel 178–81
　　stomach 167–71
　biliary tract 218–25
　differentiation of
　　benign and malignant mass 162
　　extrinsic/intrinsic lesions 161
　　polyp and diverticulum 161
fistula
　congenital 214
　defined 196
　marker of Crohn's disease 210
fungal colitis 130, 154

G

gallbladder
　cholangiocarcinoma 222
　contrast examination 217
　diverticula 217
　inflammatory disease 220
　linear/band-like filling defects 218
　mass 220
　mucinous adenocarcinoma 36, 217
　multiple filling 220
　phrygian cap 218
　porcelain 36, 217
　round or mass-like filling defects 220
　septate 218
gallstones 36, 218
　calcifications 216
　gallstone ileus 94
　opacifications 216–17
　perforation 180, 216
Gardner's syndrome 122, 178, 184
gas
　abnormal patterns 1–29, 215–16
　　neonate 16–20
　　summary and discussion 1–3
　biliary tract 22–3, 215–16
　extraluminal
　　abscesses 26–8
　　biliary tree 22–3
　　bowel wall 22, 102
　　diffuse retroperitoneal gas 24
　　pelvic collections 26
　　perforated viscus 21
　　portal veins 22
　　postoperative 21
　　retroperitoneal
　　　diffuse 24
　　　following perforation 24
　　　pneumomediastinum 25
　　spontaneous (idiopathic) 21
　　urinary bladder 26
　　vaginal/uterine 26
　intraluminal
　　large bowel 10–14
　　small bowel 4–8, 118, 133
　normal patterns
　　adult 1
　　infant 1
gastric outlet obstruction 88–90
　see also stomach

Index

gastrin-secreting tumors 117
gastroplasty 142
genital tract, tuberculous calcifications 52
giardiasis
    duodenal signs 115
    small bowel signs 118, 148
granuloma, suture 192
granulomatous disease
    eosinophilic 202
    esophagitis 196
    gastritis 142, 200
    mediastinitis 166

H

Hampton line 200
hemangiomas
    calcification 48
    multiple 122, 133, 178
hepatic artery, chemotherapy effects on stomach 142
hepatic portal system
    gas 215–16
    lymphoma 222
    see also liver
hernias 6–9
    anterior abdominal 72
    Bochdalek's (diaphragmatic) 8, 57, 58, 64, 76
        neonate 18
    femoral 6, 72
    hiatus 64
    incarcerated 6
    indirect inguinal 6
    internal abdominal 6
    large bowel 158
    lesser sac 72
    Morgagni 8, 64
    obstructed inguinal, neonate 20
    obturator 72
    paraduodenal 6, 72
    paraesophageal 8, 64
    pericecal 74
    pleuroperitoneal 60
    Richter's 6
    small bowel, external/internal 94, 150
    Spigelian 72
    transmesenteric 6
    traumatic diaphragmatic 8
    umbilical 6
herpes zoster colitis 130, 155
Hirschsprung's disease 13, 18, 104, 152
histoplasmosis 122, 130
hydropneumoperitoneum, neonate 57
hypothyroidism 104

I

ileocecal valve, incompetence 96
ileum see small bowel
ileus
    adynamic
        colon cut-off sign 100
        generalized 97, 102, 124
    adynamic localized (sentinel loop) 2, 8, 9, 83, 97
        mimicking small bowel obstruction 97
    colonic (Ogilvie's syndrome) 14, 102
    gallstone 94
    meconium 18
    paralytic 14
    reflux 2
iliac fossa mass 74

infant, normal gas patterns 1
intraperitoneal abscess 28
intussusception 6, 96, 170, 174, 180, 192

J

jejunoileal bypass 12, 102
jejunum
    atresia 16
    diverticula 209
    wall pattern 1
    see also small bowel
juvenile gastrointestinal polyposis 122, 133, 184

K

Kaposi's sarcoma 180, 209
kidney
    abnormal position 60–2
    abscess 26
    calcifications 38–44
        cystic (curvilinear) 44
        disseminated cortical 42
        focal parenchymal 42
        medullary 40
        nephrocalcinosis 40
        nephrolithiasis 38–9
        pyramidal 40
    horse-shoe 63
    normal position 55
Klatskin tumors 222

L

lactase deficiency 124
large bowel
    adhesions 102, 158, 192
    air—fluid levels, and obstruction 83
    amebiasis 128, 129, 154, 188, 211
    amyloidosis 104, 130
    anastomotic stricture 152
    artifacts and foreign bodies 131
    calcifications 38, 186
    carcinoid syndrome 152, 186
    carcinoma 4, 152, 186, 212
    cecum
        carcinoma 4
        displacement 74
        volvulus 10, 100, 101
    coffee bean sign 100, 101
    colitis
        amebic 128, 129
        cathartic colon 156
        caustic 130, 156
        cystica profunda 133, 192
        cystica superficialis 133
        cytomegalovirus 130, 155
        fungal 130
        herpes zoster 130, 155
        ischemic 14, 102, 128–9, 156, 190, 211
        pseudomembranous 130, 156, 192
        radiation-induced 130, 158, 211
        tuberculous 128
        ulcerative 126–127, 156, 190, 211
        see also Crohn's disease
    colon cut-off sign, pancreatitis and strictures 100
    colonic lipomatosis 133
    diarrhea, air—fluid levels 84, 92
    distension, causes 10–14, 98–104

    diverticula 211–14
        vs polyps 162
        pseudodiverticula 212
    diverticulitis, diverticulosis 99, 104, 130, 154, 188, 212
    duplication cyst 182
    endometrioma 178, 182
    endometriosis 152, 178, 182
    enlargement of retrorectal space 80
    filling defects 182–93
    fistulas 211–14
    hemangiomas, multiple 133
    hernia see hernias
    ileocecal valve 182
    inflammatory pseudotumor 190
    intussusception 192
    inverted appendix 182
    ischemia 14, 102
    lipoma 182
    lymphoma 152, 186
    megacolon 12, 14, 98
        toxic megacolon 102
    metastases 152, 186, 212
    mucosae, abnormal patterns 108, 126–33
    multiple hamartoma syndrome 133
    narrowing 152–9
        endometriosis 152
        extracolonic inflammatory process 154
        transient localized spasm 152
    nodular lymphoid hyperplasia 131, 184
    normal position 55
    obstructive lesions 10–14, 99–104
        pseudoobstruction 102
    parasitic infections 118, 120, 148, 180, 192
    polyp, vs diverticulum appearances 162
    polyposis syndromes 133, 122, 167, 182–4
        adenomatous polyps 182
        pneumatosis cystoides coli 184
        pseudopolyps 184
    radiation enteritis 130, 158, 211
    salmonellosis 128
    schistosomiasis 128, 154, 192
    separation or displacement of loops 74–81
        descending colon 76
        hepatic flexure 76
        malrotation 74
        retroperitoneal cyst 75
        retroperitoneal fibroma 75
        sigmoid 78
        sigmoid volvulus 10, 100, 101
        splenic flexure 76
        transverse colon 76
    shigellosis 128
    staphylococcal enterocolitis 128
    strictures 102
    trichuriasis 128
    ulcers 211–14
        nonspecific, benign 130, 212
    urticaria 131, 192
    villous adenoma 184
    wall, extraluminal gas patterns 22, 102
    wall pattern 1
    see also ileus; volvulus
laryngectomy, cricopharyngeal achalasia 83
left atrial enlargement 163
leiomyoma, leiomyosarcoma
    filling defects
        esophagus 164, 206
        small bowel 178, 209
    gas bubbles 29
    gastric 200

lesser sac abscess 28
linitis plastica 140–3
lipiodol embolisation, liver 33
liver
　abscess 26, 176, 215, 226
　calcifications 32–3
　hepatic fibrosis 226
　mass 176
　normal/abnormal position 57
liver flukes 224
lymphangiectasia, intestinal 116, 118, 122
lymphogranuloma venereum 100, 130, 155, 211
lymphoid hyperplasia, nodular 107, 122, 131, 172, 178
lymphoma
　duodenum 115
　esophagus 136, 163
　large bowel 152, 186
　porta hepatis 222
　small bowel 117, 118
　stomach 112

M

macroglobulinemia 122
male genital tract, calcifications 50–2
malrotation, neonate 16
mastocytosis 116, 120
Meckel's diverticulum 96, 178
meconium ileus 18, 96
meconium peritonitis 18, 52, 96
meconium plug syndrome 18
mediastinitis 166
megacolon *see* large bowel
Ménétrier's disease, with hypoproteinemia 112, 117, 118, 170
mercury poisoning 130
mesenteric artery, superior m. a. syndrome 146, 174
mesenteric ischemia
　infarction 98
　and small bowel obstruction 92, 96, 98
　see also small bowel
mesenteric mass 70
mesenteritis, retractile 148
meteorism 4
midgut volvulus, neonate 16
Mirizzi syndrome 222
Morrison's pouch abscess 76
moulage sign 124
mucormycosis 130
mucosae, abnormal patterns 105–33
mucoviscidosis 116
muscular dystrophy, colonic dilatation 104

N

narrowing in GI tract 135–59
　see also specific regions
necrotizing enterocolitis *see* ischemic bowel disease
neonate
　abnormal gas patterns 16–20
　　double bubble sign 144
　　triple bubble sign 96
　adrenal and retroperitoneal calcifications 44
　annular pancreas 16
　Bochdalek's (diaphragmatic) hernia 18
　intramural duplication cyst 18
　ischemic bowel disease 18
　microcolon 152
　midgut volvulus 16
　normal gas patterns 1
　obstructed inguinal hernia 20
　omphalocele 72
　peritoneal bands 16
　pneumoperitoneum 20, 57
　pyloric stenosis 16, 88–89
nephrocalcinosis 40
nephrolithiasis 38
neurofibromatosis 122
neuromuscular disorders, esophageal motility dysfunction 87
nodular lymphoid hyperplasia 107, 122, 131, 172, 178, 184

O

Ogilvie's syndrome 14, 102
ovarian calcifications 50–2

P

pancreas
　abscess 28
　annular
　　adult diagnosis 144, 172
　　neonate 16
　calcifications 34–6
　carcinoma
　　duodenal appearances 115, 144, 176
　　abnormal position 68
　　gallbladder filling defect 222
　　gastric signs 112
　ectopic 172, 178, 202
　islet-cell tumor 115
　normal position 55
　pseudocyst 146
pancreatitis
　chronic 224
　colonic signs 130
　duodenal displacement 68, 115
　gastric signs 112
　strictures, colon cut-off sign 100
parasitic infections 118, 120, 148, 180, 192
pelvic abscess
　colonic involvement 99
　extraluminal gas 26
pelvic calcifications 48–53
　female 50
　male 50
pelvic lipomatosis, colonic involvement 158
pelvic mass 158
peptic ulcer *see* ulcers
perforated viscus, signs 21
periappendicular abscess 28
peritoneal bands, neonate 16
peritonitis
　ascites 70, 97, 102
　tuberculous calcifications 52
Peutz—Jeghers syndrome 6, 122, 167, 172, 178, 184
pharyngeal dysfunction 83–4
pharyngeal venous plexus 163
phleboliths 48
pneumatosis cystoides coli 192
pneumatosis intestinalis 118, 133, 180
pneumomediastinum
　esophageal trauma 198
　retroperitoneal gas 25
pneumoperitoneum, neonate 20, 57
polyp, differention from diverticulum 162
polyposis syndromes
　adenomatous polyps 182
　　duodenum 116
　　familial 122, 133, 167, 178, 182
　　juvenile 122, 133, 184
　　large bowel 133, 122, 167, 182–4
　　stomach 114
portal veins, extraluminal gas 22
pseudolymphoma, stomach 112
pseudomembraneous colitis 130, 156, 192
　see also large bowel, colitis
pyloric stenosis
　adult 88, 204
　neonate 16, 88–89, 204
pylorus, double 202

R

radiation enteritis
　large bowel 130, 158, 211
　small bowel 117, 122, 150
　stomach 142
rectum
　hemorrhoids 108, 192
　Morgagni columns 108
　mucosae, abnormal patterns 108, 126–33
　solitary rectal ulcer syndrome 130, 155, 211
　valves of Houston 108
　see also large bowel
retroperitoneal compartments
　calcifications 44–7
　　in the neonate 44
　cyst 75
　fibroma 75
　gas 24, 25
　mass 176
　space 2–3
retrorectal space, enlargement space 80
Rokitansky—Aschoff sinuses 217, 219, 220

S

salmonellosis (typhoid fever) 120, 128
schistosomiasis 128, 154, 192
scleroderma 87, 97, 104
sclerosing cholangitis 226
sentinel loop (localized/adynamic ileus) 2, 8, 9
sexually transmitted disease
　gonorrheal proctitis 128
　see also lymphogranuloma venereum
shigellosis, large bowel 128, 154
sigmoid volvulus 10, 100, 101
sinus tract 196, 211
small bowel
　adenocarcinoma 178
　adhesions 148
　amyloidosis 117, 118, 119
　anastomotic stricture 148
　atresia 16, 147
　calcifications 38
　carcinoid syndrome 147, 178, 209
　carcinoma 147
　dermatomyositis 124
　diarrheal pattern, air—fluid levels 84, 92
　differentiation of polyp and diverticulum 162
　dilatation 92–8
　　non-obstructive 97
　distension, causes 4–8
　diverticula 209
　　Meckel's diverticulum 209
　drug effects 124

edema 118, 119
eosinophilic gastroenteritis 117, 118, 122
filling defects 178–81
    leiomyoma, leiomyosarcoma 178
fistulas 209–10
    cholecystoenteric fistula 22, 215
    and diverticulitis 210
hemangiomas, multiple 133
hematoma 180
hernia *see* hernias
inflammatory pseudotumor 180
intussusception 6, 96, 180
ischemic bowel disease 117, 124
    elderly patient 98
    hemorrhagic disease 117
    neonate 18
    and small bowel obstruction 92, 96, 98, 150
Kaposi's sarcoma 180, 209
leiomyoma, leiomyosarcoma 178, 209
lipoma 182
lymphoma 117, 118, 148, 180, 209
metastases 122, 147, 180
    melanoma 209
mucosae, abnormal patterns 107, 117–25
    dilatation and normal folds 124
    'granularity' 122–3
    irregular folds without dilatation 118–22
    polyposis 122
    'stack of coins' 117
    thickened folds and dilatation 117
    thickened folds and gastric involvement 117
    thickened irregular folds 117–18
narrowing 147–51
    adjacent inflammation 147
nodular lymphoid hyperplasia 122, 178
normal position 55
obstruction 83, 92
    causes 4
    diagnosis 2, 5
    with/without vascular compromise 94–6
parasitic infections 118, 120, 148, 180, 192
pneumatosis intestinalis 118, 133, 180
polyps and benign tumors 178
radiation enteritis 117, 122, 150
scleroderma 124
separation or displacement of loops 70–3
strangulation 4, 5, 96
thickening 70
ulcers 209
volvulus 96, 100, 144, 150
wall, extraluminal gas 22
wall pattern 1
see also specific conditions
spleen
    abnormal position 58
    absence 58
    calcifications 34
    normal position 55
    posttraumatic splenomegaly 78
sprue, non-tropical (celiac disease) 115, 124
staphylococcal enterocolitis 128
stenotic lesions 135–159
    see also specific regions
stomach
    abnormal position 64–6
        exogastric mass 142
    amyloidosis 112, 142
    areae gastricae, enlargement 105, 114
    artifactual surface patterns 106
    bezoar 170

carcinoma 112, 140, 164, 168
    malignancy criteria 200, 202
caustic gastritis 142
dilatation 88–90
diverticula 200–5
double pylorus 202
duplication cyst 167
ectopic pancreas 167
eosinophilic gastritis 112, 142
eosinophilic granuloma 202
erosive gastritis 114, 200, 202
extrinsic mass 168
filling defects 167–71
fistulas 200–5
functional disturbance without obstruction 90
gastric dilatation 88–90
gastric intussusception 170, 174
gastric outlet obstruction 88–90
gastric volvulus 88
granulomatous gastritis 142
hypertrophic gastritis 111
lymphoma 112, 140, 168
    pseudolymphoma 200
Ménétrier's disease 112
metastases 140, 168
mucinous adenocarcinoma 38
mucosae, abnormal patterns 105, 111–14
narrowing (linitis plastica) 140–3
normal position 55
and pancreatitis 112
phlegmonous gastritis 142
polyposis syndromes 114
polyps and benign tumors 167
pseudolymphoma 112
radiation injury 142, 200
sarcoma 168
scarring 112–13
ulcers 111, 115, 142, 170, 200–5
    benign vs malignant 200, 202
varices 112, 170
villous adenoma 168
volvulus 88, 142
web 167
strongyloidiasis
    large bowel appearances 154
    small bowel appearances 120, 148
subhepatic abscess 176
subphrenic abscess 26, 57

T

Thorotrast injection deposits 33, 34
thumbprinting 102, 103
thyroid enlargement 164
toxic megacolon 14
tracheobronchial rest 136
trichuriasis, large bowel 128
tuberculosis 117, 188
tuberculous calcifications
    cystitis 48
    genital tract 52
    peritonitis 52
tuberculous colitis 128
    M. bovis vs *M. tuberculosis* 128
Turcot syndrome 184
typhlitis 14
typhoid fever
    large bowel appearances 128
    small bowel appearances 120

U

ulcerative colitis 126–127, 156, 190, 126–127, 156, 190, 211
ulcers 111, 115, 142, 170, 174
    aphthoid 211
    Hampton line 200
    malignant vs benign 195
    nonspecific 130
    postbulbar, duodenum 144
    solitary rectal ulcer syndrome 130, 155, 211
    see also Crohn's disease; *specific organs and conditions*
uremia
    duodenal signs 115
    gastric signs 112
ureters, calcifications 44
urinary bladder
    calculi 48
    displacement 56
    normal position 56
    tuberculous calcifications 48
    wall, calcifications 48
urinary fistulas 214
urticaria pigmentosa (mastocytosis) 116, 120

V

vagotomy 124
valvulae conniventes
    absence, causes 4
    distribution 107
varices
    duodenum 116
    esophagus 110, 166
    stomach 112, 170
volvulus
    cecal 10, 100, 101
        coffee bean sign 100, 101
    gastric 88, 142
    large bowel including sigmoid 10, 100, 101, 158
    mesenteroaxial 64
    midgut 144
    neonate 16
    pseudovolvulus 100
    small bowel 96, 100, 150

W

Whipple's disease 116, 117, 118, 122

Y

Yersinia enterocolitica
    large bowel 211
        children 128
    small bowel 120
        healing 122

Z

Zollinger—Ellison syndrome 111, 115, 117, 206